Benign Prostatic Hyperplasia: Clinical Urology

Benign Prostatic Hyperplasia: Clinical Urology

Edited by Lucy Mitchel

hayle
medical

New York

Hayle Medical,
750 Third Avenue, 9th Floor,
New York, NY 10017, USA

Visit us on the World Wide Web at:
www.haylemedical.com

ISBN: 978-1-63241-916-3

Cataloging-in-Publication Data

Benign prostatic hyperplasia : clinical urology / edited by Lucy Mitchel.
   p. cm.
Includes bibliographical references and index.
ISBN 978-1-63241-916-3
1. Benign prostatic hyperplasia. 2. Benign prostatic hyperplasia--Treatment.
3. Prostate--Hypertrophy. 4. Prostate--Aging. 5. Urology. I. Mitchel, Lucy.
RC899 .B46 2020
616.65--dc23

Table of Contents

Preface

Benign prostatic hyperplasia (BPH) is a clinical condition marked by an increase in size of the prostate gland. Frequent urination, inability to urinate and loss of bladder control are certain symptoms of BPH. The underlying mechanism responsible for the appearance of these symptoms is the enlarged prostate pressing on to the urethra. This makes the passage of urine out of the bladder difficult. Obesity, type 2 diabetes, family history and erectile dysfunction are certain risk factors. If BPH is not resolved, it may lead to urinary tract infections. The diagnosis of BPH is based on a rectal exam, a history of lower urinary tract symptoms, and an exclusion of other conditions with similar symptoms. Kidney function tests and prostate specific antigen allows kidney damage and prostate cancer to be evaluated. The management of this condition requires certain lifestyle alterations, such as moderating the consumption of caffeine products and alcohol, decreasing fluid intake before bedtime, increasing physical activity, among others. If the problem is not solved through medication, a transurethral resection of the prostate or a prostatic artery embolization may be needed. This book elucidates the concepts and innovative models around prospective developments with respect to diagnosis and treatment of benign prostatic hyperplasia. Through this book, we attempt to further enlighten the readers about the new concepts in clinical urology.

Various studies have approached the subject by analyzing it with a single perspective, but the present book provides diverse methodologies and techniques to address this field. This book contains theories and applications needed for understanding the subject from different perspectives. The aim is to keep the readers informed about the progresses in the field; therefore, the contributions were carefully examined to compile novel researches by specialists from across the globe.

Indeed, the job of the editor is the most crucial and challenging in compiling all chapters into a single book. In the end, I would extend my sincere thanks to the chapter authors for their profound work. I am also thankful for the support provided by my family and colleagues during the compilation of this book.

Editor

Dutasteride plus Tamsulosin fixed-dose combination first-line therapy versus Tamsulosin Monotherapy in the treatment of benign prostatic hyperplasia: a budget impact analysis in the Greek healthcare setting

Maria Geitona[1†], Pinelopi Karabela[2*†], Ioannis A Katsoulis[3†], Hara Kousoulakou[3†], Eleni Lyberopoulou[2†], Eleftherios Bitros[2†], Loukas Xaplanteris[2†] and Sotiria Papanicolaou[3†]

Abstract

Background: The purpose of this study was to explore the budget impact of dutasteride plus tamsulosin fixed-dose combination (DUT + TAM FDC) versus tamsulosin monotherapy, in the treatment of patients with benign prostatic hyperplasia (BPH) from the perspective of the Greek healthcare insurance system.

Methods: A Microsoft Excel-based model was developed to estimate the financial consequences of adopting DUT + TAM FDC within the Greek healthcare setting. The model, compared six mutually exclusive health states in two alternative treatment options: current standard of care and the introduction of DUT + TAM FDC in the market. The model used clinical inputs from the CombAT study; data on resource use associated with the management of BPH in Greece were derived from expert panel, and unit cost data were derived from official reimbursement tariffs. A payer perspective was taken into account. As patient distribution data between public and private sectors are not available in Greece two scenarios were investigated, considering the whole eligible population in each scenario. A 4 year time horizon was taken into account and included treatment costs, number of transurethral resections of the prostate (TURPs) and acute urinary retention (AUR) episodes avoided.

Results: The clinical benefit from the market adoption of DUT + TAM FDC in Greece was 1,758 TURPs and 972 episodes of AUR avoided cumulatively in a four year period. The increase in total costs from the gradual introduction of DUT + TAM FDC to the Greek healthcare system ranges from €1.3 million in the first year to €5.8 million in the fourth year, for the public sector, and €1.2 million to €4.0 million, for the private sector. This represents an increase of 1.91% to 7.94% for the public sector and 1.10% 3.29% in the private sector, during the 4-year time horizon.

Conclusions: Budget impact analysis (BIA) results indicated that the gradual introduction of DUT + TAM FDC, would increase the overall budget of the disease, however providing better clinical outcomes. DUT + TAM FDC drug acquisition cost is partly offset by the reduction in the costs associated with the treatment of the disease.

Keywords: Benign prostate hyperplasia, Dutasteride plus tamsulosin fixed-dose combination, Budget impact, Costs, Health resources

* Correspondence: pinelopi.a.karabela@gsk.com
†Equal contributors
[2]GlaxoSmithKline, Athens, Greece
Full list of author information is available at the end of the article

Background

Benign prostatic hyperplasia (BPH), a common benign neoplasm in men, is a chronic condition with an age dependent epidemiology. It is associated with progressive lower urinary tract symptoms (LUTS) and affects 75% of men older than 70 [1]. Although many epidemiological clinical studies have been conducted worldwide over the last 20 years, the prevalence of clinical BPH remains difficult to determine. A broadly accepted clinical definition of BPH is lacking, and thus performance of adequate epidemiological studies is hampered [2]. A commonly occurring condition in men with underlying BPH is acute urinary retention (AUR). AUR is an uncomfortable and potentially life-threatening condition characterized by a sudden inability to urinate associated with intense suprapubic discomfort. Medical intervention is often required in order to relieve the severe discomfort experienced by patients with AUR [3]. Overall, the common clinical manifestations attributed to BPH include LUTS, urinary tract infection, incomplete bladder emptying, acute and chronic urinary retention, chronic renal insufficiency, urosepsis, and hematuria [1].

Therapeutic interventions for LUTS, due to BPH, provide sustained improvement in clinical symptoms and quality of life (QoL), while inhibiting progression of the condition [4]. The two main pharmacological agents for the management of BPH/LUTS are 5-alpha-reductase inhibitors (5-ARIs) and alpha-blockers. Dutasteride is a 5-ARI and works by blocking the conversion of testosterone to dihydrotestosterone, thus reducing cellular growth and in turn reducing the size of the prostate [5]. Tamsulosin is an uroselective alpha-blocker and exerts its activity by relaxing bladder neck muscles and prostate muscle fibres that in turn improve in urine flow rate [6]. Combination therapy was significantly superior to both monotherapies at reducing the relative risk of BPH clinical progression, as concluded by the Combination of Avodart™ (dutasteride) and Tamsulosin (CombAT) study. CombAT was a randomised, multicentre, double-blind, parallel-group study in 4,844 men of 50 years or older with a clinical diagnosis of BPH for the treatment of moderate to severe BPH that spanned over 4 years [7].

The increasing use of pharmacological agents, during the past twenty years, has transformed the management of BPH as shown by a dramatic decrease in the use of transurethral prostatectomy (TURPs), inpatient hospitalization, length of hospital stay and an increase in the number of outpatient visits for the condition, in the US [8]. In 2000, the direct cost of BPH treatment in the US was estimated to be US$1.1 billion exclusive of outpatient pharmaceuticals [8]. Another study conducted in UK estimated the annual economic burden of BPH ranged between £62 million and £91 million, excluding the intangible costs [9].

Recent economic evaluations have been undertaken with a specific focus on pharmaceutical intervention related to treatment of BPH. Specifically for the DUT + TAM FDC vs. tamsulosin monotherapy, economic analyses have been conducted in the UK [10], Canada [11], Spain [12], and Scandinavia [13], where the fixed-dose combination therapy was shown to be cost-effective compared to tamsulosin monotherapy.

The aim of this study was to assess the budget impact of the fixed dose combination dutasteride and tamsulosin (DUT + TAM FDC) versus tamsulosin monotherapy for the treatment of moderate to severe BPH in Greece.

Methods

A budget impact analysis was conducted based on a Markov decision model for the treatment of moderate to severe BPH comparing DUT + TAM FDC combination therapy over tamsulosin monotherapy. The model was populated with local healthcare resource utilisation estimates, unit costs and epidemiological data. Clinical efficacy data was retrieved from the ComBAT study. Univariate sensitivity was conducted by examining changes in the prevalence of BPH, number of patients based on prostate volume, and success rate of TURPs.

Model description

The pharmacoeconomic analysis was conducted based on a Markov decision model developed with Microsoft Excel. Using data from the CombAT study [7] the analysis was based on a Markov stochastic process with 6 mutually exclusive health states iterated over 3 month cycles for a total of 4 years (Figure 1 Markov model structure and health states). A Markov model is a decision analytic technique that allows simulation of disease progression during a defined period of time, and is particularly suitable to model medical conditions that involve uncertainty over a long time horizon and/or recurrent events [14].

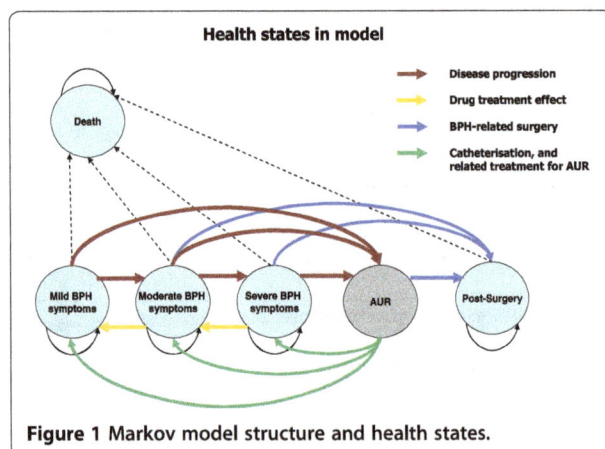

Figure 1 Markov model structure and health states.

The six discrete health states (or 'Markov states') which simulated each possible clinical event and described disease progression, were the following: 'mild', 'moderate', 'severe' BPH, based on IPSS symptom severity as defined in the CombAT trial, AUR, post-surgery and death [10]. The AUR was modelled as a temporary health state. Successful treatment of AUR with emergency catheterization or trial without catheter (TWOC) would return the patients to the previous health state.

Unsuccessful treatment would lead to the post-surgery health state with the implication of a BPH-related surgery.

The model characteristics have been based on the Walker et al. study [10]. Although there are a number of surgical options for BPH, the model assumed all patients have TURP when surgery is indicated. The use of TURP has been the gold standard for decades [15] and the American Urological Association guidelines consider this intervention as the benchmark for surgical therapies [16], while the European Urological Association guidelines report TURP as the preferred treatment for prostate sizes ranging from 30 to 80 mL [2]. Patients undergoing TURP enter the post-surgery health state, where they remain until the end of the 4-year time horizon or death. A patient can undergo up to two TURP procedures (after failure of the first procedure or relapse).

Assumptions regarding the progression of the condition over time and BPH events, such as AUR, surgery or death had to be made for the model. Transition probabilities between health states [10] were derived directly from the CombAT study individual patient-level data [7] and the clinical study report. Patient-level data related to the mild, moderate and severe 'Markov' health states were available from follow-up visits every 3 months and accordingly probabilities for transitions between each of these health states were derived. For AUR and post-surgery health states, the three-month transition probabilities were calculated from the number of yearly events using standard methods as described by Briggs et al. [17]. For patients who experienced AUR, the care pathway was not reported in the CombAT trial. thus, the model assumed that 50% of TWOC procedures are successful based on a clinical review by Emberton et al. [18]. Furthermore, patients who underwent BPH-related surgery followed the care pathway that is published in international literature [19].

The European Urology Association BPH treatment guidelines helped inform the probability of any adverse event associated with TURP [2]. This total probability was applied to all patients in the post-surgery state, regardless of the success or failure of the procedure. Adverse events (AEs) associated with medical therapy were based on the CombAT trial. However, since the percentage of patients experiencing serious drug-related AEs was <1% in all treatment arms of the CombAT trial, these were excluded from the analysis.

Overall, the model simulated and compared:

- Standard of Care (SoC): Patients are treated with tamsulosin only, representing current standard care.
- DUT + TAM FDC: Gradual introduction of DUT + TAM FDC therapy in the treatment of BPH, with defined market share gains over time.

In each of the treatments compared, the health costs allocated to each discrete state were accumulated, through the 4-year time horizon [10].

The Markov model was designed assuming that treatment switching only occurred at the end of each year and that patients remained on DUT + TAM FDC therapy upon regression to mild BPH symptoms. This is a plausible clinical assumption as according to a study from Toren et al. [20], preventive administration of 5-ARI could decrease the incidence of BPH clinical progression, which was validated during the expert panel. The model assumed 100% compliance with pharmacotherapy and that patients incur different resource use and costs according to the severity of their symptoms. The patients who entered the model had an initial urology consultation at a higher cost. The costs described in Table 1 only applied to patients entering the model from year two onwards, since patients in the model in year one were assumed to have already had their initial urologist consultation. The AUR 'Markov' state was modelled as a tunnel state which occurred at mid-cycle length and no patients were assumed to be in the AUR state at the beginning of each cycle. Non AUR patients were only assumed to undergo TURP procedures from the 'moderate' and 'severe' symptom severity health states. No patients were assumed to die while undergoing treatment for AUR; all-cause mortality was applied to patients at the beginning of each cycle. Patients who developed AUR, following immediate catheterization, underwent TWOC. If this was successful, they returned to their previous symptom severity 'Markov' state. The AUR state was modelled in this way to reflect that successful catheterization and TWOC had no effect on disease progression.

The post-surgery 'Markov' state was modeled according to Figure 2 Post surgery pathway, with the assumption that patients underwent only one type of BPH surgery, a TURP.

Furthermore, patients were assumed to undergo a TURP procedure when the TWOC procedure failed. Patients undergoing a TURP procedure entered a 'Post surgery' health state and followed the pathway shown in Figure 2. In this decision diagram 'failure' was defined when patients did not achieve >50% reduction in the IPSS score after surgery.

Model inputs

Patient population

A cohort of Greek male patients aged ≥50 years, diagnosed with moderate to severe BPH, as defined by an

Table 1 Unit costs by healthcare sector

Exam/laboratory test	Scenario	Unit cost (€)	Reference
Consultation			
Cost per follow up urologist visit	Public	10.00	National Organization for the Provision of Healthcare Services (EOPYY) (www.eopyy.gov.gr) accessed 1 October 2012
	Private	50.00	Average price confirmed by expert panel consensus.
Cost per serum creatinine test	Public	4.05	Social Security Institution IKA* tariff (PD157/55)
	Private	16.00	Biomedicine SA price (provided 1 October 2012)**
Cost per urodynamic test	Public	18.99	Social Security Institution IKA tariff (PD157/55)
	Private	268.50	Average price from pricelists of two major private hospitals in Athens ('Hygeia' hospital and 'Iaso' general hospital)
Cost per flexible cystoscopy	Public	4.05	Social Security Institution IKA tariff column A (PD 15766 surgical)
	Private	650.00	Average price from pricelists of two major private hospitals in Athens (Hygeia hospital and Iatriko Athinon hospital)
Procedure			
Cost of prostate related surgery without complications	Public	1,007.00	DRG list FEK 946 -12Mar2012 (DRG B02X)
	Private	1,000.00	DRG list FEK 946 -12Mar2012 (DRG Y05X)
Cost of prostate related surgery with complications	Public	2,127.00	Average of DRGs Y05M (cost of prostate related surgery with complications) and B02M (cost of prostate related surgery with complications) (FEK 946 -12Mar2012).
	Private	2,848.00	DRG Y05M (FEK 946–12 Mar2012)
Cost per episode of AUR (non-elective)	Public	7.63	Social Security Institution IKA tariff for catheterization (PD 157/3, 157/65 surgical)
	Private	50.00	Average price confirmed by expert panel consensus

*IKA Social Security fund.
**Biomedicine SA is a leading primary healthcare services provider in Greece.

International Prostate Symptom Score (IPSS) populated the model in order to resemble the population characteristics of the CombAT study. Due to lack of national epidemiological data on BPH, the internationally accepted prevalence of BPH in the aforementioned age group was used and set at 30%, while the proportion of patients diagnosed with moderate to severe BPH was 63%, as

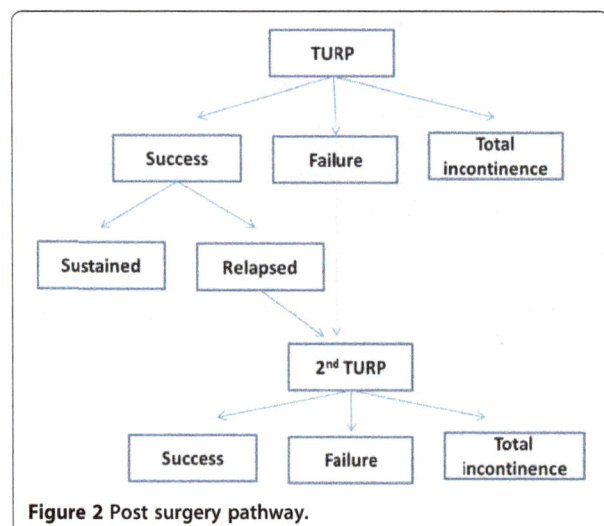

Figure 2 Post surgery pathway.

documented in international and European studies [21-23]. Based on the 2001 Greek population census, the men population aged over 50 was 1,724,867 and consequently, the estimated number of men entering the model was set at 326,000 (=1,724,867*0,3*0,63).

The initial distribution of patients in each of the BPH symptom health states that have entered the model was defined by the baseline IPSS of the CombAT trial. Specifically, 7% of patients had improved to mild symptoms (IPSS <12) before starting treatment and the remaining 93% of patients would be considered as moderate to severe condition (63% and 30% moderate and severe, respectively) [11]. The IPSS range for mild symptoms is 0–7, moderate 8–19 and severe 20–35. The model allowed new patients to enter based on BPH incidence in accordance with the International Society of Pharmacoeconomics and Outcomes Research (ISPOR) guidelines [24].

Clinical data
The CombAT trial was a 4-year randomized double-blind parallel group study in 4,844 men ≥50 yrs. of age with clinically diagnosed moderate to severe BPH, IPSS ≥12, prostate volume ≥30 ml, and serum prostate specific antigen (PSA) 1.5–10 ng/ml [7].

The most common aetiology of male LUTS is BPH, thus the incidence of BPH was estimated from the incident of recorded male LUTS in the Netherlands, according to the Verhamme *et al.* study [23]. Based on this study, the calculated incidence in men aged older than 50 years (2,090) was divided by the number of man-years (110,321) equalling 18.94 per 1,000 man-years.

For the overall mortality weighing, the mortality rates were calculated from the World Health Organization (WHO) health statistics and health information system interim life tables [25]. The annual risk of death in 2009 was extracted for Greek men aged >50 years.

Resource utilization data

The medical resource use regarding the management of patients with BPH in Greece was not available from existing literature or valid national data sources, thus this information was retrieved from a local expert panel and use of the Delphi technique [26]. A panel of 9 clinical experts in urology was assembled in order to collect primary data regarding patient management patterns for BPH in the local healthcare setting. The synthesis of the panel was geographically representative and consisted of urologists from academic institutions and major city hospitals in Greece. The questions related to the medical resource use were projected on a screen and the expert panel was asked to enter their estimates using a handheld tele-voting system. Consensus was achieved using the Delphi method with up to two iterations of open discussion followed by re-voting from the panellists. The average of the experts' answers was then included in the model grouped by routine care of patients with BPH, treatment of AUR and TURP consultations.

No Ethics Committee approval was requested for the primary research component of the study, as the conduct of interviews with physicians and experts' panels are not subject to any approval according to the Greek legislation.

Cost data

Costs used in the model are in nominal 2013 Euros and were not discounted nor inflated, as recommended by international guidelines for BIA [24].

Drug costs for tamsulosin and DUT + TAM FDC were based on the retail prices (Price Bulletin 15 February 2013, ΥΥΚΑ 2013/2). Specifically DUT + TAM FDC was priced at €30.02 and tamsulosin at €12,42 (which is the volume-weighted average price of originator and generics according to market share data provided by IMS Health Greece (www.imshealth.com).

As serious drug-related AEs were <1%,% in all treatment arms of the CombAT trial, these were excluded from the analysis.

Costs of consultations, procedures and laboratory tests were taken from officially published public tariffs and

private hospitals in Athens. Hospitalization costs were based on the DRG list from the Greek Ministry of Health, (official government gazette March 2012 [27]).

The unit costs for the private and public sector setting are presented in Table 1.

Market data

DUT + TAM FDC has been available in Greece since 2011, thus market share data (provided by IMS Health Greece) were used as input for the model for the first two and a half years of the analysis.

Market uptake of DUT + TAM FDC was defined as the percentage of the total first-line treatment BPH market that is gained every year. In particular, DUT + TAM FDC gained 2.0%, 4.0%, 4.5% and 11.0% of market share in the 4-years' time horizon used in the model. Moreover, the percent of moderate to severe BPH patients, who switched from SoC to DUT + TAM FDC, at the end of every year, was set to 3.0%, 4.0%, and 5.5%.

Perspective of analysis

The study was conducted from the payer perspective, and in particular two different scenarios were investigated: the public sector scenario, which includes the costs reimbursed by social insurance funds, and the private sector scenario, which includes the costs incurred by patients and private health insurance. Because there are no published estimates of the percentages of the respective sectors in the total healthcare setting, these two were explored separately as two extreme scenarios.

Model outputs

The model estimated the following outputs thought the 4-year time horizon from the introduction of DUT + TAM FDC in the Greek market. Clinical outcomes refer to the number of TURPS or number of episodes of AUR avoided as well as the incremental cost per AUR avoided. Economic outputs include total costs (i.e., costs of drug treatment, costs of consultations, costs of AUR and costs of BPH related surgery).

Results
Resource utilization

Table 2 shows the resource utilisation of BPH patients, which the expert panel affirmed was consistent across both the social and private healthcare setting. Patients are treated and followed up directly by urologists for all prostate related complication, while visits to GPs are limited to remote areas.

Table 2 Routine care for patients with BPH

Resource use	Average results
Patients with 'Mild' IPSS score	
Number of GP visits in first year	1.22
Number of GP visits per year	0.44
Number of urologist visits per year in subsequent years	1.11
Patients with 'Moderate' IPSS score	
Number of urologist visits in first year	2.22
Number of GP visits per year	2
Number of urologist visits per year in subsequent years	2.39
Patients with 'Severe' IPSS score	
Number of urologist visits in first year	2.56
Number of GP visits per year	0
Number of urologist visits per year in subsequent years	2.78
Number of flexible cystoscopies per year	0.39
Proportion of patients undergoing flexible cystoscopy	7%
Successful TURP	
Number of peri-operative urologist consultations	2.67
Number of follow up urodynamic tests	0.06
Unsuccessful TURP	
Number of peri-operative urologist consultations	3.89
Number of follow up urodynamic tests	0.06
Patients with total and permanent incontinence	
Number of urologist visits per year	4.56
Procedures with complications	
Number of follow up urologist visits	3.44
All procedures	
Number of peri-operative flexible cystoscopies	1.1

Abbreviations: *IPSS* International Prostate Symptom Score, *GP* general practitioner.

Model results
Clinical outcomes
Table 3 presents the clinical outcomes of the gradual introduction of DUT + TAM FDC, in the 4-year time horizon of the model.

Cost outputs
Public sector scenario
Table 4, presents the total economic impact from the gradual introduction of DUT + TAM FDC to the various cost components of BPH disease managment (i.e., consultations, surgery, AUR costs, drug costs) in the public sector.

Private sector scenario
Table 5 presents the total economic impact of gradual introduction of DUT + TAM FDC to the various cost components of BPH disease managment (i.e., consultations, surgery, AUR costs, drug costs) in the private sector.

Sensitivity analysis
In order to assess the impact of uncertainty of various model inputs on the results of the study, univariate sensitivity analyses were conducted on two variables that contributed to the cost of treatment: eligible patient population and higher success rates of TURPs.

The prevalence of BPH was allowed to vary by ±10% in one-way sensitivity analyses, in order to reflect the uncertainty due to lack of local epidemiological data (Table 6).

A separate analysis estimated the budget impact from the introduction of DUT + TAM FDC when the eligible population included only patients with a baseline prostate volume > 50 mL (Table 6) which according to clinical practice is viewed as enlarged.

Additionally the success rate of surgical procedures in terms of symptoms improvement was allowed to vary by +11% and +22% in order to present the variation of clinical practice [28-30]. These adjustments are aligned with the assumption that no surgical re-treatment would be required after initial operation.

Sensitivity analysis results indicate that the overall budget for the treatment of BPH increases with use of DUT + TAM FDC compared to tamsulosin monotherapy during the 4 year study period (Table 6), for either of the two scenarios (private and public sector).

Table 3 Clinical results

Year	Tamsulosin monotherapy (SoC)		Tamsulosin monotherapy & gradual introduction of DUT + TAM FDC		Number avoided	
	TURP	AUR episodes	TURP	AUR episodes	TURPS	AUR episodes
1	7,145	5,786	7,102	5,726	42	60
2	12,507	6,366	12,147	6,198	360	168
3	9,637	5,943	9,215	5,702	422	241
4	11,475	7,183	10,541	6,679	934	503
Total	**40,763**	**25,277**	**39,006**	**24,305**	**1,758**	**942**

Table 4 Cost analysis of public sector

Year	Consultation costs (€)	Surgery costs (€)	AUR costs (€)	Drug costs (€)	Total costs (€)	Total budget impact (%)
SoC: Tamsulosin monotherapy						
1	11,497,557	8,628,675	44,144	47,577,203	67,747,579	-
2	11,527,061	15,104,305	48,573	47,785,803	74,465,743	-
3	11,260,338	11,638,737	45,344	47,734,616	70,679,036	-
4	11,412,776	13,858,461	54,803	47,798,059	73,124,100	-
Tamsulosin monotherapy & gradual introduction of DUT + TAM FDC						
1	11,492,585	8,577,613	43,687	48,930,196	69,044,082	-
2	11,404,330	14,669,865	47,289	50,606,379	76,727,862	-
3	11,102,755	11,128,827	43,506	52,334,084	74,609,173	-
4	11,173,679	12,730,920	50,963	54,976,669	78,932,231	-
Budget impact						
1	−4,972	−51,061	−457	1,352,994	1,296,503	1.91
2	−122,731	−434,440	−1,284	2,820,575	2,262,120	3.04
3	−157,583	−509,909	−1,838	4,599,467	3,930,137	5.56
4	−239,097	−1,127,541	−3,840	7,178,610	5,808,131	7.94

Discussion

The present study is the first to estimate the budget impact from the introduction of DUT + TAM FDC therapy in the treatment of moderate to severe BPH, in the Greek health care setting. The study estimated that the gradual introduction of DUT + TAM FDC would result in avoidance of 1,758 TURPs and 972 AURs, in total over the 4-year time horizon, compared with tamsulosin monotherapy. In terms of BIA, the study showed that the introduction of the new therapeutic intervention would increase the disease management budget by 1.9% in year one, up to 7.9% in year four from the public sector perspective, and by 1.1% to 3.3% respectively from the private sector perspective. The observed increase is driven from pharmaceutical costs which are partly offset by the reduction in the costs associated with the overall treatment of the disease. In particular, savings associated with the use of combination therapy arise from the reduction in consultations, surgeries and AURs. These savings are estimated at €1.13 and €1.95 million in the public and private sector scenarios, respectively.

Table 5 Cost analysis of private sector

Year	Consultation costs (€)	Surgery costs (€)	AUR costs (€)	Drug costs (€)	Total costs (€)	Total budget impact (%)
SoC: Tamsulosin monotherapy						
1	49,924,365	14,706,649	289,282	47,577,203	112,497,498	-
2	50,090,297	25,743,665	318,303	47,785,803	123,938,068	-
3	48,962,652	19,836,976	297,142	47,734,616	116,831,388	-
4	49,630,480	23,620,258	359,129	47,798,059	121,407,926	-
Tamsulosin monotherapy & gradual introduction of DUT + TAM FDC						
1	49,898,950	14,619,620	286,287	48,930,196	113,735,054	-
2	49,458,768	25,003,208	309,888	50,606,379	125,378,243	-
3	48,142,186	18,967,890	285,101	52,334,084	119,729,260	-
4	48,397,466	21,698,485	333,965	54,976,669	125,406,586	-
Budget impact						
1	−25,415	−87,028	−2,995	1,352,994	1,237,555	1.10
2	−631,529	−740,457	−8,415	2,820,575	1,440,175	1.16
3	−820,467	−869,086	−12,042	4,599,467	2,897,873	2.48
4	−1,233,014	−1,921,773	−25,163	7,178,610	3,998,659	3.29

Table 6 Sensitivity analysis of net budget impact of DUT + TAM FDC (€)

Year	1	2	3	4
Public sector	1,296,503	2,262,120	3,930,137	5,808,131
Prevalence of BPH				
20%	864,336	1,553,230	2,752,483	4,195,474
40%	1,728,671	2,971,017	5,107,791	7,420,837
Only BPV > 50 cc	537,096	1,142,338	1,886,053	2,934,517
Probability that first and second TURPs are successful				
88%	1,300,878	2,299,356	3,973,923	5,904,891
99%	1,305,243	2,336,509	4,017,601	6,001,441
Private sector	1,237,555	1,440,175	2,897,873	3,998,659
Prevalence of BPH				
20%	825,037	993,147	2,031,237	2,892,582
40%	1,650,074	1,887,239	3,764,509	5,104,980
Only BPV > 50 cc	422,530	719,264	1,263,342	2,003,231
Probability that first and second TURPs are successful				
88%	1,245,058	1,504,091	2,973,305	4,165,148
99%	1,252,516	1,567,598	3,048,198	4,330,599

The biggest challenge in the present study was to estimate model inputs, due to lack of local data in published literature. Clinical data were based on the pivotal trial (the ComBAT study), incidence, prevalence of BPH and LUTS [29] data were extracted from European sources [22,23], and were subsequently confirmed by the expert panel. Our analysis was performed with inclusion of all patients, regardless of pre-treatment prostate volume (326,000 men estimation). Resource utilisation data were collected via the expert panel with the use of the Delphi technique, while local unit cost data were collected through publicly available sources.

Among the parameters examined in the sensitivity analyses, prevalence data had the highest impact in the results, due to the change of eligible patients number that enter the model.

There are certain limitations in the current study. The analysis was performed with a computer based model, which raised the need for adoption of simplifications and assumptions that may have not reflected real life data and may have created uncertainties. However, these uncertainties were minimized through the use of expert opinion. Due to lack of strong supporting evidence, such as registries or officially published sources, expert opinions were used to gather data regarding health resource utilization.

In addition, the lack of data on the patient distribution between the public and private sector in Greece has not allowed the generation of a weighted average for the

total costs. Therefore, to overcome this limitation two extreme scenarios of public and private sectors and the relevant unit costs, were estimated separately. The differences observed between the two sectors' unit cost data are due to the fact that public sector reimbursement rates do not reflect real cost, as they have not been updated since 1992 [31]. The two scenarios aimed at providing a range within which true costs lie.

Our findings may be used to inform the development of health policy resource allocation decisions regarding the pharmaceutical treatment of BPH. However, further research and additional empirical data are necessary in order to estimate more accurately the cost of DUT + TAM FDC, and also incorporate quality of life estimates that these patients experience compared to the currently administered monotherapies, in the Greek healthcare setting. Especially in the environment of economic recession that Greece is experiencing, economic evaluation studies that would reveal the value-for-money of new therapies can help policy decision makers rely on evidence based treatments and achieve health insurance fund sustainability.

Conclusions

BIA results indicated that the gradual introduction of DUT + TAM FDC, increases the overall budget of the disease while providing better clinical outcomes in terms of avoidance of 1,758 TURPs and 972 AUR episodes. These results can be used in the decision-making process for resource allocation purposes. Further research on patient reported outcomes and additional economic evaluation studies that would incorporate the incremental monetary effect with the quality-adjusted life year that BPH patients gain from DUT + TAM FDC, compared to the currently administered monotherapies, would reveal the value-for-money estimate of the fixed-dose combination therapy in the Greek healthcare system.

Competing interests

Funding for the research and preparation of this article was provided by GlaxoSmithKline, which approved the study design and manuscript. At the time of the analysis, Pinelopi Karabela, Eleni Lyberopoulou, Eleftherios Bitros and Loukas Xaplanteris were full- time employees of GlaxoSmithKline. Hara Kousoulakou, Ioannis Katsoulis, and Sotiria Papanicolaou were employees of PRMA Consulting, a consultant to GlaxoSmithKline.

Authors' contributions

PK, HK, EL, LX and SP participated in the design and coordination of the study and the analysis and interpretation of the data, and drafted the manuscript. EB revised the manuscript critically for important intellectual content. MG, PK, IAK, HK, LX and SP participated in the expert panel for the validation of the data on medical resource utilization and contributed to the manuscript preparation. All authors read and approved the final manuscript.

Acknowledgments

The authors would like to thank Dr. Stavros Gravas Assistant Professor of Urology at University Hospital of Larissa, Dr. Dimitrios Hatzichristou Professor of Urology, Medical School, Aristotle University of Thessaloniki, Dr. Aristidis Karagiannis Director of Urology Department at Euroclinic, Dr. Charilaos Katsifotis Director of Urology Department at Polykliniki hospital, Dr. Dimitrios Malovrouvas Director of Urology Department at Evangelismos hospital,

Dr. Dionissios Mitropoulos Professor of Urology, Medical School, University of Athens, Dr. Petros Perimenis Professor of Urology, Medical School, University of Patras, Dr. Fragiskos Sofras Professor of Urology, Medical School, University of Crete, and Dr. Anastasios Thanos Director of Urology Department at St. Savvas hospital for their participation in the expert panel.

Author details
[1]School of Social Sciences, University of Peloponnese, Corinth, Greece. [2]GlaxoSmithKline, Athens, Greece. [3]PRMA consulting, Athens, Greece.

References

1. Kirby R, McConnel JD, Fitzpatrick JM, Roehrborn CG, Boyle P: *Textbook of Benign Prostatic Hyperplasia*. 2nd edition. Oxon, UK: CRC Press; 2004.
2. de la Rosette J, Alivizatos G, Madersbacher S, Sanz CR, Nordling J, Emberton M, Gravas S, Michel MC, Oekle M: Guidelines on benign prostatic hyperplasia. *Eur Assoc Urol* 2006, Retrieved from http://www.uroweb.org/fileadmin/user_upload/Guidelines/11%20BPH.pdf on May 19, 2014.
3. Lepor H: Managing and preventing acute urinary retention. *Rev Urol* 2005, 7(Suppl 8):S26–S33.
4. Gravas S, de la Rosette JJ: Investigational therapies targeted to the treatment of benign prostatic hyperplasia. *Expert Opin Investig Drugs* 2013, 22(3):357–368.
5. Roehrborn CG, Boyle P, Nickel JC, Hoefner K, Andriole G: Efficacy and safety of a dual inhibitor of 5-alpha-reductase types 1 and 2 (dutasteride) in men with benign prostatic hyperplasia. *Urology* 2002, 60(3):434–441.
6. Lepor H: Alpha blockers for the treatment of benign prostatic hyperplasia. *Rev Urol* 2007, 9(4):181–190.
7. Roehrborn CG, Siami P, Barkin J, Damiao R, Major-Walker K, Nandy I, Morrill BB, Gagnier RP, Montorsi F: The effects of combination therapy with dutasteride and tamsulosin on clinical outcomes in men with symptomatic benign prostatic hyperplasia: 4-year results from the CombAT study. *Eur Urol* 2010, 57(1):123–131.
8. Wei JT, Calhoun E, Jacobsen SJ: Urologic diseases in america project: benign prostatic hyperplasia. *J Urol* 2008, 179(5 Suppl):S75–S80.
9. Drummond MF, McGuire AJ, Black NA, Petticrew M, McPherson CK: Economic burden of treated benign prostatic hyperplasia in the United Kingdom. *Br J Urol* 1993, 71(3):290–296.
10. Walker A, Doyle S, Posnett J, Hunjan M: Cost-effectiveness of single-dose tamsulosin and dutasteride combination therapy compared with tamsulosin monotherapy in patients with benign prostatic hyperplasia in the UK. *BJU Int* 2013, 112(5):638–646.
11. Ismaila A, Walker A, Sayani A, Laroche B, Nickel JC, Posnett J, Su Z: Cost-effectiveness of dutasteride-tamsulosin combination therapy for the treatment of symptomatic benign prostatic hyperplasia: a Canadian model based on the CombAT trial. *Can Urol Assoc J* 2013, 7(5–6):E393–E401.
12. Antonanzas F, Brenes F, Molero JM, Fernandez-Pro A, Huerta A, Palencia R, Cozar JM: Cost-effectiveness of the combination therapy of dutasteride and tamsulosin in the treatment of benign prostatic hyperlasia in Spain. *Actas Urol Esp* 2011, 35(2):65–71.
13. Bjerklund Johansen TE, Baker TM, Black LK: Cost-effectiveness of combination therapy for treatment of benign prostatic hyperplasia: a model based on the findings of the combination of avodart and Tamsulosin trial. *BJU Int* 2012, 109(5):731–738.
14. Brennan A, Chick SE, Davies R: A taxonomy of model structures for economic evaluation of health technologies. *Health Econ* 2006, 15(12):1295–1310.
15. El-Hakim A: TURP in the new century: an analytical reappraisal in light of lasers. *Can Urol Assoc J* 2010, 4(5):347–349.
16. McVary KT, Roehrborn C, Avins LA, Barry MJ, Bruskewitz RC, Donnel RF, Foster HE, Gonzalez CM, Kaplan SA, Penson DR, Ulchaker JC, Wei JT: American Urological Association Guideline: Management of Benign Prostatic Hyperplasia (BPH). 2010 Retrieved from http://www.auanet.org/common/pdf/education/clinical-guidance/Benign-Prostatic-Hyperplasia.pdf, on May 19, 2014.
17. Briggs A, Claxton K, Sculpher M: *Decision Modelling for Health Economic Evaluation*. UK: Oxford: Oxford University Press; 2006.
18. Emberton M, Anson K: Acute urinary retention in men: an age old problem. *BMJ* 1999, 318(7188):921–925.
19. Harding C, Robson W, Drinnan M, Sajeel M, Ramsden P, Griffiths C, Pickard R: Predicting the outcome of prostatectomy using noninvasive bladder pressure and urine flow measurements. *Eur Urol* 2007, 52(1):186–192.
20. Toren P, Margel D, Kulkarni G, Finelli A, Zlotta A, Fleshner N: Effect of dutasteride on clinical progression of benign prostatic hyperplasia in asymptomatic men with enlarged prostate: a post hoc analysis of the REDUCE study. *BMJ* 2013, 346:f2109.
21. Emberton M, Cornel EB, Bassi PF, Fourcade RO, Gomez JM, Castro R: Benign prostatic hyperplasia as a progressive disease: a guide to the risk factors and options for medical management. *Int J Clin Pract* 2008, 62(7):1076–1086.
22. Trueman P, Hood SC, Nayak US, Mrazek MF: Prevalence of lower urinary tract symptoms and self-reported diagnosed 'benign prostatic hyperplasia', and their effect on quality of life in a community-based survey of men in the UK. *BJU Int* 1999, 83(4):410–415.
23. Verhamme KM, Dieleman JP, Bleumink GS, van der Lei J, Sturkenboom MC, Artibani W, Begaud B, Berges R, Borkowski A, Chappel CR, Costello A, Dobronski P, Farmer RD, Jimenez Cruz F, Jonas U, MacRae K, Pientka L, Rutten FF, van Schayck CP, Speakman MJ, Sturkenboom MC, Tiellac P, Tubaro A, Vallencien G, Vela Navarrete R: Incidence and prevalence of lower urinary tract symptoms suggestive of benign prostatic hyperplasia in primary care–the Triumph project. *Eur Urol* 2002, 42(4):323–328.
24. Mauskopf JA, Sullivan SD, Annemans L, Caro J, Mullins CD, Nuijten M, Orlewska E, Watkins J, Trueman P: Principles of good practice for budget impact analysis: report of the ISPOR Task Force on good research practices–budget impact analysis. *Value Health* 2007, 10(5):336–347.
25. World Health Organization website: Life-tables for Greece. 2013 Retrieved from http://apps.who.int/gho/data/?theme=main&vid=60640 on October 11, 2013.
26. Nuijten MJ, Mittendorf T, Persson U: Practical issues in handling data input and uncertainty in a budget impact analysis. *Eur J Health Econ* 2011, 12(3):231–241.
27. Greek official government gazette FEK 946 -12Mar2012. 2012 Retrieved from http://www.et.gr/index.php/2010-01-21-13-05-53/2010-01-21-14-09-50/50-products/fek/73-fek-issue-b on October 11, 2013 (in Greek).
28. Madersbacher S, Lackner J, Brossner C, Rohlich M, Stancik I, Willinger M, Schatzl G: Reoperation, myocardial infarction and mortality after transurethral and open prostatectomy: a nation-wide, long-term analysis of 23,123 cases. *Eur Urol* 2005, 47(4):499–504.
29. Milonas D: Significance of operative parameters on outcomes after transurethral resection of the prostate. *Medicina (Kaunas)* 2010, 46(1):24–29.
30. Reynard JM, Shearer RJ: Failure to void after transurethral resection of the prostate and mode of presentation. *Urology* 1999, 53(2):336–339.
31. Greek Official Government Gazette FEK 62 30-4-91 issue A. PD 157/91. 2013 Retrieved from http://www.et.gr/index.php/2010-01-21-13-05-53/2010-01-21-14-09-50/50-products/fek/72-fek-issue-a on October 11, 2013 (in Greek).

2

Determinants of peri-operative blood transfusion in a contemporary series of open prostatectomy for benign prostate hyperplasia

Mathew Y. Kyei[*], George O. Klufio, James E. Mensah, Samuel Gepi-Attee, Kwabena Ampadu, Bernard Toboh and Edward D. Yeboah

Abstract

Background: The objective of this study was to determine the factors responsible for peri-operative blood transfusion in a contemporary series of open prostatectomy for benign prostate hyperplasia and thus offer a guide for blood product management for the procedure.

Methods: This was a prospective study of 200 consecutive patients who underwent open prostatectomy for BPH from January 2010 to September 2013 at the Korle Bu Teaching Hospital, Accra. The data analyzed included the pre-operative blood haemoglobin level (Hb), presence of co-morbidities, the case type, indication for the surgery, ASA score, anaesthetic method used, systolic blood pressure, status of the operating surgeon, duration of surgery and the operative prostate weight. The transfusion of blood peri-operatively was also documented.

Results: The mean age of the patients was 69.1 years. Elective cases formed 83.5 % with refractory retention of urine being the commonest indication for surgery (68.0 %). The mean pre-operative Hb was 12.1 g/dl. Consultants performed 56.0 % of the prostatectomies. Transvesical approach was used in 90.0 % of the cases. The mean operative time was 101.3mins (range 35.0–240.0) with a mean operative prostate weight of 110.8 g (range 15–550 g). Most of the patients (82.0 %) had spinal anaesthesia. The blood transfusion rate was 23.5 %. The transfusion rate was significantly higher in patients with anaemia ($p = .000$), emergency cases ($p = .000$), the use of general anaesthesia ($p = .002$), a resident as the operating surgeons ($p = .034$), prostate weight >100 g ($p = .000$) and duration of surgery ($p = .011$). In a multivariable logistic regression analysis however only the pre-operative Hb ($p = .000$. OR 0.95, 95 % CI [0.035–0.257]) and the duration of surgery ($p = .025$, OR 1.021, 95 % CI [1.003–1.039]) could predict blood transfusion in open prostatectomy for BPH in this series.

Conclusions: A 'group and save' policy should be the preferred blood ordering procedure for patients with Hb ≥ 13.0 g/dl scheduled for an elective open prostatectomy for BPH under spinal anaesthesia. A long operative time however may increase the need for blood transfusion.

* Correspondence: matkyei@yahoo.com
Department of Surgery and Urology, School of Medicine and Dentistry,
College of Health Sciences, University of Ghana, P. O. Box 4236, Accra, Ghana

Background

Open prostatectomy for the surgical management of benign prostate hyperplasia (BPH) is now rarely used in most developed countries except for large prostates [1, 2]. This exclusive indication for the procedure in these countries is currently being shared with newer modalities of treatment like the holmium laser resection of the prostate [3]. However in resource poor countries, open prostatectomy remains the main mode of surgical management of benign prostate hyperplasia irrespective of the prostate size [4]. The surgical outcomes of open prostatectomy for BPH continue to be the basis for comparing and evaluating the effectiveness and safety of the newer methods of surgical management of large prostates [5]. This is because of the excellent clinical outcomes with improvement in lower urinary tract symptoms and an observed lower failure rate [5]. Thus a report on contemporary series of open prostatectomy in this era of newer treatment modalities may provide useful information in relation to blood transfusion requirements as we evaluate these newer techniques.

A frequently encountered challenge in open prostatectomy compared to the newer methods of surgical management of BPH is peri-operative bleeding requiring blood transfusion. The reported blood transfusion rates in open prostatectomy for BPH range from 3.3 % to 36.8 % [2, 5–8]. Blood transfusion carries risk of transfusion reactions and disease dissemination [9, 10] and there is substantial economic cost associated with allogeneic transfusions [11]. In developing countries where open prostatectomy is currently mostly practiced, assess to blood for transfusion is limited as there are only few voluntary blood donors. These surgeries are sometimes unduly delayed on account of lack of acceptable blood donors. An understanding of the factors that determine the transfusion rate in a contemporary series of open prostatectomy for BPH may form the basis for deciding pre-operatively, the likelihood of needing blood transfusion in a particular operation. This will enable a more rational ordering of blood products for the procedure as part of a blood management strategy. It will also bring to light modifiable factors that when addressed, could potentially make the transfusion rate in open prostatectomy comparable to the newer minimally invasive methods of prostatectomy for BPH.

Methods

This was a prospective study on the management of 200 consecutive patients who had consented in writing to undergo open prostatectomy for benign prostate hyperplasia at the Urology Unit of the Korle Bu Teaching Hospital in Accra. The study period was from January 2010 to September 2013 and approved by the Ethical and Protocol committee of the Korle Bu Teaching Hospital under the Medical Directorate. The diagnosis of BPH was made on the basis of the patient's clinical presentation and the finding of a prostate with benign features on digital rectal examination. Patients noted to have abnormal digital rectal examination or elevated total PSA had transrectal ultrasound guided prostate biopsy (12 cores) for histological confirmation of BPH.

Four consultant urologists and three senior urology residents carried out the operations in this study. The total number of open prostatectomy for BPH that had been performed by the consultants prior to the study ranged from 80–600 while that of the residents was 10–25 cases.

The surgical method used was either a transvesical open prostatectomy or Millins retropubic prostatectomy as described in Campbell Urology 7th Edition (2007) [12].

For the technique of the transvesical prostatectomy, the patient is positioned in the supine position and the suprapubic area shaved. The lower abdomen and external genital area are prepped and draped. A 22 or 24-Fr Foley urethra catheter is inserted into the bladder and the bladder filled with 250 mL of saline and the catheter removed. A lower midline incision is made and deepened through the subcutaneous tissue. The linea alba is incised, and the rectus abdominis muscles separated in the midline. The transversalis fascia is incised to expose the space of Retzius. The peritoneum is swept cephalad to develop the prevesical space. A self-retaining Balfour retractor is placed in the incision to retract the rectus muscles laterally. The anterior bladder wall is identified, and two 2–0 Vicryl stitches are placed on each side of the midline below the peritoneal reflection. A vertical cystotomy is then made with an electrocautery and using a pair of Metzenbaum scissors, the cystotomy is extended cephalad and caudally to within 1 cm of the bladder neck. Several pairs of stay sutures are placed using 2–0 Vicryl on each side of the midline to facilitate exposure. A figure-of-eight suture using 0 Vicryl is placed and tied at the most caudal position of the cystotomy to prevent further extension of the cystotomy incision during blunt finger dissection of the adenoma. This suture is subsequently used to close the cystostomy as the first layer. After inspecting the bladder, a Millins retractor is placed in the bladder and used to further expose the trigone bringing the bladder neck and prostate into view. The ureteric orifices are identified and using electrocautery, a circular incision is made in the bladder mucosa distal to the trigone. Care is taken not to injure the ureteric orifices. With the use of a pair of Metzenbaum scissors, the plane between the prostatic adenoma and prostatic capsule is developed at the 6-o'clock position and once well-established plane is created posteriorly, the prostatic adenoma is enucleated using blunt dissection. At the apex, the prostatic urethra is transected using a pinch action of the two fingertips avoiding excessive traction so as to avoid avulsing the urethra and injuring the sphincteric mechanism. The prostatic adenoma is removed from the prostatic fossa. The prostatic fossa is then examined for discrete bleeding sites that are controlled with 3–0 vicryl suture ligatures. In addition, a 0-vicryl suture is used to place two figure-of-eight sutures to advance the bladder mucosa into the prostatic fossa at the 5-o'clock and 7-o'clock positions at the prostatovesical junction to ensure control of the main arterial blood supply to the prostate. These maneuvers lead to complete hemostasis.

A 22 or 24 -Fr 3-way Foley urethral catheter with a 30-mL balloon is passed through the urethra into the bladder and the cystotomy incision closed in two layers. The first layer of closure is performed using the figure-of-eight suture of 0 Vicryl that was placed and tied at the most caudal position of the cystotomy using it as a running suture. The previously placed 2–0 Vicryl stay-sutures are tied over the first layer of closure to complete the two-layer closure completing a watertight bladder closure. Thirty milliliters of saline is placed in the balloon to ensure that the catheter balloon remains in the bladder and does not retract into the prostatic fossa. The urethral catheter is irrigated to confirm a watertight closure and to verify that haemorrhage is minimal. A small wound drain is placed via a separate stab incision lateral to the bladder and exits the skin. The rectus fascia is closed with vicryl 1 suture in a running fashion. The skin is closed with nylon 3–0. The drain is then secured to the abdominal wall. Continuous bladder irrigation is initiated to prevent clot formation. The urethral catheter is removed on post operative day 7 and the patient discharged with the skin stitches removed on post operative day 10.

For the operative technique in the retro-pubic open prostatectomy, the patient is positioned supine with the table placed in a mild Trendelenburg position without extension. The suprapubic area is shaved, prepped, and draped maintaining sterility. A 22 or 24-Fr Foley urethral catheter with a 30-mL balloon is passed into the bladder and connected to a sterile closed drainage system, and the balloon is inflated with 30 mL of saline. For the patients with refractory retention of urine, the urethral catheter is maintained for the procedure. A lower midline incision from the umbilicus to the pubic symphysis is made and deepened through the subcutaneous tissue. The linea alba is incised and the rectus abdominis muscles separated in the midline. The transversalis fascia is incised sharply exposing the space of Retzius. The peritoneum is mobilized cephalad starting at the pubic symphysis. A self-retaining Balfour retractor is placed in the incision and widened and a well-padded, malleable blade is connected to the retractor and used to displace the bladder posteriorly and superiorly. The anterior surface of the bladder and prostate are exposed. The preprostatic adipose tissue is gently removed to expose the superficial branch of the dorsal

vein complex and the puboprostatic ligaments with coagulation of the superficial branch of the dorsal vein. Next, we gain complete control of the dorsal vein complex as well as the lateral pedicles at the bladder neck, the main arterial blood supply to the prostate gland. This is achieved by firstly incising the endopelvic fascia laterally and partial transection of the puboprostatic ligaments. A 3–0 Monocryl suture on a 5/8-inch circle-tapered needle is passed in the avascular plane between the urethra and the dorsal vein complex at the apex of the prostate and tied. The lateral pedicles at the prostatovesical junction are ligated using figure-of-eight suture (vicryl 0) deep into the prostatovesical junction thus securing the main arterial blood supply to the prostate adenoma. With a sponge stick on the bladder neck to depress the bladder posteriorly, a No. 15 blade on a long handle is used to make a transverse capsulotomy in the prostate 2.0 cm distal to the bladder neck. The incision is deepened to thelevel of the adenoma and extended laterally in each direction to permit complete enucleation. A pair of Metzenbaum scissors is used to dissect the overlying prostatic capsule from the underlying prostatic adenoma. Once a well-defined plane is sufficiently developed, the index finger is inserted between the prostatic adenoma and the capsule to further develop the plane laterally and posteriorly allowing for enucleation and removal of the prostate adenoma with preservation of a strip of posterior prostatic urethra. The prostatic fossa is carefully inspected to ensure that all of the adenoma has been removed and that hemostasis is complete. A 22 or 24 -Fr, three-way Foley catheter with a 30-mL balloon is inserted through the anterior urethra and prostatic fossa into the bladder and the prostatic capsule closed using viryl 2–0 in two layers water tight with the sutures beginning laterally and meeting in the midline. Thirty milliliters of water is then placed in the balloon to ensure that the catheter balloon remains in the bladder and does not retract into the prostatic fossa. The bladder is then irrigated with saline to ensure continued hemostasis and to test the capsular closure for leakage. A suction drain is placed via a separate stab incision lateral to the prostate and bladder on one side to prevent hematoma and urinoma formation. The pelvis is irrigated with copious amounts of normal saline solution, and the rectus fascia is re-approximated with a size 1 vicryl suture. The skin is closed with interrupted nylon 3.0 sutures. The drain is secured to the abdominal wall, and traction applied to the catheter by placing gauze bandaged around the urethral catheter. Bladder irrigation is instituted until the urine become clear of blood. The urethral catheter is removed on post operative day 7 and the patient discharged with removal of the skin stitches on the 10th post operative day.

The data collected and entered into a proforma included the pre-operative haemoglobin level(Hb), presence of comorbidities and the case type (elective or emergency). Emergency prostatectomy was performed for patients who presented with severe haematuria due to BPH or sepsis from indwelling/stuck catheters as part of their resuscitation. The other parameters documented included the indication for the surgery, the anaesthetic method used, the systolic pressure at start of the operation, the status of the operating surgeon (i.e. consultant or resident), the duration of surgery, the operative prostate weight and the estimated blood loss. The requirement of blood transfusion including the units of blood transfused was documented.

The decision to transfuse blood intra-operatively was based on pallor of the mucous membranes, blood pressure instability and difficulty maintaining oxygen saturation intra-operative and/or haemoglobin levels determined by using the HemoCue. For the post-operative assessment of the haemoglobin level, Standard laboratory determined haemoglobin levels using a BC-6800 hematology Analyzer by Mindray was used with haemoglobin level less than 8.0 g/dl serving as a trigger for blood transfusion post operatively. The enucleated prostate specimens were submitted for histopathological examination.

The data was analyzed using the statistical package for the social sciences (SPSS) version 21 with the results presented as percentages and mean with standard deviation. Categorical variables were analyzed by chi-square. A significant statistical difference was accepted whenever $p < .05$. Blood transfusion and pre-operative haemoglobin, were evaluated as categorical data.

A multivariable logistic regression analysis was performed using the variables pre-operative haemoglobin level, duration of surgery, age, ASA score, systolic blood pressure, type of anaesthesia, status of the operating surgeon and operative prostate weight.

Results

Patient characteristics

Two hundred patients who had open prostatectomy for BPH were studied.

The majority of the patients 136 (68.0 %) had refractory retention of urine as the indication for surgery (Table 1).

The mean age of the patients was 69.1 ± 9.1 year (range 48–92 years) with mean body weight of 70.8 ± 12.6 kg. The mean pre-operative haemoglobin level was 12.0 ± 2.4 g/dl and that of the systolic blood pressure at the start of surgery was 152.2 ± 21.8 mmHg (range 102–219 mmHg). The mean surgery time (duration of Surgery) was 101.3 ± 32.5mins with that of the estimated blood loss being 365.8 ± 226.1 mls. The mean operative prostate weight was 110.5 ± 90.5 g (Table 2).

Ninety (45 %) of the patients had associated co-morbidities comprising hypertension 75 (37.5 %) [Including one person with hypertension and asthma], diabetes mellitus alone 4 (2.0 %), hypertension with diabetes mellitus 10 (5.0 %) and bronchial asthma 1 (0.5 %).

One hundred and sixty-seven (83.5 %) of the cases were elective cases while 33 (16.5 %) were emergencies.

Eighty-eight of the surgeries (44.0 %) were performed by senior residents in urology while 112 (56.0 %) were carried out by consultant urologists. Open transvesical prostatectomy was the operative method used in 180 (90.0 %) of the cases whilst retropubic prostatectomy was in 20 (10.0 %). Spinal, general and epidural anaesthesia were used in 164 (82.0 %), 28 (14.0 %) and 8 (4.0 %) of the operations respectively. Forty-seven (23.5 %) 0f the cases were transfused while 153 (76.5 %) were not (Table 3).

A total of 95 units of blood were transfused with an overall transfusion rate of 23.5 % (47/200) (Table 4).

After histological review of the enucleated prostate specimen, two cases (1 %) had foci of adenocarcinoma but the rest were confirmed as benign prostate hyperplasia. None of the patients with foci of adenocarcinoma was transfused.

Relationship between the blood transfusion rate and various patient characteristics

Certain individual parameters had varied influence on the transfusion rate. The transfusion rate was significantly higher in patients with anaemia ($p = .000$), emergency cases ($p = .000$), the use of general anaesthesia ($p = .002$), a resident as the operating surgeons ($p = .034$), prostate weight > 100 g ($p = .000$) and duration of surgery ($p = .011$) (Tables 5, 6 and 7).

Table 1 Indications for open prostatectomy

Indication for open prostatectomy	Number of patients (%)
Refractory retention of urine	136 (68.0)
Haematuria due to BPH	45 (22.5)
Lower urinary tract symptoms	10 (5.0)
BPH with associated bladder calculi	4 (2.0)
BPH with associated mild renal dysfunction	2 (1.0)
Refractory retention of urine with stuck urethral catheter	3 (1.5)
Total	200 (100)

Table 2 Patients characteristics

	Age (yrs)	Pre-operative Hb (g/dl)	Systolic Blood pressure (mmHg)	Surgery Time (duration of surgery) [mins]	Estimated blood loss (ml)	Operative prostate weight (g)
Mean	69.0859	11.9943	152.1632	101.3100	365.7895	110.5094
Median	69.0000	12.6000	150.0000	95.0000	300.0000	80.0000
Mode	75.00	13.30	140.00(a)	90.00	300.00	60.00
Std. Deviation	9.14562	2.36919	21.75062	32.49003	226.11000	90.45363
Range	44.00	13.30	117.00	205.00	900.00	535.00
Minimum	48.00	3.10	102.00	35.00	100.00	15.00
Maximum	92.00	16.40	219.00	240.00	1000.00	550.00

Table 3 Patients characteristics (categories)

VARIABLE	Number of patients	%
Blood Transfusion		
Transfused	47	23.5
Not-transfused	153	76.5
Age ($n = 198$)		
≤70 yrs	109	55.1
>70 yrs	89	44.9
Co-Morbidities		
No comorbidities	110	55.0
Presence of comorbidities	90	45.0
Case Type		
Elective	167	83.5
Emergency	33	16.5
Status of Surgeon		
Consultant	112	56.0
Resident	88	44.0
Anaestheisa used		
Spinal anesthesia	164	82.0
General anaesthesia	28	14.0
Epidural	8	4.0
Operative Method used		
Transvesical prostatectomy	180	90.0
Millins retropubic prostatectomy	20	10.0
Operative Prostate weight		
Prostate weight ≤ 100 g	130	65.0
Prostate weight >100 g	70	35.0
Duration of surgery		
Surgery time ≤ 90mins	95	47.5
Surgery time > 90mins	105	52.5
Total	200	

For patients with severe anaemia (pre-operative blood haemoglobin level <8.0 g/dl), the transfusion rate was 92.3 % while the transfusion rate for those with normal pre-operative blood haemoglobin level ≥ 13.0 g/dl was 5.5 % (Table 6). The patients with Hb < 8 that were not transfused were emergency cases who underwent the procedure without blood being available in the blood bank. They however kept their haemodynamic stability after the procedure and hence no further transfusions were offered them.

Multivariable logistic regression

In a multivariable logistic regression analysis using the variables pre-operative haemoglobin level (evaluated as categorical), duration of surgery, age, ASA score, systolic blood pressure, type of anaesthesia, status of the operating surgeon and operative prostate weight, only the pre-operative haemoglobin level(as categorical data) ($p = .000$, Odds Ratio (OR) = 0.95, 95 % Confidence Interval (CI) [0.035–0.257]) and duration of surgery (as a continuous data) ($p = .025$, Odds Ratio (OR) = 1.021, 95 % Confidence Interval (CI) [1.003–1.039]) could predict the likelihood of blood transfusion in open prostatectomy for BPH (Table 8).

Discussion

Peri-operative blood transfusion is common in open prostatectomy for BPH and that remains a significant disadvantage. The reported peri-operative blood transfusion rate has ranged widely from 3.3 % to 36.8 % being 3.3 % in a report by Zargooshi J (Iran) [6], 24.5 % by Elshai

Table 4 Number of units of blood transfused

Units of blood transfused	Number of patients (%)
0	153(76.5)
1	13 (6.5)
2	25 (12.5)
3	5 (2.5)
≥4	4 (2.0)
Total	200 (100)

Table 5 Blood transfusion against age, systolic blood pressure and enucleated prostate weight

			Blood Transfusion		Total	p-value
			Not-transfused	Transfused		
Patient age	Age ≤ 70 yrs	Count	83	26	109	
		% within transfusion	55.0 %	55.3 %	55.1 %	
	Age >70 yrs	Count	68	21	89	
		% within transfusion	45.0 %	44.7 %	44.9 %	
Total		Count	151	47	198	0.551
Systolic blood pressure	Systolic blood pressure ≤ 140 mmHg	Count	56	17	73	
		% within transfusion	36.6 %	36.2 %	36.5 %	
	Systolic blood pressure > 140 mmHg	Count	97	30	127	
		% within transfusion	63.4 %	63.8 %	63.5 %	
Total		Count	153	47	200	0.551
Enucleated Prostate weight	Prostate weight ≤ 100 g	Count	111	19	130	
		% within transfusion	72.5 %	40.4 %	65.0 %	
	Prostate weight > 100 g	Count	42	28	70	
		% within transfusion	27.5 %	59.6 %	35.0 %	
Total		Count	153	47	200	
		% within transfusion	100.0 %	100.0 %	100.0 %	0.000

et al (Egypt) [7] and 36.8 % by Ngugi et al (Kenya) [8]. The blood transfusion rate of 23.5 % in the present study compares with some of these reports.

Different factors have been reported to play a role in determining the need for blood transfusion in open prostatectomy for BPH. Previous reports have indicated that patient factors such as age above 70 years, increasing ASA scores and a systolic blood pressure above 140 mmHg might contribute to the need for blood transfusion in open prostatectomy [8]. These factors were not observed to be significant in this study. Of interest though is the finding of an increased transfusion rate in ASA3 by Torres-Claramunt R et al in a study on the predictors of blood transfusion in patients undergoing elective surgery for degenerative diseases of the spine [13].

This study found the presence of anaemia to be associated with a significantly higher blood transfusion rate. Using the WHO definition for anaemia, (http://www.who.int/vmnis/indicators/haemoglobin.pdf) patients who had severe anaemia pre-operatively were more likely to be transfused compared with those with normal blood haemoglobin levels. ($p = .000$). Hence the pre-operative blood haemoglobin level should serve as a guide to possible need for blood transfusion in open prostatectomy for BPH. Improving the blood haemoglobin level to normal levels before surgery could probably reduce the blood transfusion rate for this operation. The significantly higher blood transfusion rate in emergency cases may be partly due to inadequate pre-operative preparation before the procedure is undertaken in these rather ill patients.

Transfusion rate of 14.4 % in the elective cases is comparable to that of 8.2 % reported by Serrata et al. [14].

There was an observed lower blood transfusion rate in patients with co-morbidities as compared to patients without any co-morbidities ($p = .051$). The reason for this was not obvious. A possible explanation could be that those with co-morbidities had a more rigorous pre-operative preparation before surgery.

A significantly higher blood transfusion rate was observed in the operations performed under general anaesthesia. ($p = .002$) It is noteworthy that an increased use of blood transfusion associated with general anaesthesia has been observed in relation to total hip arthroplasty by Maurer et al. [15].

Although no significant difference was found between the two standard operative techniques for open prostatectomy in this study ($p = .345$), Dall'Oglio et al reported a reduced transfusion rate in an improved technique of Millin's retropubic prostatectomy compared to a classical transvesical prostatectomy [16].

The availability of surgeons specially trained in the procedure of open prostatectomy for BPH is not uniform across countries and even within a particular country. In some developing countries open prostatectomy is carried out by general surgeons [5] and in others, a significant proportion of the procedures are done by residents in training [7]. The attendant differences in experience and expertise of these categories of surgeons in performing open prostatectomy may partly be responsible for the wide variation in the reported transfusion rates for the procedure from

Table 6 Blood transfusion against Hb, case type and co-morbidities

			Blood Transfusion		Total	p-value
			Not-transfused	Transfused		
Hb Level	Severe Anaemia (Hb < 8.0 g/dl)	Count	1	12	13	
		% within transfusion	.7 %	25.5 %	6.5 %	
	Moderate Anaemia (Hb 8.0–10.9 g/dl)	Count	23	21	44	
		% within transfusion	15.0 %	44.7 %	22.0 %	
	Mild Anaemia (11.0–12.9 g/dl)	Count	43	9	52	
		% within transfusion	28.1 %	19.1 %	26.0 %	
	Normal (≥13.0 g/dl)	Count	86	5	91	
		% within transfusion	56.2 %	10.6 %	45.5 %	
Total		Count	153	47	200	0.000
Case type	Elective	Count	143	24	167	
		% within transfusion	93.5 %	51.1 %	83.5 %	
	Emergency	Count	10	23	33	
		% within transfusion	6.5 %	48.9 %	16.5 %	
Total		Count	153	47	200	0.000
Co-morbidities	No co-morbidity	Count	76	34	110	
		% within transfusion	49.7 %	72.3 %	55.0 %	
	Hypertension	Count	66	9	75	
		% within transfusion	43.1 %	19.1 %	37.5 %	
	Diabetes Mellitus	Count	3	1	4	
		% within transfusion	2.0 %	2.1 %	2.0 %	
	Hypertension with diabetes Mellitus	Count	7	3	10	
		% within transfusion	4.6 %	6.4 %	5.0 %	
	Asthma	Count	1	0	1	
		% within transfusion	.7 %	0.0 %	.5 %	
Total		Count	153	47	200	
		% within transfusion	100.0 %	100.0 %	100.0 %	0.051

different parts of the world. The present study showed that in our centre, the blood transfusion rate was significantly higher in the residents with less experience compared to that of the consultants with more experience in performing this surgery (30.7 % vrs 17.9 % [p = .034].

The finding of a significant association between the blood transfusion rate and the duration of surgery is indicative of an increased likelihood of transfusion with a longer duration of surgery. Comparing the blood transfusion rate and the mean prostate weight in various series showed no pattern of an increased blood transfusion with increasing mean prostate weights. Blood transfusion rates of 12.7 %, 6.8 %, 36.8 % and 8.2 % have been reported in procedures with mean prostate weights of 88.7 g, 104.5 g, 66.9 g and 75 g respectively [1, 4, 8, 14]. In this study a blood transfusion rate of 23.5 % was observed corresponding to a mean prostate weight of 110.5 g. Suer et al reported an increased blood transfusion rate of 19.2 % for prostates greater than 100 g compared

to those with prostate weight less than 100 g (9.4 %) [4]. Elshai et al upon stratification found no increase in blood transfusion rates between prostate weights greater than or less than 120 g [7]. This study confirmed the findings of Suer et al as the blood transfusion rate was significantly higher in prostates > 100 g (40.0 %) compared with prostate weights ≤ 100.0 g (14.6 %) [p = .000]. Even though there are currently methods for surgical resection of large prostates such as HoLEP, ThuLRP and PVP which have been found safe and effective and probable requiring less blood transfusion, [3] open prostatectomy is still used for large prostates in low resource countries like Ghana due to unavailability of these other treatment modalities.

Of the various factors which were found to be associated significantly with increased blood transfusion rate, only the pre-operative blood haemoglobin level (as categorical data) (p = .000, OR 0.95, 95 % CI [0.035–0.257]) and the duration of surgery (as continuous data) (p = .025, OR 1.02, 95 % CI[1.003–1.039]) could predict the likelihood of

Table 7 Blood transfusion against type of anaesthesia, status of surgeon, operative method and duration of surgery

			Blood Transfusion		Total	p-value
			Not-transfused	Transfused		
Anesthesia	Spinal	Count	132	32	164	
		% within transfusion	86.3 %	68.1 %	82.0 %	
	Ga	Count	14	14	28	
		% within transfusion	9.2 %	29.8 %	14.0 %	
	Epidural	Count	7	1	8	
		% within transfusion	4.6 %	2.1 %	4.0 %	
Total		Count	153	47	200	0.002
Status of operating surgeon	Consultant	Count	92	20	112	
		% within transfusion	60.1 %	42.6 %	56.0 %	
	Resident	Count	61	27	88	
		% within transfusion	39.9 %	57.4 %	44.0 %	
Total		Count	153	47	200	0.034
Operative method	Transvesical	Count	136	44	180	
		% within transfusion	88.9 %	93.6 %	90.0 %	
	Retropubic	Count	17	3	20	
		% within transfusion	11.1 %	6.4 %	10.0 %	
Total		Count	153	47	200	
		% within transfusion	100.0 %	100.0 %	100.0 %	0.345
Duration of Surgery	Surgery time ≤ 90mins	Count	80	15	95	
		% within transfusion	52.3 %	31.9 %	47.5 %	
	Surgery time > 90mins	Count	73	32	105	
		% within transfusion	47.7 %	68.1 %	52.5 %	
Total		Count	153	47	200	
		% within transfusion	100.0 %	100.0 %	100.0 %	0.011

Table 8 Multivariable logistic regression analysis

Variables in the Equation

Predictor Variables	B	S.E.	Wald (chi-square)	df	p-value	odd ratio	95 % C.I.for odd ratio	
							Lower	Upper
Pre-operative Hb (Anaemia)	−2.352	.507	21.517	1	.000	.095	.035	.257
Surgery time (Duration of surgery)	.020	.009	5.021	1	.025	1.021	1.003	1.039
Age category	−.212	.616	.119	1	.730	.809	.242	2.705
ASA score	−.369	.475	.605	1	.437	.691	.273	1.753
Systolic blood pressure	−.120	.334	.128	1	.720	.887	.461	1.708
Anesthesia	.585	.648	.814	1	.367	1.794	.504	6.390
Status of operating surgeon	1.039	.618	2.828	1	.093	2.827	.842	9.489
Operative prostate weight	.003	.004	.524	1	.469	1.003	.996	1.010
Constant	1.651	2.384	.479	1	.489	5.211		

Therefore, the multivariable logistic regression is given by

Log (transfused) = $1.651 - 2.352X_1 + 0.020X_2 - 0.212X_3 - 0.369X_4 - 0.120X_5 + 0.585X_6 + 1.039X_7 + 0.003X_8$

Variable(s) entered on step 1: hb (anaemia), surgery time, age category, ASA score, systolic, anaesthesia, status of surgeon, operative prostate weight blood transfusion in open prostatectomy for BPH following a multivariable logistic regression analysis.

Conclusions

Various factors were found to be associated significantly with increased blood transfusion rate in open prostatectomy for BPH. These included the presence of anaemia, emergency cases, use of general anaesthesia, prostate weight > 100 g, duration of surgery and a resident as the operating surgeon. However, only the pre-operative blood haemoglobin level and the duration of surgery could predict the likelihood of blood transfusion in open prostatectomy for BPH.

For patients with normal blood haemoglobin level (Hb $\geq$ 13.0 g/dl), a 'group and save' policy should be the preferred blood ordering procedure if undergoing an elective open prostatectomy for BPH, which preferably should be performed under spinal anaesthesia.

Competing interests
There are no financial or non- financial competing interests to declare.

Authors' contributions
MYK- was involved in conception and design of the study, contributed surgical expertise, involved in data collection and drafting of the final manuscript. GOK- was involved in conception and design of the study, contributed surgical expertise and offered a critical review of the manuscript for intellectual content. JEM- was involved in conception and design of the study, offered surgical expertise and also data collection. SGA- contributed surgical expertise and offered a critical review of the manuscript for intellectual content. KA- offered surgical expertise and data collection. BT- offered surgical expertise and data collection. EDY: Offered a critical review of the manuscript for intellectual content. All the authors have read and approved the final version of the manuscript.

Acknowledgements
We want to acknowledge Mr Yao Ahonon of the Public Health Department of the Korle Bu Teaching Hospital for his assistance with the statistical analysis. No external funding was obtained for this work.

References
1. Varkarakis I, Kyriakakis Z, Delis A, Protogerou V, Deliveliotis C. Long-term results of open transvesical prostatectomy from a contemporary series of patients. Urol. 2004;64:306–10.
2. Oelke M, Bachmann A, Descazeaud A, Emberton M, Gravas S, Michel MC, N'Dow J, Nordling J, de la Rossette JJ: EAU Guidelines on the treatment and follow-up of Non-neurogenic Male Lower Urinary Tract Symptoms including Benign Prostatic Obstruction. Eur Urol. 2013;64:118-140 [http://dx.doi.org/10.1016/j.eururo.2013.03.004].
3. Kuntz RM, Lehrich K, Ahyai SA. Holmium laser enucleation of the prostate versus open prostatectomy for prostates greater than 100 g: 5- year follow up results of a randomized clinical trial. Eur Urol. 2008;53:160–6.
4. Suer E, Gokce I, Yaman O, Anafarta K, Gogus O. Open prostatectomy is still a valid option for large prostates: a high-volume, single-center experience. Urol. 2008;72:90–4.
5. Tubaro A, de Nunzio C. The current role of open surgery in BPH. EAU-EBU Update series. 2006;I4:191–201.
6. Zargooshi J. Open prostatectomy for benign prostate hyperplasia: short-term outcome in 3000 consecutive patients. Prostate Cancer Prostatic Dis. 2007;10:374–7.
7. Elshai AM, El-Nahas AR, Barakat TS, Elsaadany MM, El-Hefnawy AS. Transvesical open prostatectomy for benign prostate hyperplasia in the era of minimally invasive surgery: peri-operative outcomes of a contemporary series. Arab J Urol. 2013;11:362–8.
8. Ngugi PM, Saula PW. Open simple prostatectomy and blood transfusion in Nairobi. East African Med J. 2007;84 suppl 9:12–23.
9. Hendrickson JE, Hillyer CD. Noninfectious serious hazards of transfusion. Anaesth Analg. 2009;108:759–69.
10. Perkins HA, Busch MP. Transfusion-associated infections: 50 years of relentless challenges and remarkable progress. Transfusion. 2010;50:2080–99.
11. Whitaker BI, Green J, King MR, Leibeg LL, Mathew SM, Schlumpf KS, Schrieber GB: The 2007 national blood collection and utilization survey report. Washington: Department of Health and Human services; 2007. www.hhs.gov/ash/bloodsafety/2007nbcus_survey.pdf.
12. Han M, Partin AW. Retropubic and Suprapubic Open Prostatectomy. In: Kavoussi LR, Novick AC, Partin AW, editors. Campbell-Walsh Urology9th Edition. Philadelphia: Saunders Elsevier; 2007. p. 2845–53.
13. Torres-Claramunt R, Ramírez M, López-Soques M, Saló G, Molina-Ros A, Lladó A, Cáceres E: Predictors of blood transfusion in patients undergoing elective surgery for degenerative conditions of the spine. Arch Orthop Trauma Surg. 2012;132:1393–8.
14. Serretta V, Morgia G, Fondacaro L, Curto G, Lo bianco A, Pirritano D, Melloni D, Orestano F, Motta M, Pavone-Macaluso M: Open prostatectomy for benign prostatic enlargement in southern Europe in the late 1990s: a contemporary series of 1800 interventions. Urol. 2002;60:623–7.
15. Maurer SG, Chen AL, Hiebert R, Pereira GC, Di Cesare PE. Comparison of outcomes of using spinal versus general anesthesia in total hip arthroplasty. Am J Orthop. 2007;36:E101–6.
16. Dall'Oglio MF, Srougi M, Antunes AA, Crippa A, Cury J. An improved technique for controlling bleeding during simple retropubic prostatectomy: a randomized controlled study. BJU Int. 2006;98:384–7.

3

Is absorption of irrigation fluid a problem in Thulium laser vaporization of the prostate? A prospective investigation using the expired breath ethanol test

Livio Mordasini[1*†], Dominik Abt[1†], Gautier Müllhaupt[1], Daniel S Engeler[1], Andreas Lüthi[2], Hans-Peter Schmid[1] and Christoph Schwab[1]

Abstract

Background: Benign prostatic hyperplasia (BPH) is a prevalent entity in elderly men. If medical treatment fails, monopolar transurethral resection of the prostate (TUR-P) is still considered as the standard treatment. The proportion of high-risk patients with cardiac comorbidities increases and TUR-P goes along with a relevant perioperative risk. Especially large volume influx of irrigation fluid and transurethral resection syndrome (TUR syndrome) represent serious threats to these patients. Using isotonic saline as irrigation fluid like in transurethral laser vaporization (TUV-P), TUR syndrome can be prevented. However, no prospective trial has ever assessed occurrence or extent of irrigation fluid absorption in Thulium Laser TUV-P.

Methods/Design: This is a single-center prospective trial, investigating, if absorption of irrigation fluid occurs during Thulium Laser TUV-P by expired breath ethanol test. The expired breath ethanol technique is an established method of investigating intraoperative absorption of irrigation fluid: A tracer amount of ethanol is added to the irrigation fluid and the absorption of irrigation fluid can be calculated by measuring the expiratory ethanol concentrations of the patient with an alcohol breathalyzer.

Fifty consecutive patients undergoing TUV-P at our tertiary referral center are included into the trial. Absorption volume of irrigation fluid during Thulium Laser TUV-P is defined as primary endpoint. Pre- to postoperative changes in bladder diaries, biochemical and hematological laboratory findings, duration of operation and standardized questionnaires are assessed as secondary outcome measures.

Discussion: The aim of this study is to assess the safety of Thulium Laser TUV-P in regard to absorption of irrigation fluid.

Keywords: Prostate, Benign prostatic hyperplasia, Transurethral laser vaporization of the prostate, Transurethral resection syndrome, Absorption irrigation fluid, Expired breath ethanol test

* Correspondence: livio.mordasini@icloud.com
†Equal contributors
[1]Department of Urology, Cantonal Hospital St. Gallen, Rorschacherstrasse 95, 9007 St. Gallen, Switzerland
Full list of author information is available at the end of the article

Background

Benign prostatic hyperplasia (BPH) is a prevalent entity, affecting over 50% of men older than 60 years [1]. The clinical picture of the disease includes lower urinary tract symptoms such as interrupted and weak urinary stream, nocturia, urgency, leaking and even sexual dysfunction in some individuals [2]. Medical therapy is usually the first-line treatment [3]. However, the efficacy of drugs like alpha-blockers is limited, and as disease progresses, more invasive treatment options have to be taken into consideration.

In cases with moderate to severe lower urinary tract symptoms (LUTS) monopolar transurethral resection of the prostate (TUR-P) is still the standard treatment. Especially in frail patients, conventional TUR-P is associated with relevant and potentially deleterious complications [4-6].

The proportion of elderly patients on anticoagulation or antiplatelet therapy with cardiac comorbidities increases. Especially major bleeding and transurethral resection syndrome (TUR syndrome) put these high-risk patients at a relevant perioperative risk.

TUR syndrome is caused by absorption of electrolyte-free irrigating fluid (which has to be used in monopolar TUR-P), and consists of symptoms of the circulatory and nervous systems. Mild forms are common and often go undiagnosed, while severe forms of the TUR syndrome are potentially life-threatening [7].

Using isotonic saline, like in bipolar TUR-P and TUV-P, TUR syndrome can be prevented. Moreover, these techniques were thought to completely prevent influx of irrigation fluid into the vascular system due to their excellent coagulation properties [8-11].

However, significant intraoperative fluid absorption has been demonstrated in bipolar TUR-P and with the Greenlight-Laser. The authors concluded, that these techniques should be used with caution in patients with significant cardiovascular comorbidities [12,13].

Ethanol monitoring was first used in the late 1980's as an alternative to traditional methods of measuring fluid absorption (i.e. measuring volumetric fluid balance and serum sodium concentration). These techniques, however, are bothersome and must be carried out meticulously to yield a valid Figure of absorption [14]. If ethanol is added to the irrigation fluid as a tracer, the volume of fluid absorbed can be estimated from the amount of ethanol measured in the patient's exspired breath.

The expired breath ethanol technique is an established method of investigating intraoperative absorption of irrigation fluid [15]. Isotonic 0.9% saline including 1% of ethanol is used for intra-operative irrigation. The absorption of irrigation fluid can be estimated by measuring the expiratory ethanol concentrations with an alcohol breathalyzer.

During the last years, the Thulium laser has emerged as an alternative to other types of lasers, combining the best features for performing vaporization techniques: Thulium laser has a wavelength of 2013 nm, and its target chromophore is water. The energy of the Thulium laser has a high tissue absorption rate, producing effective vaporization with scant depth in the remaining tissue. As the properties of water remain unaltered until it reaches boiling point, the effect of the laser on the tissue remains constant throughout the surgical procedure [11].

The short-term complication rate with the Thulium laser is similar to the rate described after vaporization with other laser systems [16-21] and less than that with TUR-P. Thus, Thulium vaporization of the prostate has established as a standard procedure in many urological departments including ours.

Despite recent publications on the safety and complications of Thulium vaporization of the prostate, to our knowledge, no prospective trial has assessed occurence and extent of irrigation fluid absorption in TUV-P using Thulium Laser.

We therefore aim to investigate the relevance of irrigation fluid absorption during Thulium Laser vaporization of the prostate by expired breath ethanol test.

Methods and design
Study design and location
This is a single-center prospective trial conducted at the urological department of Cantonal Hospital St. Gallen, St. Gallen, Switzerland.

Study population and recruitment
Recruitment of the study participants is performed at the urological outpatient clinic of Cantonal Hospital St. Gallen by the principle investigator (PI). The PI will check for inclusion and exclusion criteria (Table 1) by reviewing the patient's medical record and by patient-doctor conversation. Study participants are thoroughly informed about the study and included into the trial if informed consent is given.

Study procedures
Age, height, weight, free uroflowmetry, post void residual urine, co-medication, bladder voiding diary, International

Table 1 Inclusion and exclusion criteria

Inclusion criteria	Exclusion criteria
• Men older than 40	• Mild symptoms (IPSS <8)
• Patient must be a candidate for TUV-P	• Urethral stenosis
• Refractory to medical therapy or patient is not willing to consider further medical treatment	• Bladder diverticulum (>100 ml)
	• Former alcoholic or chronic liver
• Written informed consent	• disease

Prostate Symptom Score (IPSS) and ASA Score are determined preinterventionally in all study participants (Figure 1). The intervention is performed in an inpatient setting.

TUV-P

Before the operation starts, prostate size is assessed by transrectal ultrasound measurement (TRUS).

In the trial setting, TUV-P is only performed by surgeons with an experience of more than 100 transurethral interventions.

A Thulium continuous wave laser is employed (Revolix Duo 120 W, 2 micron thulium continuous wave laser; LISA laser products OHG, Katlenburg, Germany).

Application is carried out with a 24-Chr. continuous flow cystoscope (Karl Storz Endoskope; Anklin AG, Binningen, Switzerland) and a 550-µm front-firing laser fiber. The procedure begins at 80-W. In the first phase of the surgery, the bladder neck is opened and the median lobe vaporized. The lateral lobes are then vaporized until a working channel is created in the prostate. A power of 120-W is used from then on, completing vaporization of the median and lateral lobes. At the

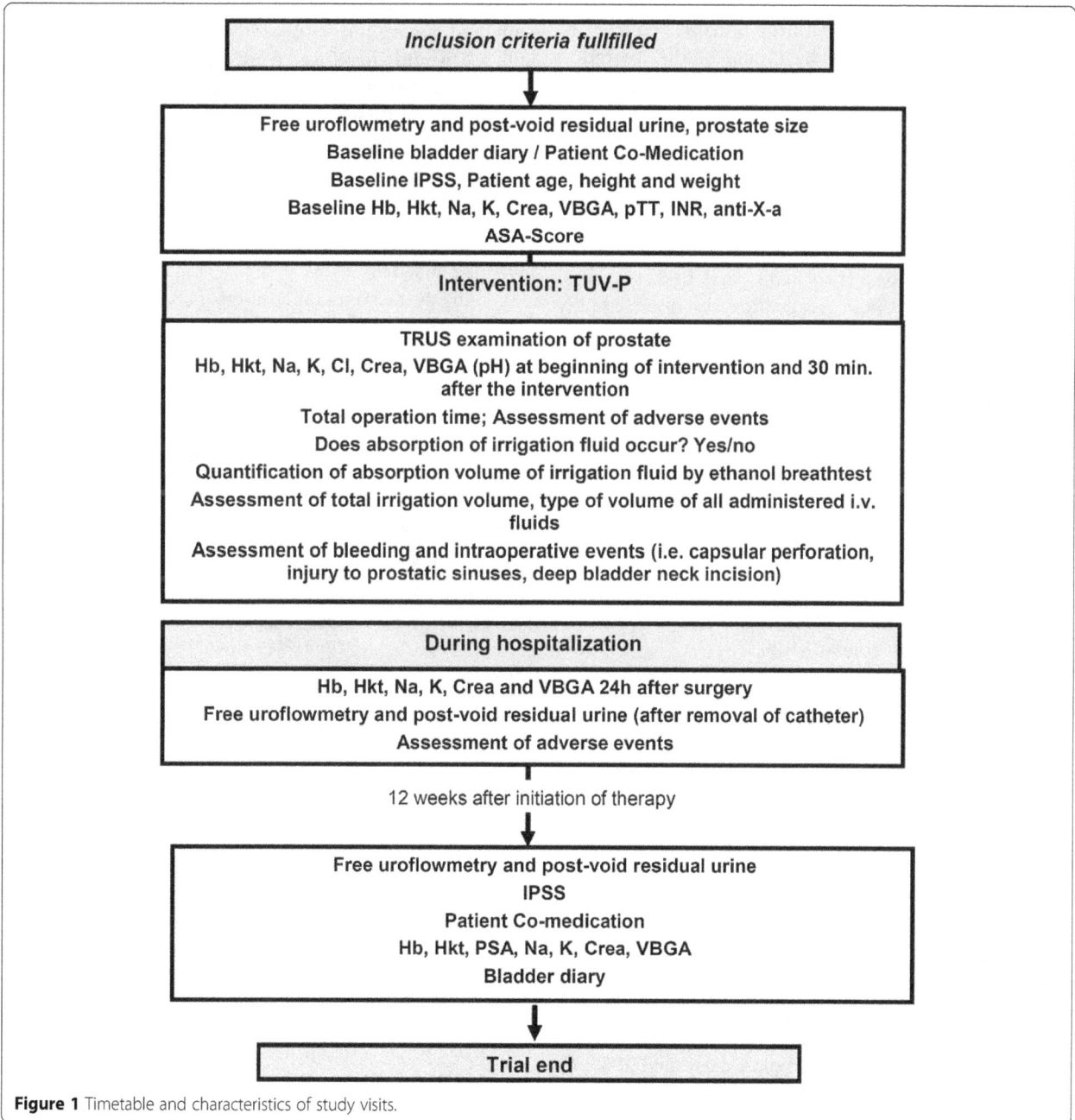

Figure 1 Timetable and characteristics of study visits.

end of surgery, a three-way 20-Chr. silicone urethral catheter will be inserted and continuous bladder irrigation with saline solution is maintained. Surgery will be performed under spinal or general anesthesia, according to anesthetist's and patient's preferences.

Bleeding or other intraoperative events such as capsular perforation, injury to prostatic sinuses or deep bladder neck incision are documented by the surgeon.

Expired breath ethanol test
Bladder irrigation is performed with conventional isotonic 0.9% saline with 1% ethanol added (Somanol® irrigation fluid Ecobag 5000 ml, Braun Medical AG, Sempach, Switzerland). The end-expiratory ethanol concentrations are measured at the beginning of the operation and at regular 10-min intervals (5-min intervals if ethanol is detected) throughout the procedure using an electrochemical AlcoQuant 6020 alcohol breathalyzer (Envitec GmbH, Wismar, Germany).

The values obtained represent the corresponding blood ethanol concentrations in mg/mL. A blood ethanol concentration of 0.05 mg/mL corresponds to ~150 mL fluid absorption. If patients are under general anesthesia, the alcohol breathalyzer is intermittently connected to the endotracheal tube via an adapter (this adapter is included in the AlcoQuant 6020 breathalyzer kit) after insufflation of the lungs with a resuscitation bag. The passively expired air is then used for the measurements. Patients under spinal anesthesia are asked to expire directly into the alcohol breathalyzer.

Hahn's mathematical formula (pre-programmed on a pocket calculator) will be used for the quantification of the total absorption volume intraoperatively [22].

$$Abs_{tot} = \sum 7007 \, EB\text{--}ethanol_i \times \Delta EB\text{--}ethanol + 632 \, EB\text{--}ethanol_i + 202$$

Blood analysis
After their baseline assessment on the day before the operation, hemoglobin, hematocrit, sodium, potassium, creatinine and a venous blood gas analysis are repeated at the beginning of the intervention, 30 minutes and 24 hours after the intervention to document possible electrolyte shifts.

Study outcome measures
Characteristics and timing of visits
After hospital discharge, a regular follow-up control is planned after 12 weeks assessing free uroflowmetry, post void residual, bladder voiding diary and IPSS. In addition, hemoglobin, hematocrit, sodium, potassium, creatinine and a venous blood gas analysis are determined.

Primary and secondary endpoints
Absorption volume of irrigation fluid during the Thulium laser TUV-P intervention was defined as primary endpoint. Secondary study endpoints are shown in Table 2.

Statistics, study sample size and power calculation
Determination of sample size
According to Wettstein et al., approximately 44% of patients showing a positive ethanol test were supposed. Among those, median fluid absorption was 1249 ml (138 – 2452 ml) [13]. This would indicate a mean fluid absorption of approximately 1250 ml, with standard deviation 579 ml. To estimate a 95% confidence interval for fluid absorption with width no larger than +/– 250 ml, we would therefore require 23 patients showing a positive ethanol test, indicating approximately evaluable 50 patients in total must be recruited.

For the secondary endpoint of rate of positive ethanol tests, the 95% confidence interval should therefore be no wider than +/– 14%.

Planned analyses
All study participants undergoing TUV-P will be considered in the final data analysis.

Primary analysis
Fluid absorption will be summarized as mean (95% confidence interval), including only those patients with a positive ethanol test.

Table 2 Primary and secondary endpoints

Primary endpoint	• Absorption volume of irrigation fluid during TUV-P
Secondary endpoints	• Duration of surgery
	• Assessment of bleeding and relevant intraoperative events (capsular perforation, injury to prostatic sinuses or deep bladder neck incision) by the surgeon
	• Amount of laser energy used intraoperatively (kilojoules)
	• Pre- to postoperative (30 min after intervention) changes in serum biochemical and hematological variables (creatinine, sodium, potassium, chloride), venous pH, hemoglobin
	• Pre- to postoperative changes (12 weeks after intervention) in flow and residual urine
	• Total irrigation volume and volume of all administered i.v. fluids
	• Duration of hospitalization post procedure
	• Duration of post procedure catheterization
	• Pre- to postoperative changes (12 weeks after intervention) in the IPSS
	• Pre- to postoperative changes (12 weeks after intervention) in bladder diary

Secondary analyses

The rate of positive ethanol tests will be summarized as n (%). Continuous secondary endpoints will be estimated as mean (95% CI), unless they are clearly non-normally distributed, in which case median (range) will be reported. Comparison of endpoints by prostate size, age and duration of symptoms will be examined using regression (linear or logistic, depending on the endpoint).

Regulatory issues

Ethical approval

Study was approved by the local ethical committee (EKSG 14/035) and is performed in consideration of the World Medical Association Declaration of Helsinki [23], the guidelines for GCP [24], and the guidelines of the Swiss Academy of Medical Sciences [25]. Handling of all personal data will strictly comply with the federal law of data protection in Switzerland [26].

Quality control, quality assurance and confidentiality

Trial-related monitoring, audits and regulatory inspections from the ethical committee (EKSG) will be permitted by the principal investigator, providing direct access to source documents. Data collection is performed using electronic case report forms (SecuTrial) programmed by Clinical Trials Unit St. Gallen. Insight into the data collected in this trial will only be provided to the involved investigators and the experts of the ethical committee responsible for the monitoring.

Missing data

In the case of patients with no follow-up at 12 weeks, baseline and earlier post-operative characteristics will be analyzed, as 12 week control is only a control of functional outcome and does not influence primary study endpoint.

Safety

The breathalyzer measures ethanol levels on a 10-min interval. New samples will be taken at a 5-min interval if ethanol is detected. The surgeons are blinded to the results of the ethanol measurements but are informed by the anesthetist, if the critical absorption volume of 2 liters is exceeded. This limit will be adopted according to the individual patient's health condition according to pre- and intraoperative recommendations of the anesthetist. If more than 2 liters of irrigation fluid are absorbed and the patient develops symptoms of cardiopulmonary stress, the operation will be finished and proceeded another day, if infravesical desobstruction was not complete.

Discussion

The aim of this study is to assess whether absorption of irrigation fluid occurs during TUV-P by expired ethanol breath test. Although different studies have been conducted, using ethanol breath test, the methodology of this monitoring method varies considerably between the studies. Protocol publications such as ours might help to standardize future trial settings.

Using a prospective single-center trial setting with clearly defined endpoints, as well as inclusion and exclusion criteria and study performance according to well-defined quality standards, data will help to assess safety of TUV-P in regard to potentially dangerous absorption of irrigation fluid. Assessment of urinary flow, post void residual and IPPS 12 weeks after the intervention are intended to ensure sufficient operative quality of TUV-P.

Moreover, potential advantages as well as problems of TUV-P can be analyzed. In addition, the study allows comparison to TUR-P data, still representing the gold standard of infravesical desobstruction.

Trial status

The trial is in the recruiting phase at the time of manuscript submission.

Abbreviations

BPH: Benign prostate hyperplasia; TUR-P: Transurethral resection of the prostate; TUV-P: Transurethral laser vaporization of the prostate; TUR syndrome: Transurethral resection syndrome; CI: Confidence interval; GCP: Good clinical practice; IPSS: International Prostate Symptom Score; PI: Principle investigator; TRUS: Transrectal ultrasound.

Competing interests

The authors declare that they have no competing interests.

Authors' contributions

All authors participated in creating the study design. LM and DA drafted the manuscript. GM, AL, HPS, DE, CS provided a critical revision of the manuscript. LM, DA, DE, HPS and CS obtained the funding of this study. All the authors read and approved the final manuscript

Acknowledgements

We would like to acknowledge Clinical Trial Unit St. Gallen for technical and financial support. Sarah Haile PhD performed the statistical analysis.

Funding

The study is funded by a grant (Nr. 14/08) from the CTU commission of Cantonal Hospital St. Gallen.

Author details

[1]Department of Urology, Cantonal Hospital St. Gallen, Rorschacherstrasse 95, 9007 St. Gallen, Switzerland. [2]Department of Anaesthesiology, Cantonal Hospital St. Gallen, Rorschacherstrasse 95, 9007 St. Gallen, Switzerland.

References

1. Levy A, Samraj GP. Benign prostatic hyperplasia: when to 'watch and wait', when and how to treat. Cleve Clin J Med. 2007;74 Suppl 3:S15–20.
2. Eckhardt MD, van Venrooij GE, van Melick HH, Boon TA. Prevalence and bothersomeness of lower urinary tract symptoms in benign prostatic hyperplasia and their impact on well-being. J Urol. 2001;166(2):563–8.
3. Michel MC, Mehlburger L, Bressel HU, Schumacher H, Schafers RF, Goepel M. Tamsulosin treatment of 19,365 patients with lower urinary tract symptoms: does co-morbidity alter tolerability? J Urol. 1998;160(3 Pt 1):784–91.
4. Hahn RG. Fluid absorption in endoscopic surgery. Br J Anaesth. 2006;96(1):8–20.

5. Mebust WK, Holtgrewe HL, Cockett AT, Peters PC. Transurethral prostatectomy: immediate and postoperative complications. a cooperative study of 13 participating institutions evaluating 3,885 patients. J Urol 2002. 1989;167(2 Pt 2):999–1003. discussion 1004.

6. Reich O, Gratzke C, Bachmann A, Seitz M, Schlenker B, Hermanek P, et al. Morbidity, mortality and early outcome of transurethral resection of the prostate: a prospective multicenter evaluation of 10,654 patients. J Urol. 2008;180(1):246–9.

7. Hahn RG. The transurethral resection syndrome. Acta Anaesthesiologica Scandinavica. 1991;35(7):557–67.

8. Geavlete B, Georgescu D, Multescu R, Stanescu F, Jecu M, Geavlete P. Bipolar plasma vaporization vs monopolar and bipolar TURP-A prospective, randomized, long-term comparison. Urology. 2011;78(4):930–5.

9. Geavlete B, Multescu R, Dragutescu M, Jecu M, Georgescu D, Geavlete P. Transurethral resection (TUR) in saline plasma vaporization of the prostate vs standard TUR of the prostate: 'the better choice' in benign prostatic hyperplasia? BJU Int. 2010;106(11):1695–9.

10. Reich O, Schlenker B, Gratzke C, Tilki D, Riecken M, Stief C, et al. Plasma vaporisation of the prostate: initial clinical results. European Urology. 2010;57(4):693–7.

11. Herrmann TR, Liatsikos EN, Nagele U, Traxer O, Merseburger AS. Eau Guidelines Panel on Lasers T: EAU guidelines on laser technologies. European Urology. 2012;61(4):783–95.

12. Hermanns T, Fankhauser CD, Hefermehl LJ, Kranzbuhler B, Wong LM, Capol JC, et al. Prospective evaluation of irrigation fluid absorption during pure transurethral bipolar plasma vaporisation of the prostate using expired-breath ethanol measurements. BJU Int. 2013;112(5):647–54.

13. Hermanns T, Grossmann NC, Wettstein MS, Fankhauser CD, Capol JC, Poyet C, et al. Absorption of irrigation fluid occurs frequently during high power 532 nm laser vaporization of the prostate. J Urol. 2015;193:211–6.

14. Olsson J, Rentzhog L, Hjertberg H, Hahn RG. Reliability of clinical assessment of fluid absorption in transurethral prostatic resection. European Urology. 1993;24(2):262–6.

15. Hahn RG. Ethanol monitoring of irrigating fluid absorption. Eur J Anaesthesiol. 1996;13(2):102–15.

16. Bouchier-Hayes DM, Van Appledorn S, Bugeja P, Crowe H, Challacombe B, Costello AJ. A randomized trial of photoselective vaporization of the prostate using the 80-W potassium-titanyl-phosphate laser vs transurethral prostatectomy, with a 1-year follow-up. BJU Int. 2010;105(7):964–9.

17. Pereira-Correia JA, de Moraes Sousa KD, Santos JB, de Morais PD, Lopes-da-Silva LF, Krambeck RL, et al. GreenLight HPS 120-W laser vaporization vs transurethral resection of the prostate (<60 mL): a 2-year randomized double-blind prospective urodynamic investigation. BJU Int. 2012;110(8):1184–9.

18. Al-Ansari A, Younes N, Sampige VP, Al-Rumaihi K, Ghafouri A, Gul T, et al. GreenLight HPS 120-W laser vaporization versus transurethral resection of the prostate for treatment of benign prostatic hyperplasia: a randomized clinical trial with midterm follow-up. European Urol. 2010;58(3):349–55.

19. Capitan C, Blazquez C, Martin MD, Hernandez V, de la Pena E, Llorente C. GreenLight HPS 120-W laser vaporization versus transurethral resection of the prostate for the treatment of lower urinary tract symptoms due to benign prostatic hyperplasia: a randomized clinical trial with 2-year follow-up. European Urol. 2011;60(4):734–9.

20. Lukacs B, Loeffler J, Bruyere F, Blanchet P, Gelet A, Coloby P, et al. Photoselective vaporization of the prostate with GreenLight 120-W laser compared with monopolar transurethral resection of the prostate: a multicenter randomized controlled trial. European Urology. 2012;61(6):1165–73.

21. Horasanli K, Silay MS, Altay B, Tanriverdi O, Sarica K, Miroglu C. Photoselective potassium titanyl phosphate (KTP) laser vaporization versus transurethral resection of the prostate for prostates larger than 70 mL: a short-term prospective randomized trial. Urology. 2008;71(2):247–51.

22. Hahn RG. Calculation of irrigant absorption by measurement of breath alcohol level during transurethral resection of the prostate. Br J Urol. 1991;68(4):390–3.

23. World Medical Association: Declaration of Helsinki - ethical principles for medical research involving human subjects. 1964, [http://www.wma.net/en/30publications/10policies/b3/]

24. International conference on harmonisation: Good clinical practice guideline. http://www.ich.org/products/guidelines/efficacy/article/efficacy-guidelines.html.

25. Swiss Academy of Medical Sciences: Guideline - concerning scientific research involving human beings. 2009, http://www.samw.ch/dms/en/Publications/Guidelines/e_Leitfaden_Forschung_def.pdf.

26. The Federal Authorities of the Swiss Confederation: Bundesgesetz über den Datenschutz (DSG) vom 19. Juni 1992, Stand. 01.01.2014. 1992, http://www.admin.ch/opc/de/classified-compilation/19920153/201401010000/235.1.pdf.

4

Patient's adherence on pharmacological therapy for benign prostatic hyperplasia (BPH)-associated lower urinary tract symptoms (LUTS) is different: is combination therapy better than monotherapy?

Luca Cindolo[1]*, Luisella Pirozzi[2], Petros Sountoulides[3], Caterina Fanizza[2], Marilena Romero[2], Pietro Castellan[4], Alessandro Antonelli[5], Claudio Simeone[5], Andrea Tubaro[6], Cosimo de Nunzio[6] and Luigi Schips[1]

Abstract

Background: *Recent studies showed that the non-adherence to the pharmacological therapy of patients affected by BPH-associated LUTS increased the risk of clinical progression of BPH.* We examined the patients adherence to pharmacological therapy and its clinical consequences in men with BPH-associated LUTS looking at the differences between drug classes comparing mono vs combination therapy.

Methods: A retrospective, population-based cohort study, using prescription administrative database and hospital discharge codes from a total of 1.5 million Italian men. Patients ≥40 years, administered alpha-blockers (AB) and 5alpha-reductase inhibitors (5ARIs), alone or in combination (CT), for BPH-associated LUTS were analyzed. The 1–year and long term adherence together with the analyses of hospitalization rates for BPH and BPH-related surgery were examined using multivariable Cox proportional hazards regression model and Pearson chi square test.

Results: Patients exposed to at least 6 months of therapy had a 1-year overall adherence of 29 % (monotherapy AB 35 %, monotherapy 5ARI 18 %, CT 9 %). Patient adherence progressively declined to 15 %, 8 % and 3 % for AB, 5ARI, and CT, respectively at the fifth year of follow up. Patients on CT had a higher discontinuation rate along all the follow-up compared to those under monotherapy with ABs or 5ARIs (all $p < 0.0001$). Moreover, CT was associated with a reduced risk of hospitalization for BPH-related surgery (HR 0.94; $p < 0.0001$) compared to AB monotherapy.

Conclusions: Adherence to pharmacological therapy of BPH-associated LUTS is low and varies depending on drugs class. Patients under CT have a higher likelihood of discontinuing treatment for a number of reasons that should be better investigated. Our study suggests that new strategies aiming to increase patient's adherence to the prescribed treatment are necessary in order to prevent BPH progression.

Keywords: Patient adherence, Drug therapy, Benign prostatic hyperplasia, Lower urinary tract symptoms, Alpha blockers, 5alfa reductase inhibitors, Administrative databases, Dutasteride, Finasteride, record-linkage analysis

* Correspondence: lucacindolo@virgilio.it
[1]Department of Urology, "S.Pio da Pietrelcina" Hospital, via San Camillo de Lellis, 1-66054 Vasto, Italy
Full list of author information is available at the end of the article

Background

Benign prostatic enlargement (BPE) is caused by a very common histopathological condition in aging men; benign prostatic hyperplasia (BPH). Clinical manifestations of BPH include lower urinary tract symptoms (LUTS), signs and sequelae of bladder outlet obstruction caused by BPE [1]. The prevalence of moderate-to-severe LUTS is high, increasing from 22 % among 50–59 year-old men to 45 % among those in the seventh decade of life. However only 19 % of men suffering from BPH-associated LUTS seek medical treatment and only 10.2 % receive pharmacological treatment [2–4].

Pharmacological therapy for BPH-associated LUTS aims at improving the patient's quality of life by relieving urinary symptoms and to a certain extent, by preventing the development of BPH-related complications. International guidelines agree that patients with moderate-to-severe LUTS are initially best managed with pharmacological therapy [5, 6].

Five classes of drugs are usually prescribed for the treatment of BPH-associated LUTS: alpha blockers (AB), 5-alpha reductase inhibitors (5ARI), phosphodiesterase-5 (PDE-5) inhibitors, antimuscarinics/beta3 agonists, and phytotherapeutics. Combination therapy (CT) with ABs and 5ARIs has been shown to be beneficial in terms of symptom control and disease progression [7–9].

Although pharmacological treatment of BPH is considered a success story among urologists, daily practice suggests that several patient's needs remain unmet. Whether or not this is due to drug's limitations, inappropriate patient management or low patient adherence to drug therapy remains unclear[4,10, 11]. Drug prescription trends and patterns for BPH-associated LUTS show a wide variation amongst countries, this variation is attributed to geographical, societal and cultural differences, cost of medications and different health policies.

A recent paper from our group showed that in "real life" practice the adherence to long-term treatment for BPH-associated LUTS significantly impacts BPH progression [12]. Data on adherence are of importance in order to understand possible unmet needs, explore patient preferences and identify areas for intervention for the health care systems [13]. In this specific issue, data from other areas of medicine confirmed that multiple medications (pills/day) could impact on patient adherence, suggesting that a fixed dose combination (more than a 2-pill therapy) can yield important improvements in patient drug adherence [14].

The aim of this study is to evaluate the patient adherence to pharmacological therapy for BPH-associated LUTS, and to analyze the adherence among drug regimens (CT vs monotherapy) together with long-term effects of drugs discontinuation.

Methods

A population-based cohort study was conducted using record-linkage analysis of three databases: drug prescriptions database, civil registry and hospital discharge records (HDR) (data on 6.5 million subjects across 22 local Italian Health Authorities).

All Italian citizens have access to health care services; medical and pharmaceutical services are provided for free or at a minimum charge as part of the National Health Service (NHS).

The Italian national drug database includes the prescriptions reimbursed by the Italian NHS; drugs are coded according to the Anatomical Therapeutic Chemical (ATC) Classification [15] and qualified with respect to dosage, and the date of the first and subsequent prescriptions from which data on adherence can be derived.

This cohort was linked with HDR which includes information on primary diagnoses and up to 5 coexisting conditions, performed procedures, dates of hospital admission and discharge. Diagnoses are classified according to the International Classification of Diseases-Ninth Revision, Clinical Modification (ICD9-CM) [16].

The Italian civil registry provides demographic information.

This study's methodology has been widely used to produce reliable epidemiological surveys [12,17, 18]. The analysis was carried out in strict compliance with the national Italian regulations for the full protection of the privacy rights of the subjects included in the databases. According to the Italian law, no ethical approval is required to perform this type of analysis and no informed consent from patients is needed. LP, CF and MR had the full access to the prescription database.

As reported in the previous paper [12] the sample population consisted of men ≥40 years who had been prescribed medications for BPH-associated LUTS during the index period (January[1st] 2004-December[31st] 2006).

Only ABs and 5ARIs were considered in the analysis (ATC codes: G04CA and G04CB, respectively). During the study period, the first prescription of a drug was considered as "index date" for including a patient. Patient adherence to therapy was estimated only for patients receiving treatment for a minimum of 6 months during the index period. Two different levels of exposure to drugs were set: at ≥ 6 months and at ≥12 months. Patients on treatment for more than 12 months during the index period were followed-up for 4 years (median time). Patients who: a) stopped one of the three regimens (AB monotherapy, 5ARI monotherapy or CT) for at least 2 consecutive months during the first year of treatment and at least 4 months/yearly during the follow-up period, or b) switched regimen were considered as "treatment discontinuation".

Patients were followed until hospitalization or surgery for BPH occurred or until their last follow-up. Patients were excluded when they were diagnosed with urethral stricture, prostate cancer in the 12 months preceding the index day.

Hospital admissions were recorded for patients receiving ≥1 year of pharmacological therapy and they were considered "BPH-related" when hospital records included a primary diagnosis and/or a surgical procedure related to BPH.

The presence of the ICD9-CM 600.xx code as primary diagnosis without surgical procedures was considered as a "BPH-related hospitalization". In the absence of clear and universally agreed upon indications for BPH-related hospitalization we included in the analyses all the hospitalizations for haematuria, urinary tract infection, urinary retention, bladder stones, and renal failure due to urinary tract obstruction caused by BPH.

The presence of ICD9-CM codes 57.0,57.91,57.92,60.21, and 60.29,60.3,60.4 as primary or secondary surgical procedures with any primary diagnoses was considered hospitalization for "BPH-related surgery".

Statistical analysis

For patients with at least 12 months of treatment, the characteristics were reported using descriptive statistics. Differences between patient treatment subgroups were assessed using a standardized difference (SD). Crude incidence rates (IRs) per 1000 men/year and incidence rate ratios (IRRs) with 95 % confidence intervals (CIs) were calculated with the Poisson regression model.

A multivariable Cox proportional hazards regression model was used to account for differences in follow-up and in baseline characteristics among groups. In all Cox models, the associations between groups and all outcomes were adjusted for co-variates known to be of prognostic importance to the outcomes: age and previous hospitalization for BPH, history of BPH-related surgery, and previous pharmacological treatment. Results were expressed as hazard ratios (HRs) and 95 % CIs. Adjusted event-free survival curves were calculated using the corrected group prognosis method. Discontinuation rate according to treatment group was compare using Pearson chi square test.

All reported that p-values are two tailed, and a p-value less than 0.05 was considered statistically different.

Analyses were conducted using SAS Statistical Package Release9.3 (SAS Institute, Cary, NC, USA).

Results

From the initial cohort of about 6.5 million individuals, men ≥40 years old were 1,447,074. Among these, only 28,273 received prescriptions for 12 months for BPH-associated LUTS, and this group was followed (median follow up 4 years, IQR 2–5.3) and represented our study cohort.

General characteristics of the group are summarized in Table 1. ABs was the most frequently prescribed drug class (87.1 %), followed by 5ARIs (8.1 %) and CT (4.7 %) that was prescribed in older patients.

Drug adherence

Patients who received prescriptions for ≥6 months were 97,407, and decreased to 61298 (63 %) at 10 months and to 28,273 (29 %) at 12 months. Patients who continued taking their drugs for up to 12 months were 35 %, 18 % and 9 % for ABs, 5ARIs and CT, respectively. These rates decreased to 15 %, 8 % and 3 % at 60 months (Fig. 1).

In men who received drug prescription for at least 12 months, the 5-year adherence was 42 % (Fig. 1). Patients who remained under pharmacological therapy for the entire follow-up period (median 4 years) represented 13 % of those identified in the index period.

Patients under CT showed a higher discontinuation rate all along the follow-up ($p < 0.0001$) compared to either monotherapy (Fig. 1).

During the follow-up period, only 12270 patients continued their prescribed pharmacological therapy. The discontinuation rate was statistically significant higher in patients under CT (discontinued vs adherent patients: SD % 19.87) (Table 2).

Hospitalization rates

During the follow-up period, the hospitalization rates for BPH and BPH-related surgery were 9.04 (95 % CI 8.49–9.62) per 1000 patient/year and 12.6 (95 % CI 11.96–13.28) per 1000 patient/year, respectively (Table 3).

As previously shown [12], the multivariate analysis confirmed that the use of 5ARIs was associated with a reduced risk of hospitalization due to BPH and BPH-related surgery (HR 0.46, 95 % CI 0.33–0.65 and HR 0.23, 95 % CI 0.15–0.35; $p < 0.0001$).Drug discontinuation on multivariate analysis was an independent risk factor for either BPH-related hospitalization or BPH surgery regardless of the therapeutic group (HR 1.65, 95 % CI 1.43–1.89 and HR 2.80, 95 % CI 2.59–3.03; $p < 0.0001$), as already reported [12].

Discussion

BPH represents a major public health issue because of its increasing prevalence, progressive nature and treatment costs [19–21]. Current guidelines recommend the use of ABs and 5ARIs as monotherapy or in combination for the treatment of BPH-associated LUTS [5,6]. However, a gap exists between guidelines and actual clinical practice [10,12, 21]. In "real life" the low adherence to prescribed medications is a recognized problem for chronic diseases [13]. Some studies deeply evaluated the problems of drug prescription and adherence for BPH as well as its impact on the clinical outcomes

Table 1 Patients' characteristics in relation to BPH treatment.

Variable	Baseline					
	Overall	AB	5ARI	CT	% Standardized difference *	
	28273	24626	2309	1338	5ARI vs AB	CT vs AB
	No. (%)	No. (%)	No. (%)	No. (%)		
Mean age (± SD)	70.28 (9.46)	69.55 (9.36)	75.61 (8.72)	74.49 (8.25)	66.99	58.3
Age						
40–55	1699 (6.01)	1641 (6.66)	42 (1.82)	16 (1.20)	−24.22	−28.42
56–65	7001 (24.76)	6579 (26.72)	248 (10.74)	174 (13.00)	−41.83	−34.89
66–75	11,120 (39.33)	9819 (39.87)	791 (34.26)	510 (38.12)	−11.65	−3.6
76–85	7054 (24.95)	5555 (22.56)	961 (41.62)	538 (40.21)	41.71	38.75
>85	1399 (4.95)	1032 (4.19)	267 (11.56)	100 (7.47)	27.63	14.04
Previous hospitalization for BPH	1312 (4.64)	1048 (4.26)	167 (7.23)	97 (7.25)	12.82	12.88
Previous BPH surgery	98 (0.35)	88 (0.36)	7 (0.30)	3 (0.22)	−0.94	−2.47
Previous BPH severity factors	854 (3.02)	715 (2.90)	95 (4.11)	44 (3.29)	6.58	2.22
Previous BPH related therapy	16,491 (58.33)	14,220 (57.74)	1377 (59.64)	894 (66.82)	3.84	18.8

Legend: AB: Alpha-blocker monotherapy; CT: Combination Therapy 5ARI; 5-alpha reductase inhibitors monotherapy; * Standardized difference greater than 10 % represents meaningful imbalance in explored variable between treatment groups

[12, 19, 21–23]. All showed concordant results: 1) the reported adherence in clinical trials is higher than that observed in real life; 2) the duration of treatment for BPH-associated LUTS is extremely short; 3) the adherence to treatment is generally low and 4) this might negatively influence BPH-related hospitalization rates.

By and large, patient adherence, or compliance, to a prescribed drug treatment is defined as the extent to which a person's attitude in terms of taking medication coincides with the medical or health advice he receives.

Adherence or compliance to a drug regimen is divided to primary non-compliance, for example when one receives a prescription, but does not have it made up at a pharmacy. Forms of secondary non-compliance include taking incorrect doses of the prescribed medication, taking the medication at wrong times, forgetting one or

more doses of the medication, or altogether stopping the medication, either by ceasing to take the medication sooner than the doctor recommended or failing to obtain a repeat prescription [24]. Poor adherence to a therapeutic regimen has been identified as a major public health problem that may have a major impact on clinical outcomes [25].

The lack of a valid method for measuring compliance is by itself a major barrier to compliance research. Both direct and indirect measures have been sought in order to quantify compliance, and although direct measures are considered to be the most accurate, their invasive nature makes them unacceptable and inappropriate to use. Indirect measurements are therefore more frequently reported in the literature and include measures such as interviews, diaries, tablet counts, and prescription refill dates. Interviews and

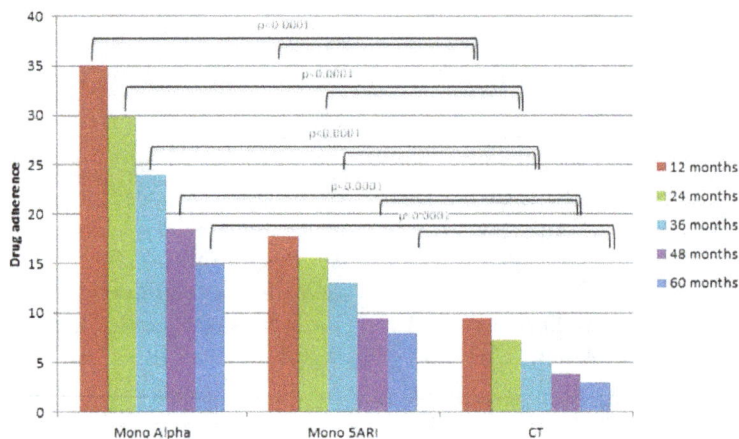

Fig. 1 Differences in adherence between different pharmacological regimens at 1, 2, 3, 4 and 5 years of follow-up

Table 2 Patients' characteristics according to drug adherence

VARIABLE	Discontinuated patients	Adherent patients	Standardized difference (%) *
Mean age (± SD)	70.15 (9.6)	70.37 (9.34)	-
Age class			
40–55	762 (6.21)	937 (5.86)	−1.4916
56–65	3131 (25.52)	3870 (24.18)	−3.0886
66–75	4784 (38.99)	6336 (39.59)	1.2350
76–85	2936 (23.93)	4118 (25.73)	4.1775
>85	657 (5.35)	742 (4.64)	−3.2957
Previous hospitalization for BPH	560 (4.56)	752 (4.70)	0.6430
Previous BPH surgery	45 (0.37)	53 (0.33)	−0.6030
Previous BPH severity factors	392 (3.19)	462 (2.89)	−1.7928
Previous BPH related therapy	7155 (58.31)	9336 (58.34)	0.0529
Therapeutic regimen			
AB	10923 (89.02)	13703 (85.63)	−10.2158
5ARI	1050 (8.56)	1259 (7.87)	−2.5140
CT	297 (2.42)	1041 (6.51)	19.8785

Legend: AB: Alpha-blocker monotherapy; 5ARI: 5-alpha reductase inhibitors monotherapy; CT: Combination Therapy; * Standardized difference greater than 10 % represents meaningful imbalance in explored variable between treatment groups

all self-report methods are vulnerable to overestimates of compliance and underestimates of non-compliance [26]. There are inherent limitations with these methods for generating valid and reliable data to give an accurate estimate of extent of patient adherence. Data from administrative databases, used in our and in other studies, are another indirect but reliable method of estimating drug consumption and patient adherence to a certain regimen [12, 21, 22]. Patient adherence to medical treatment is generally suboptimal irrespective of the drug or the treated condition. Studies on patient adherence on pharmacological therapy for the treatment of hypertension have shown that 50 % of patients discontinue their medication while two-thirds of patients that stay on treatment seem to lower their drug doses [26].

Although data regarding pharmacotherapy for BPH-associated LUTS are limited, a recent study from France confirmed that the 1-year adherence ranges between 21 % to 26 [21]. Madershbacher in 2007, looking at the results from clinical trials, depicted a clinical scenario describing the adherence rates of different therapeutic regimens. They found that the discontinuation rates in the 5-ARIs trials were lower than in the AB trials; and

confirmed a 2-year discontinuation rate of 10–20 % of patients under 5ARIs. On the other hand, discontinuation rates were lower for combination therapy (18 %) compared to finasteride (24 %) and doxazosin (27 %) monotherapy [19]. Even more interesting, these data are in contradiction with our results: a statistically significant lower adherence for CT compared to either AB or 5ARI monotherapies. These discrepancies are probably due to different study design. Our "real life" approach shows that patients abandon CT for several reasons that should be better investigated. Moreover, we found that the prolonged use of 5ARIs and adherence to the prescribed regimen were significantly associated with a lower risk of BPH-related hospitalization and surgery.

In the BPH population the decision to adhere to pharmacological treatment is primarily based on the patient's perception of bother due to LUTS and its impact on quality of life, and definitely depends on patient expectations and beliefs. The patient's perspective towards BPH and its management play a major role in the decision to initiate, continue or abandon treatment [27]. Even if we recognize that the reasons for the lack of drug adherence are multiple and difficult to analyze

Table 3 Hospitalization rates for BPH and BPH-related surgery

Outcomes	Overall		Mono alpha		Mono 5ARI		CT	
	Events	IR (95 % CI)	Events	IR (95 % CI)	Events	IR (95 % CI)	Events	IR (95 % CI)
Hospitalization for BPH (non surgical reasons)	989	9.04 (8.49;9.62)	918	9.58 (8.98;10.22)	34	3.77 (2.69;5.27)	37	8.10 (5.87;11.18)
BPH - related surgery	1393	12.60 (11.96;13.28)	1351	13.96 (13.23;14.72)	23	2.54 (1.69;3.82)	19	4.08 (2.60;6.40)

Legend: AB: Alpha-blocker monotherapy; 5ARI; 5-alpha reductase inhibitors monotherapy; CT: Combination Therapy; IR: incidence rate for 1000 person-years (especially using this methodological approach), it is important to remember that the strategy "enhance compliance by decreasing the number of pills" has been widely demonstrated in other fields of medicine [14]. There is convincing evidence from the literature suggesting that adherence is inversely associated with the complexity of the drug regimen. In this concept, the so-called fixed-dose combination (FDC) drugs (2 or more drugs produced in a single pill/tablet) have been developed in order to treat one disease with complementary actions (e.g., diabetes mellitus, asthma) or treat multiple clinical conditions (e.g., hypertension and hyperlipidemia) [14]. A FDC regime containing 0.5 mg of dutasteride and 0.4 mg of tamsulosin in the same pill is available for the treatment of BPH-associated LUTS.

Recent reports show that the use of FDC is associated with lifestyle advice resulted in rapid and sustained improvements in men with moderate BPH-associated LUTS [28] and that FDC is a cost-effective option in a estimated lifetime budget cost model [29] .

Even though the parameters that would modify patient's adherence are multiple and complex (spanning from awareness campaigns to better patient counselling) it seems reasonable to support the use of FDC for BPH-associated LUTS in order to decrease patient withdrawal and to increase adherence to the guidelines.

Several limitations of our study should be acknowledged. Studies based on data from administrative databases cannot be considered efficacy studies and do not include clinical variables or patient reported outcomes [30]. Another serious limitation is the imbalance between regimens, but this reflects the prescription attitudes. Moreover the current analysis is specific to the Italian situation and its generalization should be done with caution.

In this study we demonstrated that in "real life" patient adherence to BPH medication is different to that reported in clinical trials and that patients under CT abandon treatment more frequently that patients under monotherapy do.

Conclusions
Patient adherence to pharmacotherapy for BPH-associated LUTS is low. The need for combining two drugs to treat BPH represents a serious obstacle to better adherence. Persistence on pharmacological treatment is associated with a lower rate of hospitalization for BPH-related reasons. The use of a fixed-dose combination drug could increase adherence to treatment and would likely prevent BPH progression.

Abbreviations
5ARIs: 5alpha-reductase inhibitors; AB: Alpha-blocker; ATC: Anatomical Therapeutic Chemical; BPE: Benign prostatic enlargement; BPH: Benign prostatic hyperplasia; CIs: Confidence intervals; CT: Combination therapy; FDC: Fixed-dose combination; HDR: Hospital discharge records; HRs: Hazard ratios; ICD9-CM: International Classification of Diseases-Ninth Revision, Clinical Modification; IRRs: Incidence rate ratios; IRs: Incidence rates; LUTS: Lower urinary tract symptoms; NHS: National Health Service; PDE-5: Phosphodiesterase-5; SD: Standardized difference.

Competing interests
Cindolo does surgical tutorship for AMS and received honoraria from GSK for presentations. Tubaro is consultant and received research grant from Allergan and Astellas; he is investigator and paid speaker for AMS; he does presentations for Ferring, GSK and Pfizer; he is consultant for Bayer; he is consultant and investigator for GSK.
Pirozzi, Fanizza, Romero, De Nunzio, Castellan, Sountolides, Simeone, Antonelli, Schips declare declare that they have no competing interests.

Authors' contributions
LC and MR worked on the study concept and design. MR collected the data. CF, LP, PC, CDN and LC analyzed and interpretated the data. LC, LP and PS drafted the manuscript. AA, CS, AT and LS contributed with critical revision of the manuscript for important intellectual content. CDN and CF performed statistical analysis. LC obtained funding. LP given administrative, technical, or material support. CS and LS have made supervision. All authors read and approved the final manuscript.

Authors' information
Not applicable.

Acknowledgments
The authors thank Kimberlee Ann Manzi for reviewing the linguistic style of the manuscript.

Funding
Glaxo SmithKline provided an unrestricted grant for this research. The sponsor played no role in the concept, the design, the discussion of the study.

Author details
[1]Department of Urology, "S.Pio da Pietrelcina" Hospital, via San Camillo de Lellis, 1-66054 Vasto, Italy. [2]Department of Clinical Pharmacology and Epidemiology, Fondazione "Mario Negri Sud", Santa Maria Imbaro, Italy. [3]Department of Urology, General Hospital of Veria, Veria, Greece. [4]Department of Urology, "SS. Annunziata" Hospital, Chieti, Italy. [5]Department of Urology, "Spedali Civili" Hospital, Brescia, Italy. [6]Department of Urology, "Sant'Andrea" Hospital, University "La Sapienza", Rome, Italy.

References
1. Irwin DE, Kopp ZS, Agatep B, Milsom I, Abrams P. Worldwide prevalence estimates of lower urinary tract symptoms, overactive bladder, urinary incontinence and bladder outlet obstruction. BJU Int. 2011;108(7):1132–8.
2. Garraway WM, Collins GN, Lee RJ. High prevalence of benign prostatic hypertrophy in the community. Lancet. 1991;338:469–71.
3. Rosen R, Altwein J, Boyle P, Kirby RS, Lukacs B, Meuleman E, et al. Lower urinary tract symptoms and male sexual dysfunction: The multinational survey of the aging male (MSAM-7). Eur Urol. 2003;44:637–49.
4. Fourcade RO, Lacoin F, Rouprêt M, Slama A, Le Fur C, Michel E, et al. Outcomes and general health-related quality of life among patients medically treated in general daily practice for lower urinary tract symptoms due to benign prostatic hyperplasia. World J Urol. 2012;30(3):419–26.
5. Oelke M, Bachmann A, Descazeaud A, Emberton M, Gravas S, Michel MC, et al. EAU guidelines on the treatment and follow-up of non-neurogenic male lower urinary tract symptoms including benign prostatic obstruction. Eur Urol. 2013;64(1):118–40.
6. McVary KT, Roehrborn CG, Avins AL, Barry MJ, Bruskewitz RC, Donnell RF, et al. Update on AUA guideline on the management of benign prostatic hyperplasia. J Urol. 2011;185:1793–803.

7. McConnell JD, Roehrborn CG, Bautista OM, Andriole Jr GL, Dixon CM, Kusek JW, et al. Medical Therapy of Prostatic Symptoms (MTOPS) Research Group. The long-term effect of doxazosin, finasteride, and combination therapy on the clinical progression of benign prostatic hyperplasia. N Engl J Med. 2003;349(25):2387–98.

8. Roehrborn CG, Siami P, Barkin J, Damião R, Major-Walker K, Nandy I, et al. The effects of combination therapy with dutasteride and tamsulosin on clinical outcomes in men with symptomatic benign prostatic hyperplasia: 4-year results from the CombAT study. Eur Urol. 2010;57:123–31.

9. Füllhase C, Chapple C, Cornu JN, De Nunzio C, Gratzke C, Kaplan SA, et al. Systematic Review of Combination Drug Therapy for Non-neurogenic Male Lower Urinary Tract Symptoms. Eur Urol. 2013;64(2):228–43.

10. Strope SA, Elliott SP, Saigal CS, Smith A, Wilt TJ, Wei JT. Urologic Diseases in America Project. Urologist compliance with AUA best practice guidelines for benign prostatic hyperplasia in Medicare population. Urology. 2011;78(1):3–9.

11. De Nunzio C, Tubaro A. BPH: unmet needs in managing LUTS - a European perspective. Nat Rev Urol. 2011;9(1):9–10.

12. Cindolo L, Pirozzi L, Fanizza C, Romero M, Tubaro A, Autorino R, et al. Drug Adherence and Clinical Outcomes for Patients Under Pharmacological Therapy for Lower Urinary Tract Symptoms Related to Benign Prostatic Hyperplasia: Population-based Cohort Study. Eur Urol 2014 Nov 20. pii: S0302-2838(14)01180-4. doi: 10.1016/j.eururo.2014.11.006. [Epub ahead of print]

13. Yeaw J, Benner JS, Walt JG, Sian S, Smith DB. Comparing adherence and discontinuation across 6 chronic medication classes. J Manag Care Pharm. 2009;15(9):728–40.

14. Pan F, Chernew ME, Fendrick AM. Impact of fixed-dose combination drugs on adherence to prescriptionmedications. J Gen Intern Med. 2008;23(5):611–4.

15. WHO Collaborating Centre for Drug Statistics Methodology. ATC Index with DDDs. Oslo, Norway: WHO; 2003.

16. US Centers for Disease Control and Prevention. International Classification of Diseases, Ninth Revision, Clinical Modification (ICD-9-CM). Last access on March the 1, 2014 http://www.cdc.gov/nchs/icd/icd9cm.htm.

17. De Berardis G, Lucisano G, D'Ettorre A, Pellegrini F, Lepore V, Tognoni G, et al. Association of aspirin use with major bleeding in patients with and without diabetes. JAMA. 2012;307(21):2286–94.

18. Cindolo L, Fanizza C, Romero M, Pirozzi L, Autorino R, Berardinelli F, et al. The effects of dutasteride and finasteride on BPH-related hospitalization, surgery and prostate cancer diagnosis: a record-linkage analysis. World J Urol. 2013;31(3):665–71.

19. Madersbacher S, Marszalek M, Lackner J, Berger P, Schatzl G. The long-term outcome of medical therapy for BPH. Eur Urol. 2007;51(6):1522–33.

20. Emberton M, Cornel EB, Bassi PF, Fourcade RO, Gómez JM, Castro R. Benign prostatic hyperplasia as a progressive disease: a guide to the risk factors and options for medical management. Int J Clin Pract. 2008;62(7):1076–86.

21. Lukacs B, Cornu JN, Aout M, Tessier N, Hodée C, Haab F, et al. Management of lower urinary tract symptoms related to benign prostatic hyperplasia in real-life practice in France: a comprehensive population study. Eur Urol. 2013;64(3):493–501.

22. Nichol MB, Knight TK, Wu J, Barron R, Penson DF. Evaluating use patterns of and adherence to medications for benign prostatic hyperplasia. J Urol. 2009;181(5):2214–21.

23. Souverein PC, van Riemsdijk MM, de la Rosette JJ, Opdam PC, Leufkens HG. Treatment of benign prostatic hyperplasia and occurrence of prostatic surgery and acute urinary retention: a population-based cohort study in the Netherlands. Eur Urol. 2005;47(4):505–10.

24. Donovan JL, Blake DR. Patient non-compliance: deviance or reasoned decision-making? Social Science and Medicine. 1992;34:507–13.

25. Vermeire E, Hearnshaw H, Van Royen P, Denekens J. Patient adherence to treatment: three decades of research. A comprehensive review. J Clin Pharm Ther. 2001;26(5):331–42.

26. Kruse W. Patient compliance with drug treatment: new perspectives on an old problem. Clinical Investigation. 1992;70:163–6.

27. Robert G, Descazeaud A, de la Taille A. Lower urinary tract symptoms suggestive of benign prostatic hyperplasia: who are the high-risk patients and what are the best treatment options? Curr Opin Urol. 2011;21:42–8.

28. Roehrborn CG, Oyarzabal Perez I, Roos EP, Calomfirescu N, Brotherton B, Wang F, et al. Efficacy and safety of a fixed-dose combination of dutasteride and tamsulosin treatment (Duodart™) compared with watchful waiting with initiation of tamsulosin therapy if symptoms do not improve, both provided with lifestyle advice, in the management of treatment-naïve men with moderately symptomatic benign prostatic hyperplasia: 2-year CONDUCT study results. BJU Int 2015 Jan 7. doi: 10.1111/bju.13033. [Epub ahead of print]

29. Sayani A, Ismaila A, Walker A, Posnett J, Laroche B, Nickel JC, et al. Cost analysis of fixed-dosecombination of dutasteride and tamsulosin compared with concomitant dutasteride and tamsulosin monotherapy in patients with benign prostatic hyperplasia in Canada. Can Urol Assoc J. 2014;8(1–2):E1–7.

30. Sarrazin MS, Rosenthal GE. Finding pure and simple truths with administrative data. JAMA. 2012;307(13):1433–5.

5

Benign prostatic hyperplasia complicated with T1DM can be alleviated by treadmill exercise—evidences revealed by the rat model

Kuan-Chou Chen[1,2], Shian-Ying Sung[3], Yi-Ting Lin[4,5], Chiu-Lan Hsieh[6], Kun-Hung Shen[7*], Chiung-Chi Peng[8*] and Robert Y. Peng[5]

Abstract

Background: Both benign prostatic hyperplasia (BPH) and Type-1 diabetes mellitus (T1DM) share similar epidemiologic features and are all associated with the insulin-like growth factor (IGF)-mediated hormonal imbalance. The purpose of this study is to understand whether exercise (EX) could alleviate DM and DM + BPH.

Methods: Sprague-Dawley rats were divided into eight groups: normal control, EX, BPH, BPH + EX, DM, DM + EX, BPH + DM, and BPH + DM + EX. T1DM was induced by intraperitoneal (ip) injection of streptozotocin (65 mg/kg) in Week 2, and BPH was induced by successive ip injections of Sustanon® (testosterone, 3.5 mg/head) plus estradiol (0.1 mg/head) from Week 3 to Week 9. Treadmill exercise training (20 m/min, 60 min per time) was performed three times per week for 6 weeks.

Results: In BPH + EX, EX maintained at a constant body weight (BW); and suppressed stromal layer thickening, collagen deposition, blood glucose (BG), levels of testosterone (Ts), 5α-reductase(5αRd), dihydrotestosterone (DHT), androgen receptor (AR), serum hydrogen peroxide, TBARs, and interleukin-6 (IL-6). EX recovered testes size and substantially increased nitric oxide (NO) levels. In DM + EX group, EX decreased BW, PW, nuclear proliferation, inflammatory cell aggregation, collagen deposition, and BG. As contrast, EX upregulated insulin, IGF, Ts, NO, 5αRd, AR, and DHT, and substantially reduced PSA. In BPH + DM + EX, EX maintained BW at a subnormal level, slightly suppressed prostate stromal inflammation, collagen deposition, and BG, moderately restored sIn and IGF. Although failed to suppress Ts, EX highly upregulated 5αRd and suppressed DHT and AR, together with highly upregulated NO resulting in substantially reduced PSA.

Conclusion: EX, by remodeling androgen and NO expressions, can effectively alleviate BPH, DM, and BPH + DM.

Keywords: Exercise, BPH, T1DM, Insulin, Androgen, Nitric oxide (NO)

Background

Benign prostatic hyperplasia (BPH) is the most common benign tumor in men. Epidemiological data have indicated that BPH may be associated with the metabolic syndrome (MetS) [1] which can substantially increase the risk of BPH and low urinary tract symptoms (LUTS) [2].

When complicated with diabetes mellitus (DM), the mechanisms that regulate reactive stroma biology in BPH can be altered anatomically, pathologically, and biochemically [3]. Prostatic volume and the anterior-posterior diameter are positively associated with the component number of MetS [1]. The possible pathophysiologic mechanisms needed to explain these relations include an increased sympathetic tone, the alterations in sex steroid hormone expression, and the induction of systemic inflammation and oxidative stress [4]. The levels of insulin-like growth factor (IGF) and IGF-binding proteins (IGFBPs) in prostate tissue and blood are associated with the risk of developing BPH,

* Correspondence: robert.shen@msa.hinet.net; misspeng@tmu.edu.tw
[7]Division of Urology, Department of Surgery, Chi-Mei Medical Center, 901 Chung Hwa Road, Yung Kang City, Tainan 701, Taiwan
[8]Graduate Institute of Clinical Medicine, College of Medicine, Taipei Medical University, 250 Wu-Shing St., Xin-Yi District, Taipei 110, Taiwan
Full list of author information is available at the end of the article

which also regulate the circulating androgen and growth hormones [2].

Regular exercise (EX) is associated with low levels of interleukin-6 (IL-6), tumor necrosis factor-α (TNF-α), and simultaneously, with increases in antiinflammatory substances, such as adiponectin, IL-4, and IL-10 [5]. Hence, moderate EX training can exert antioxidant and antiinflammatory systemic protective effects [5]. Much of the literature supports a clinically relevant, independent, and strong inverse relationship between EX and the development of BPH and LUTS [6–8]. Furthermore, running considerable distances per week may lower the BPH risk, independent of the BMI and diet [9].

EX has been shown to have beneficially improved the Type 2 DM (T2DM) [10, 11] and BPH [9]. Moreover, amounting evidences also have revealed that a close association between BPH and T2DM through a common pathogenic mechanism is possible [12]. Parsons et al. in a chort report indicated that obesity, elevated fasting plasma glucose level, and DM are risk factors for BPH [13]. Previous document even substantially pointed out that diabetic vascular damage may cause hypoxia which in turn may contribute to pathogenesis of BPH [14]. Recently, we have showed EX beneficially alleviated BPH [7], however, the documented effect of EX on patients concomitantly affiliated with BPH plus Type 1 DM (BPH + T1DM) is still lacking. We hypothesized that EX could be beneficial to BHP + T1DM subjects. In this present study we developed a BPH + DM rat model to verify whether EX could improve such a metabolic syndrome.

Methods

Chemicals

T-Pro Western Blot Stripping Reagent was obtained from BioPioneer (San Diego, CA, USA); streptozotocin (STZ), Sirius Red, bovine serum albumin (BSA), and sodium dodecyl sulfate-polyacrylamide were purchased from Sigma-Aldrich (St. Louis, MO, USA); Coomassie Brillant Blue R-250, Coomassie Brillant Blue-G, glycine, and Tris base were obtained from US Biological (USA). Bis-acrylamide solution was purchased from Serva (Germany). Sustanon® was provided by the Schering-Plough Company (Kenilworth, NJ, USA) which is an injectable testosterone medication containing four testosterone esters at concentrations: 30 mg/mL of testosterone propionate, 60 mg/mL of testosterone phenylpropionate, 60 mg/mL of testosterone isocaproate, and 100 mg/mL of testosterone decanoate. The overall androgenic potency per mL of Sustanon® is equivalent to 176 mg of testosterone. Tris (hydroxymethyl) aminomethane hydrochloride (Tris-HCl) and hydrogen peroxide were purchased from Panreac (Spain). PageRuler™ Prestained Protein Ladder was supplied by Fermentas

(Canada). TEMED, ammonium persulfate (APS), and mineral oil were products of Bio-Rad (USA).

The sources of various kits were: Rat insulin ELISA kit (Mercodia, Sweden), AssayMax mouse insulin-like growth factor-1 (IGF-1 ELISA Kit; AssayPro, USA), rat Interleukin-6 (IL-6) ELISA kit (PeproTech, USA). TBARS ELISA kit (Cayman Chemical, USA), hydrogen peroxide (H_2O_2) assay kit (BioVision, USA) testosterone EIA (Cayman Chemical, USA), and dihydrotestosterone ELISA kit (Alpha Diagnostic, USA).

While the suppliers of antibodies were: antirabbit IgG (eBioscience, USA), antimouse IgG (Jackson ImmunoResearch, USA), β-actin antibody (Novus Biologicals, USA), antigoat IgG, 5α-reductase antibody, androgen receptor antibody (Santa Cruz Co., USA), and prostatic-specific antigen (PSA) antibody (Bioss, Scotland).

Animals

This experiment was approved by the Institutional Animal Care and Ethics Committee of Taipei Medical University (Taipei, Taiwan), and adhered to the animal care standards of the American College of Sports Medicine. In brief, 64 male Sprague-Dawley rats, aged 6 weeks, weighing 250–265 g were purchased from Biolasco Co. (Taipei, Taiwan). The rats were housed in an animal room conditioned at 24 ± 2 °C, RH 70–75 %, with a 12 h/12 h light/night cycle. The access of water and chow was ad libitum. The animals were acclimated in the animal room during the first week and then divided into eight groups, with eight rats in each group: Group 1, normal control; Group 2, BPH control; Group 3, DM control; Group 4, BPH + DM; Group 5, EX control; Group 6, BPH + EX; Group 7, DM + EX; and Group 8, BPH + DM + EX. The animals were separately caged, with 2 rats in each cage. In Week 2, DM groups were induced with a single intraperitoneal (ip) injection of streptozotocin (65 mg/kg) The BPH groups were induced in Week 3 by daily ip injection with Sustanon® (testosterone, 3.5 mg/head) and estradiol (0.1 mg/head), consecutively for 8 weeks. Exercise training was conducted from Week 12 until Week 17 on a rat exercise treadmill (Fortelice, International Co., Ltd., Taiwan). according to the program: rats were allowed to sprint at 20 m/min, 60 min per time, three courses per week, this program was continued successively for a total period of 6 weeks.

Blood collection and analysis of the lipid profiles

The control biochemical data were established at the end of the first week before experiment. The control data of the DM-control was established 1 week after STZ-induction, and those of the BPH-control group was collected 8 weeks after Sustanon®-induction. Blood collection was performed at the end of Week 2 and Week 17. In

Week 17, the rats were bled from the abdominal arteriole immediately before euthanized with CO_2 anesthesia. The blood obtained was centrifuged at 4 °C at $3000 \times g$ for 10 min using a freezer-type centrifuge (1580 MGR, Gyrozen, Korea), and the serum high-density lipoprotein (HDL), serum low-density lipoprotein (LDL), serum cholesterol (CHOL), and triglyceride (TG) were determined using respective kits by following the manufacturer's instructions.

Collection of tissue specimens

After euthanized, the prostates with seminiferous vesicles and testis were excised, photoed and weighed. Half of each organ was immersed in a 10 % formalin fixation solution, and the other half was rapidly immersed into liquid nitrogen, and stored at –80 °C for further use.

Extraction of proteins

To 200 mg prostate tissues lysis buffer (1.6 mL) was added, homogenized (microquantity-type homogenizer, T10 Basic, IKA, Germany) on ice and left to react for 30 min. The homogenate was centrifuged using the freezer-type centrifuge (1580 MGR) at $12000 \times g$ at 4 °C for 20 min. The supernatant (protein lysate, PLS) was separated and stored at –80 °C for further use.

Western blot analysis of 5α-reductase

The PLS was assayed for total protein content. To PSL, a two-fold volume of Western sample loading dye (WSLD) solution was loaded. The mixture (named herein PSL-WSLD) was heated in a dry heating bath (100 °C) for 10 min, and treated as follows. PSL-WSLD containing 30 μg of protein was loaded onto 10 % SDS-PAGE and the electrophoresis was conducted in the SDS-PAGE electrophoresis chamber (Mini-Protean Tetra Cell, Bio-Rad, USA), using the SDS-PAGE electrophoresis buffer (running buffer of pH 8.3, containing 25 mM Tri-HCl, 192 mM glycine, 0.1 % SDS, and deionized water to adjust to 1 L) at 75 V for 30 min. The protein spots were electrotransferred onto the PDVF membrane using a Mini Trans-Blot (Bio-Rad, USA) at 4 °C and 75 V for 20 h. The PVDF membrane was removed and marked with the obtained molecular weight. The marked membrane was sliced according to the molecular weight, immersed in a blocking buffer, and agitated at 4 °C overnight. The membrane was rinsed with a TBST solution thrice and left to stand for 10 min. The primary antibodies were applied and left to react for 1 h at ambient temperature, and then rinsed with the TBST solution. The secondary antibodies were applied, and left to react at ambient temperature for 1 h. After rinsed with the TBST solution, enhanced chemiluminescence (ECL) was applied and left to react completely.

Protein expression was imaged using a luminescent image analyzer (LAS-4000; Fujifilm, Tokyo, Japan).

Enzyme linked immunosorbent analysis for determining serum insulin, IGF, TBARS, H_2O_2, testosterone, DHT and prostate IL-6

The blood obtained was immediately centrifuged using the freezer-type centrifuge (1580 MGR) at $3000 \times g$ and 4 °C for 10 min. The supernatant serum was separated and stored at –80 °C if not used immediately. The sera were used for determining insulin, IGF, TBARS, H_2O_2, testosterone and DHT. Prostatic tissues (100 mg) were minced into chops having size <3 mm^3 and extensively washed with PBS containing heparin to prevent potential peripheral blood contamination. The mince was incubated with 200 U/mL type I collagenase and 100 mg/mL DNase type I (Sigma Chemical Company, St. Louis, MO) in RPMI 1640 medium plus 10 % fetal calf serum and 6 % penicillin/streptomycin solution (Gibco BRL Life Technologies, Gaithersburg). The tissues were dissociated overnight at 37 °C and used for determination of IL-6. The following protocol for assay was performed following the instructions given by the manufacturers.

Pathological examination and Sirius Red staining

After CO_2-euthanized, prostate, testes, seminal vesicle, bladder, pancreas, kidneys, heart, liver, and muscles were excised, photoed and weighed. Half of each organ was fixed in 10 % formalin, paraffin-embedded, and sliced with a microtome. The specimens were forwarded to the National Laboratory Animal Center (NLAC, Taipei) to receive pathological examination.

The paraffin-embedded specimens were dewaxed with xylene, and rehydrated successively with gradient ethanol solutions (100, 95, 80, and 70 %). These specimens were first stained with the Fouchet dying agent to attain a clear contrasting background, then with Weigert's haematoxylin to stain the nuclei (to a bluish-black color), and finally with Sirius Red to stain the collagen (to red). The semifinished specimens were immediately dehydrated, mounted, and examined using an optical microscope (BX41M-ESD, Olympus, Japan).

Immunohistochemical stain for androgen receptor (AR) and prostatic specific antigen (PSA)

The paraffin-embedded tissue specimens were placed in an incubator held at 37 °C overnight, immersed in xylene for 10 min to remove the residual embedding paraffin, and successively rehydrated with gradient ethanol solutions (100, 95, 80, and 70 %). Citric acid (10 mM, pH 6.0) was added to the rehydrated specimens. After 15 min, the specimens were treated with 3 % H_2O_2 for 15 min and then rinsed twice with PBS. The primary antibodies were applied and left to react for 2 h. After rinsed twice with PBS, the secondary antibodies were applied, left to react for 30 min, and peroxidase-conjugated streptavidin was added to react for 1 h and the specimens were rinsed with PBS twice. Finally, the specimens were reacted with the coloring agent diaminobenzidine (DAB) for 30 min, rinsed twice with PBS, dehydrated with gradient ethanol solutions, and mounted.

Determination of NO

Griess reagent (20 μL) was added to 20 μL of serum (or tissue homogenate) and mixed well. Double-distilled water (160 μL) was added to the mixture to make up to a total volume 200 μL. The optical density was read at 550 nm against the blank. A calibration curve was established using 20 μL of a standard sodium nitrite solution, similarly treated with 20 μL of Griess reagent and 160 μL of double-distilled water, and finally the optical density was read at 550 nm. The nitric oxide content of the samples was calculated from the reference curve.

Statistical analysis

Data obtained in the same group were analyzed with Duncan's multiple range test, using the Statistical Analysis System software (SAS 9.0). Data were expressed as mean ± SD. Different letters indicated significant differences at a confidence level of $p < 0.05$.

Results

Body weight variation was affected by the treatments

After BPH induction, the body weight of the normal control and EX control groups steadily increased from Week 3 until Week 17, reaching 552.5 ± 68.6 g and 557.8 ± 53.4 g, respectively. The body weights of the BPH and BPH + EX groups increased for the initial 2 weeks until Week 5 to 423.7 ± 53.4 g and 433.0 ± 32.1 g, respectively, and then remained unchanged until Week 17. In the DM group, a body weight of approximately 246.0 ± 40.0 g almost remained unchanged all the way until Week 17. The body weight of the DM + EX group increased steadily to 339.5 ± 14.01 g after the EX intervention. By contrast, the BPH + DM and BPH + DM + EX groups rapidly gained weight to 395.7 ± 8.6 g and 320.0 ± 79.4 g, respectively, in Week 17 (Fig. 1).

Testes weights

Figure 2a-c reveals the testis of BPH, DM, BPH + DM, DM + EX, and BPH + DM + EX were all much smaller in size compared to the normal. Ex greatly increased the testes size in BPH group but not in groups DM, BPH + DM, and BPH + DM + EX (Fig. 2b, c).

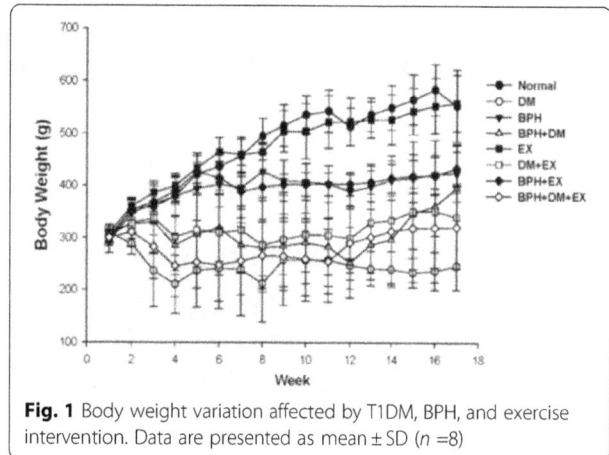

Fig. 1 Body weight variation affected by T1DM, BPH, and exercise intervention. Data are presented as mean ± SD (n =8)

Apparent prostatic size and weight were affected by the treatments

The mean prostatic weights of the normal control, EX control, BPH control, BPH + EX, DM control, DM + EX, BPH + DM, and BPH + DM + EX groups were 3.52 ± 0.76 g, 4.03 ± 0.76 g, 4.90 ± 0.65 g, 4.55 ± 0.80 g, 1.38 ± 0.89 g, 2.60 ± 1.09 g, 2.86 ± 0.67 g, and 2.43 ± 1.17 g, respectively (Fig. 3b). Compared with the normal prostatic size, the EX control exhibited a slightly enlarged prostate. The morphology and weight of the prostate in the EX and BPH + EX groups was comparable (Fig. 3a and b), but a substantial prostatic weight difference was observed between the normal and BPH groups ($p < 0.05$) (Fig. 3b). The prostate in the DM groups was severely shrunken (Fig. 3a and b). In the BPH + DM group, the extent of shrinkage was much less severe than that in the DM group. EX increased the prostatic size and weight in the DM + EX group ($p < 0.05$), but not in the BPH + DM + EX group (Fig. 3b).

Lipid profile

The level of HDL for the control, BPH, DM, and BPH + DM value without EX were 46.8 ± 10.8 mg/dL, 41.7 ± 1.7 mg/dL, 35.4 ± 16 mg/dL, and 38.5 ± 7.6 mg/dL, respectively. While EX altered the corresponding values to 49.9 ± 13.6 mg/dL, 44.3 ± 6.3 mg/dL, 37.8 ± 11.8 mg/dL, and 43.3 ± 8.9 mg/dL, respectively (Fig. 4a-b).

Likely, without EX intervention, the serum LDL level of BPH, DM, and BPH + DM were substantially raised to 13.4 ± 0.5 mg/dL, 18.2 ± 0.5 mg/dL, and 13.1 ± 1.8 mg/dL, respectively compared to the control 6.8 ± 0.8 mg/dL (Fig. 4a). EX correspondingly alleviated the values to 8.5 ± 4.4 mg/dL, 13.6 ± 3.3 mg/dL, and 10.6 ± 6.1 mg/dL, respectively, comparing with the EX control 7.3 ± 3.4 mg/dL (Fig. 4b).

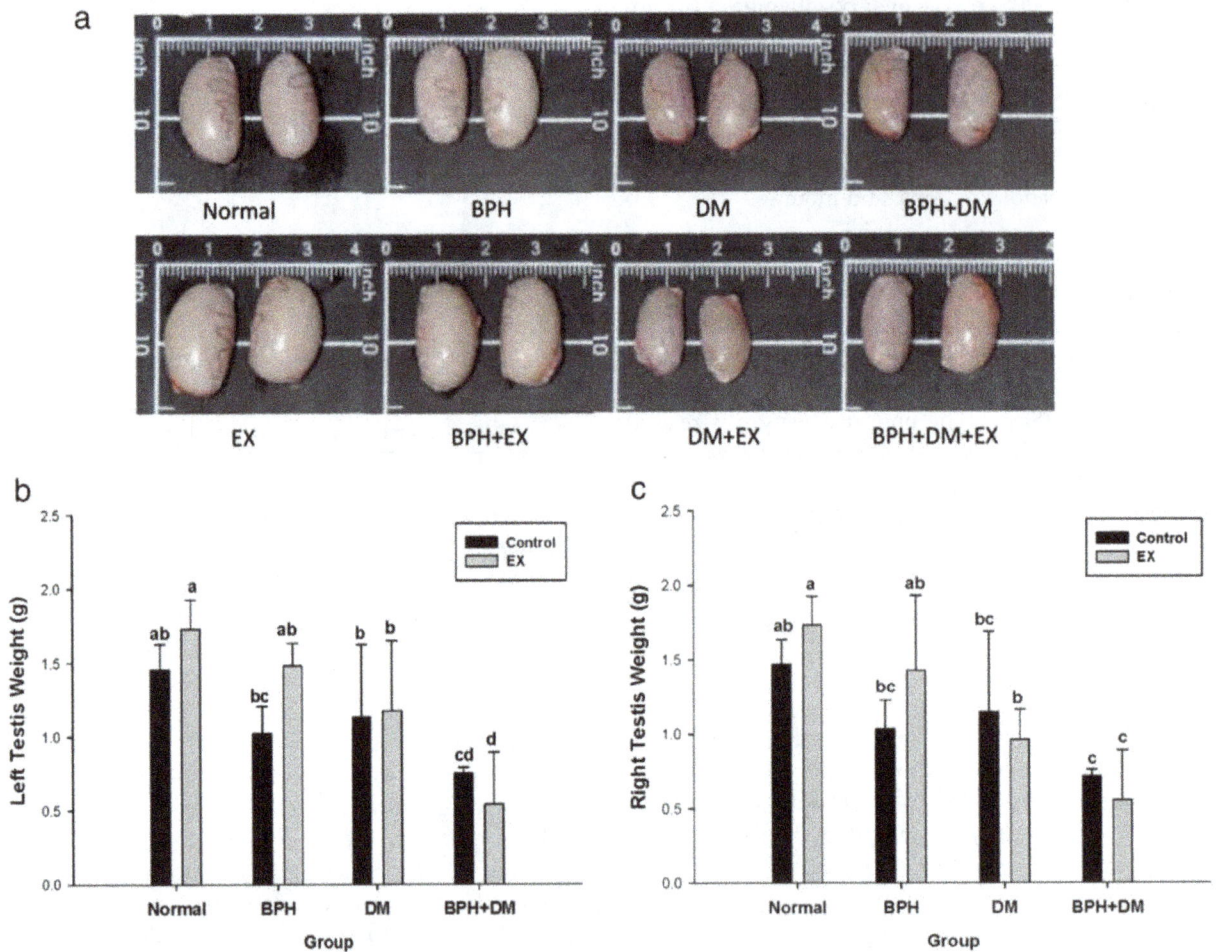

Fig. 2 The morphology and size of testis affected by T1DM, BPH, and exercise intervention. Dimensions are indicated by the real length in cm and inch (**a**). The left testes weight are indicated as mean ± SD (**b**). The right testes weight are indicated as mean ± SD (**c**). The different symbols in lower case indicate significantly different from each other (*p* < 0.05). The symbol 'a' denotes the highest data, 'b' the next, and so on

Moreover, without the EX intervention, the ratio LDL/HDL revealed to be 0.15, 0.32, 0.51, and 0.34 for groups normal, BPH, DM, and BPH + DM. As contrast, EX intervention greatly improved these ratio to 0.15, 0.19, 0.36, and 0.24, respectively.

Without EX intervention, DM and BPH + DM highly raised the serum TG levels to 200.5 ± 10.1 mg/dL, and 164.7 ± 9.4 mg/dL compared to the control 61.1 ± 9.6 mg/dL (note: The normal gross range is 26–145 mg/dL) (Fig. 4a). Although BPH had slightly raised this value to 70.7 ± 7.7 mg/dL, it still fell in normal gross range. Similarly, without EX intervention DM and DM + BPH elevated the serum CHOL level to 143.8 ± 8.2 mg/dL, and 140.7 ± 15.0 mg/dL. EX intervention slightly suppressed the CHOL levels in DM and BPH + DM to 138.4 ± 17.4 mg/dL, and 118.3 ± 15.4 mg/dL respectively, while BPH group showed 57.2 ± 18.1 mg/dL compared to the EX control 61.3 ± 9.3 mg/dL (Fig. 4b).

Hematoxylin-eosin staining

The prostatic tissues of the BPH group exhibited the manifestation of epithelial hyperplasia (epithelial cells piling-up formation)(indicated by solid arrows), as well as slight interstitial leukocytic infiltration (Fig. 5a and b). The prostate of DM rats revealed epithelial hyperplasia, moderate to severe inflammation, moderate lymphocytic infiltration (indicated by dotted arrows), and slight to moderately severe acinar atrophy (Fig. 5a and b). In BPH + DM rats, a high degree of hyperplasia and severe inflammation were observed. EX alleviated most of these pathological events (Fig. 4a and b; see BPH + EX, DM + EX, and BPH + DM + EX).

Sirius Red staining

Sirius Red stains the collagen to red, in essence underlying severe collagen deposition with inflammation of interstitial tissues. In the BPH groups, collagen

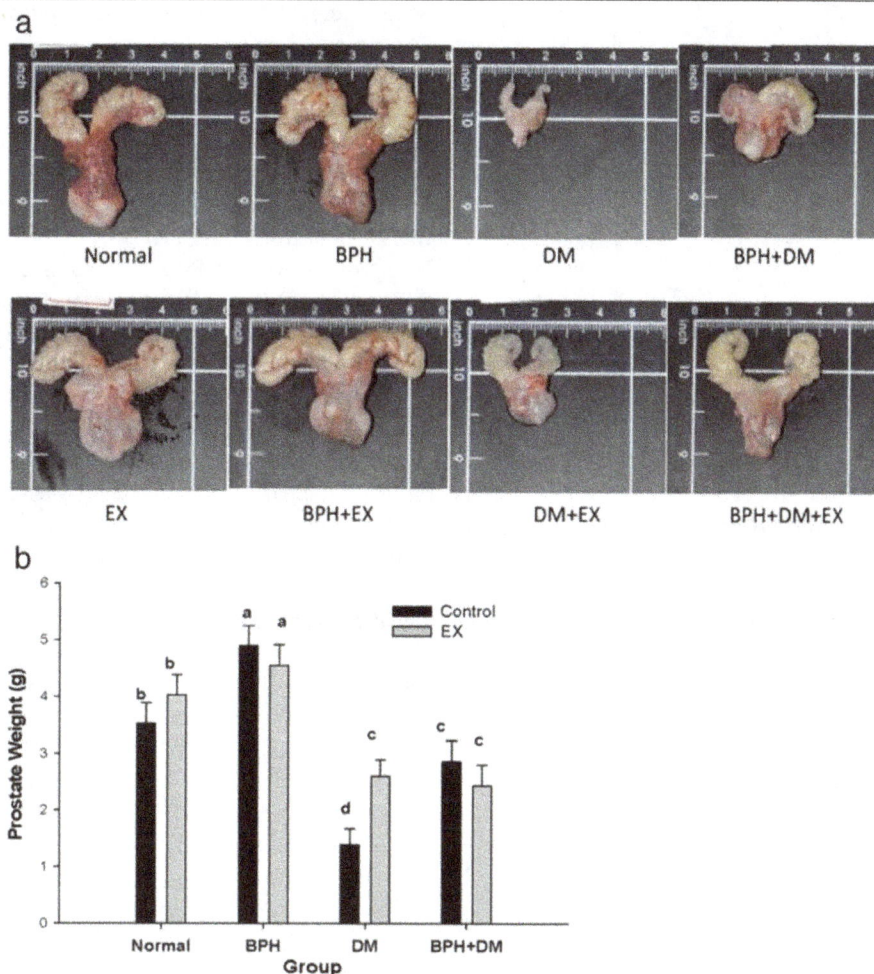

Fig. 3 Prostatic morphology (**a**) and prostatic weight (**b**) affected by T1DM, BPH, and exercise intervention. Dimensions are indicated by the real length in cm and inch (**a**). The prostatic weight are indicated as mean ± SD. The different symbols in lower case indicate significantly different from each other ($p < 0.05$). The symbol 'a' denotes the highest data, 'b' the next, and so on

deposition substantially increased to 54.32 ± 2.19 %, which was further enhanced to 333.46 ± 10.35 % in the DM groups, compared with the normal control value (10.25 ± 0.28 %). EX substantially reduced the collagen deposition to 36.37 ± 0.74 % and 308 ± 3.56 % in the BPH and DM groups, respectively ($p < 0.01$) (Fig. 5c). Remarkably, collagen deposition in the BPH + DM group, whose control exhibited an initial deposition level of 71.62 ± 2.78 %, was also substantially suppressed by EX to 37.24 ± 2.20 % ($p < 0.05$) (Fig. 5c).

Blood glucose levels were affected by BPH, DM, and EX
In Week 17, the mean blood glucose (BG) levels in the normal, BPH, EX, and BPH + EX groups were 127.0 ± 7.1 mg/dL, 119.7 ± 7.0 mg/dL, 210.5 ± 9.8 mg/dL, and 135.0 ± 12.5 mg/dL, respectively($p < 0.05$). In the DM groups (DM, BPH + DM, DM + EX, and BPH + DM + EX), the corresponding values were 600.0 ± 10.1 mg/dL, 594.1 ± 12.0 mg/dL, 525.8 ± 31.7 mg/dL, and $555.4 \pm$

24.9 mg/dL, respectively ($p < 0.01$) (Fig. 6a). Thus, DM prominently increased 4.14–4.72 folds the serum glucose levels in the DM groups. In the DM + EX and BPH + DM groups, the blood sugar levels were substantially, yet only slightly, decreased (Fig. 6a).

Serum insulin levels in the BPH, DM, and EX groups
The insulin levels in the control and BPH groups were comparable, ranging from 1.45 ± 0.13 µg/L to 1.68 ± 0.18 µg/L regardless of EX (Fig. 6b). In the DM group the insulin level was lowered to only 0.62 ± 0.06 µg/L, which was substantially improved by EX to 0.82 ± 0.05 µg/L ($p < 0.05$). A similar trend was observed in the BPH + DM group.

Insulin-like growth factor was affected by BPH, DM, and EX
The IGF in the normal control was 1087.3 ± 41.0 ng/mL, EX reduced this level to 535.2 ± 54.9 ng/mL ($p < 0.01$). In

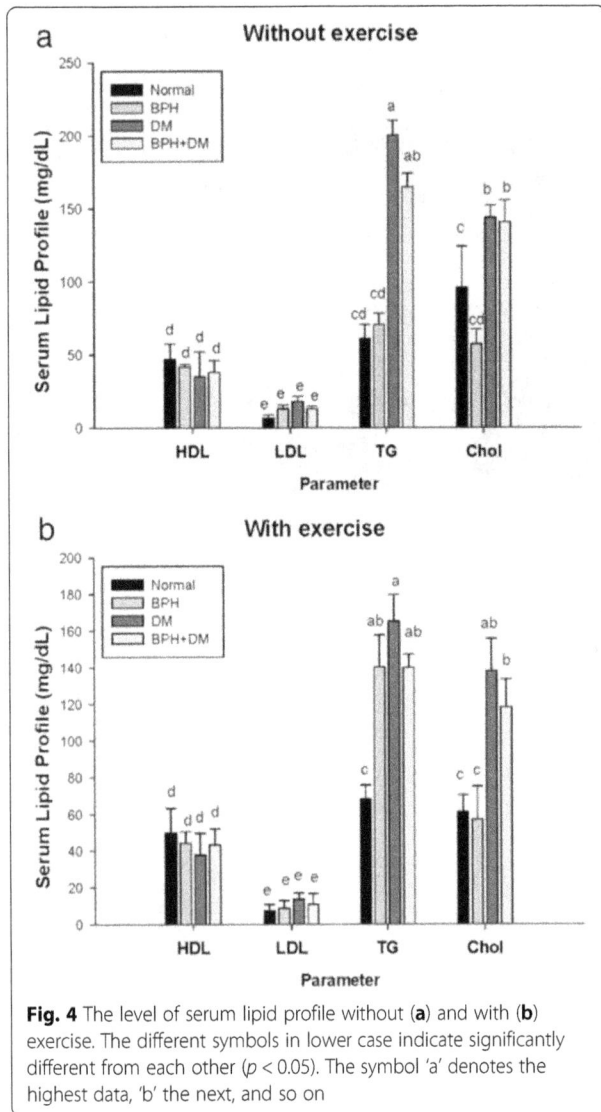

Fig. 4 The level of serum lipid profile without (**a**) and with (**b**) exercise. The different symbols in lower case indicate significantly different from each other (*p* < 0.05). The symbol 'a' denotes the highest data, 'b' the next, and so on

were increased to 889.3 ± 62.9 pg/mL and 896.1 ± 54.6 pg/mL, respectively (Fig. 7a).

5α-Reductase

In contrast with the testosterone profile, 5α-reductase exhibited a similar profile in all groups. The relative data for the normal control, EX control, BPH control, BPH + EX, DM control, DM + EX, BPH + DM, and BPH + DM + EX groups were 0.30 ± 0.07, 0.41 ± 0.12, 0.71 ± 0.05, 0.55 ± 0.04, 0.46 ± 0.10, 0.76 ± 0.07, 0.56 ± 0.07, and 0.76 ± 0.05 folds contrasting to the reference β-actin, respectively (*p* < 0.05) (Fig. 7b).

EX upregulated the 5α-reductase levels in the normal group, although the change was negligible (Fig. 7b). However, 5α-reductase activity was substantially upregulated in the DM + EX and BPH + DM + EX groups. By contrast, 5α-reductase activity was substantially inhibited in the BPH + EX group (Fig. 7b).

Dihydrotestosterone

The normal, EX and DM controls exhibited dihydro-testosterone (DHT) levels of 665.9 ± 37.7 pg/mL, 669.8 ± 76.7 pg/mL, and 122.8 ± 88.4 pg/mL, respectively (*p* < 0.01). EX did not alter the normal DHT level, whereas EX substantially raised, yet incompletely restored, the DHT level in the DM group to 351.96 ± 70.34 ng/mL (*p* < 0.01) (Fig. 7c). Because of the administration of testosterone (Sustanon®), the DHT of all BPH groups was raised to levels higher than those in the normal and DM groups (Fig. 7c). EX effectively suppressed the DHT levels in the BPH + EX and BPH + DM + EX groups. Conversely, EX increased the DHT levels in DM + EX rats (Fig. 7c).

Androgen receptor and prostate-specific antigen

The androgen receptor (AR) that was once highly expressed in BPH was substantially suppressed by EX. By contrast, AR in the DM control appeared to be more diffusely spreading due to the degenerative destruction of the tissues (Fig. 7d and e). EX effectively upregulated AR in the normal and DM groups (*p* < 0.01), but apparently lowered AR in the BPH and BPH + DM groups (*p* < 0.05) (Fig. 7d (×400) and e). In parallel, the PSA level in the normal control was slightly upregulated, and that of BPH and BPH + DM groups were significantly lowered (Fig. 7f). Interestingly, the PSA of DM rats was more apparently localized and downregulated by the EX intervention (Fig. 7f)

Pro-inflammatory factors affected by BPH, DM, and EX
Serum hydrogen peroxide

The serum hydrogen peroxide levels were highly stimulated to 17.27 ± 1.19 and 18.34 ± 0.45 μmol/mL respectively in the control groups of DM and BPH +

the BPH, DM, and BPH + DM groups, EX substantially raised the IGF, compared with each corresponding control groups (*p* < 0.05) (Fig. 6c).

Androgen-related biochemical parameters affected by BPH, DM, and EX
Testosterone

EX considerably increased the serum testosterone levels to 797.2 ± 89.6 pg/mL, compared with the control value of 508.6 ± 69.5 pg/mL. BPH increased this concentration to 972.6 ± 52.4 pg/mL (*p* < 0.01), whereas EX substantially lowered it to 856.8 ± 55.5 pg/mL (*p* < 0.05). By contrast, the testosterone level was highly suppressed in the DM control group to 115.5 ± 66.1 pg/mL, and EX restored its level to 543.7 ± 46.6 pg/mL (*p* < 0.01), being comparable to that in the normal control. In the BPH + DM and BPH + DM + EX groups, the testosterone levels

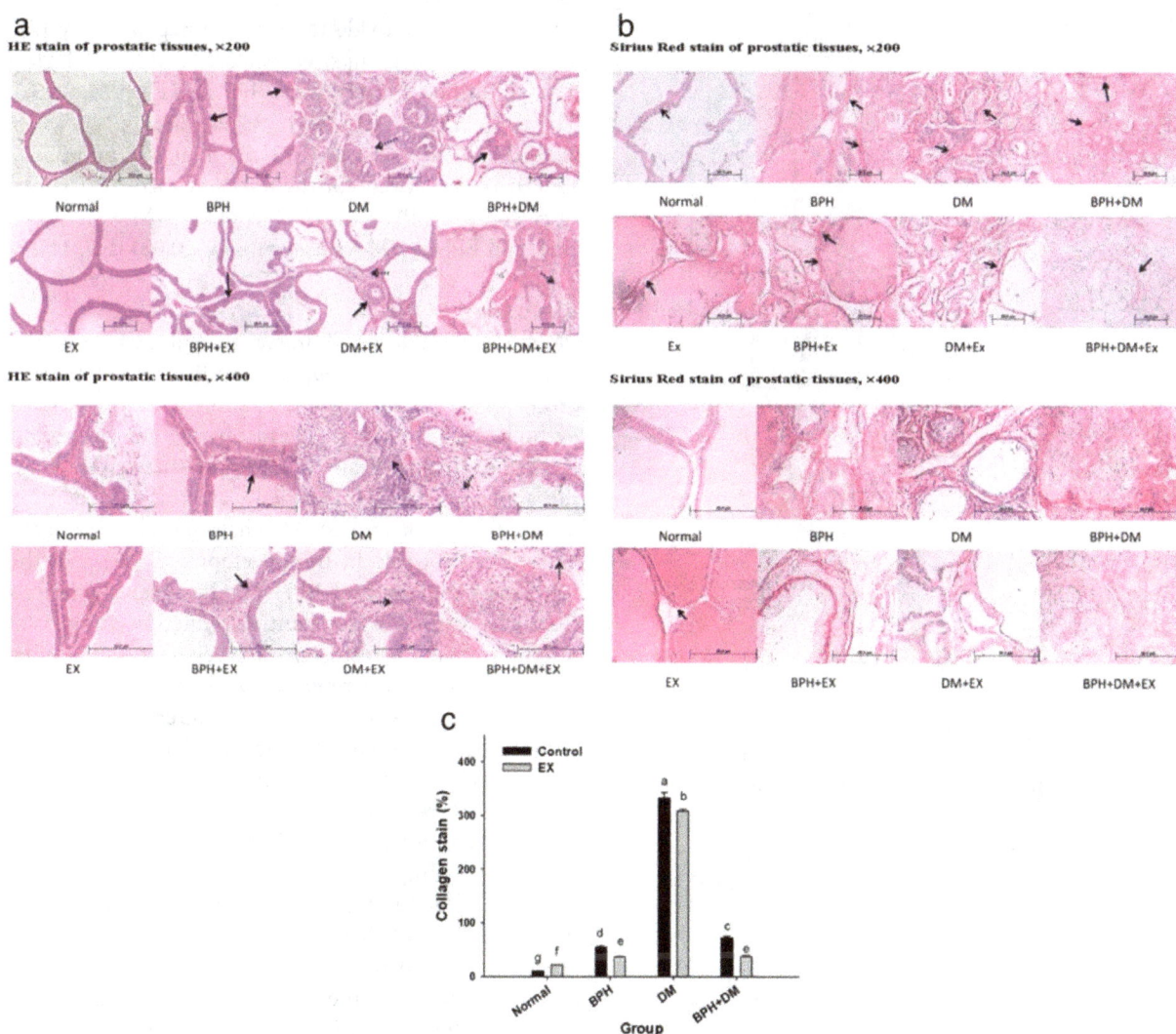

Fig. 5 Hematoxylin-eosin stain (**a**), Sirius Red stain (**b**), and collagen dposition (**c**) of prostatic tissues affected by different treatments. (in (**a**) and (**b**), magnification: upper × 200, lower panel × 400). Different symbols in lower case in the Fig. 5c indicate significantly different from each other ($p < 0.05$). The symbol 'a' denotes the highest data, 'b' the next, and so on

DM compared to the normal 9.88 ± 1.45 and the BPH control 11.75 ± 0.48 µmol/mL ($p < 0.05$) (Fig. 7). EX substantially suppressed the serum hydrogen peroxide levels to 6.25 ± 0.87, 6.96 ± 0.96, 15.18 ± 0.54, and 9.49 ± 0.68 µmol/mL, respectively for groups normal, BPH, DM, and BPH + DM ($p < 0.05$) (Fig. 8).

Serum TBARS

The serum TBARs levels were slightly suppressed in groups normal and BPH compare to each individual control. In the DM and BPH + DM controls, the serum TBARS were highly stimulated to levels 4.54 ± 0.16 µM and 4.7 ± 0.45 µM, respectively (Fig. 9). Although EX completely failed to improve the TBRAs

level in DM group, EX showed slight yet significant suppressive effect on the TBARS level in the BPH + DM rats ($p < 0.05$) (Fig. 9).

Prostate tissue IL-6

The IL-6 levels of each controls were all raised in groups BPH, DM, and BPH + DM. The levels reached 0.96 ± 0.1, 1.61 ± 0.18, and 2.35 ± 0.17 pg/mL, respectively (Fig. 10). EX slightly raised the IL-6 level to 0.68 ± 0.04 pg/mL compared to the normal. Conversely, EX slightly but significantly suppressed the IL-6 levels in groups BPH and DM. Astonishingly, EX effectively alleviated the IL-6 level from 2.4 ± 0.4 pg/mL down to 0.68 ± 0.06 pg/mL in group BPH + DM ($p < 0.01$) (Fig. 10).

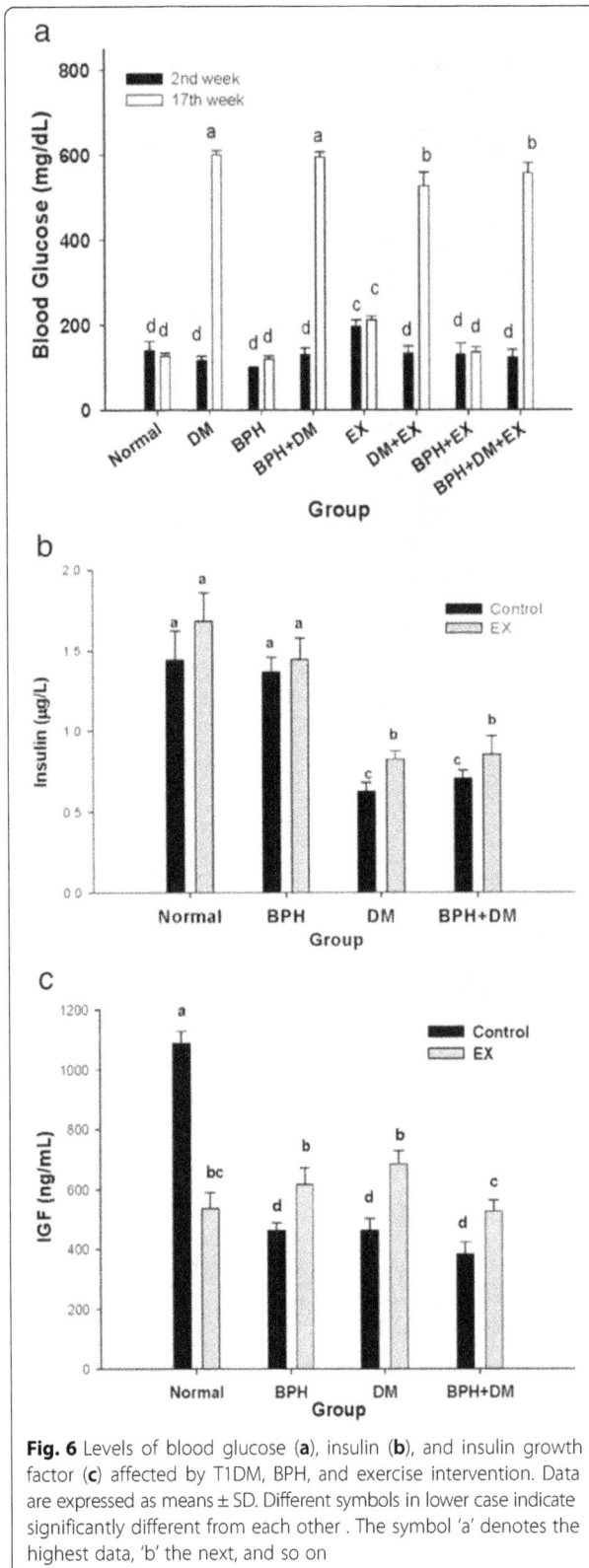

Fig. 6 Levels of blood glucose (**a**), insulin (**b**), and insulin growth factor (**c**) affected by T1DM, BPH, and exercise intervention. Data are expressed as means ± SD. Different symbols in lower case indicate significantly different from each other . The symbol 'a' denotes the highest data, 'b' the next, and so on

Serum nitric oxide

The serum nitric oxide (NO) was upregulated by EX in all experimental groups, particularly in the BPH group. The serum NO levels were 175.5 ± 11.2 μM, 243.5 ± 33.1 μM, 132.6 ± 10.5 μM, 357.6 ± 58.7 μM, 135.6 ± 25.0 μM, 248.7 ± 38.4 μM, 137.1 ± 40.0 μM, and 352.3 ± 17.9 μM, respectively for the normal control, EX control, BPH control, BPH + EX, DM control, DM + EX, BPH + DM, and BPH + DM + EX groups ($p < 0.05$) (Fig. 11).

Discussion

DM severely reduced the prostatic weight, whereas EX increased that of DM group but not that of BPH + DM group

Pathologically, BPH is characterized by hyperplastic epithelial, stromal growth [15] and tissue remodeling in the aging prostate [16], which was consistent with our findings (Fig. 5a and b). Stromal-epithelial interaction plays a critical role in the development and growth of the prostate gland and BPH [2]. Ikeda et al. indicated that DM caused a substantial reduction in prostatic weight and serum testosterone levels in rats [17]. Similar results were also reported by Porto et al. [18]. The prostate weight was substantially increased in the BPH control, compared with the normal control. EX did not substantially affect the prostatic weight (Fig. 3b). Conversely, DM remarkably reduced the prostatic weight, and EX effectively inhibited the reduction in prostatic weight (Fig. 3b).

Literature elsewhere also indicated that BPH exhibits manifestations of hypoxia and chronic inflammation [19]. We showed that EX slightly improved hyperplasia and inflammation of the dorsolateral lobe (NLAC report, not shown here) (Fig. 5a and b), and DM caused epithelial hyperplasia inflammation, lymphocytic infiltration, and acinar atrophy (NLAC report, not shown here). As contrast, EX alleviated the chronic inflammation of the DM + EX group (Fig. 5a and b).

Here some controversial arguments may arise. One may claim about the T1DM model to be characterized by some important histopathological alterations that are typical of the initial phase of BPH, including inflammation, tissue remodeling and increased stromal proliferation and more importantly, which is associated to a condition of hypogonadism as already reported by others [20] and pointed out that such a condition of hypogonadism is also associated with significant prostate alterations.

However, there in fact exists a big discrepancy between the DM model and the BPH model. As cited by Zhang et al. [20], the DM animal models could be elicited by two techniques, one by alloxan, and the other by streptozotocin (STZ). Indeed, in the DM model, a state of hypogonadism would have occurred, and supplement

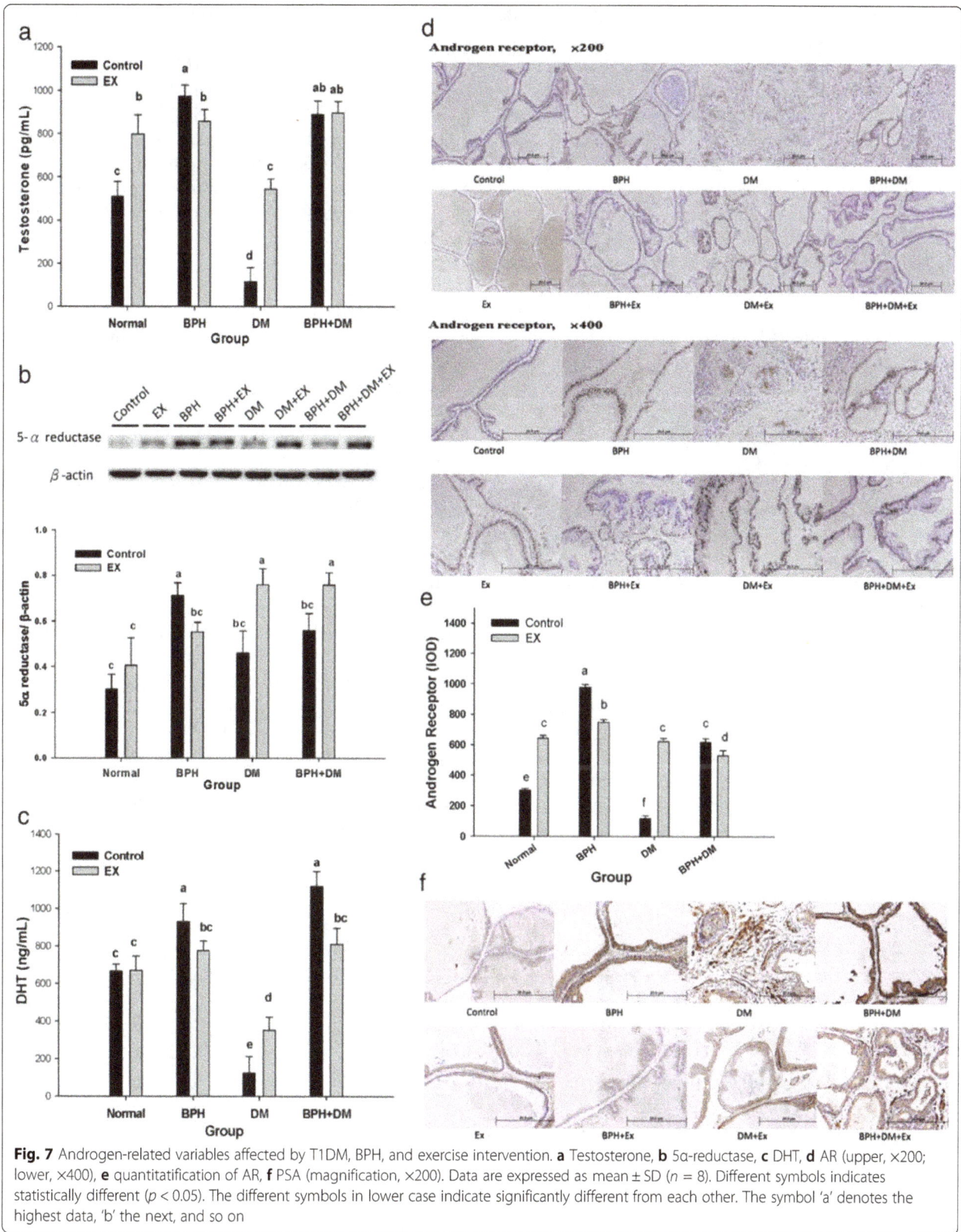

Fig. 7 Androgen-related variables affected by T1DM, BPH, and exercise intervention. **a** Testosterone, **b** 5α-reductase, **c** DHT, **d** AR (upper, ×200; lower, ×400), **e** quantitatification of AR, **f** PSA (magnification, ×200). Data are expressed as mean ± SD (n = 8). Different symbols indicates statistically different (p < 0.05). The different symbols in lower case indicate significantly different from each other. The symbol 'a' denotes the highest data, 'b' the next, and so on

with testosterone definitely would be beneficial [20]. However, we were creating a complicate animal model that is DM + BPH. DM model was induced at week 2 by STZ, and the BPH model was then induced one week later using T + E. Recently, the pathological etiology and clinical findings for BPH all are pointing to the hypertestosteronemia, dyslipidemia, and oxidative stress. In our experiment, we really have recognized the change of testis in different groups involving the DM, BPH and the DM + BPH, the testes sizes in DM and BPH were reduced slightly, as contrast, EX has apparently recovered its weight and size (Fig. 2a-c).

Increased body weight and body mass index have been confirmed to be the risk factors of prostate enlargement [21–23]. The results presented here are controversial; we demonstrated that the body weight severely decreased, suggesting pathological changes in the STZ-induced DM, testosterone-induced BPH, and innate human DM models. Previously, we demonstrated that EX was able to suppress the prostatic inflammation in BPH [7]. A similar result regarding the DM group was reported by Belotto et al. [24].

The pathological etiology of dyslipidemia of BPH is entirely different from DM

In Fig. 4a-b, we showed the dyslipidemic pattern without and/or with EX intervention in BPH rats was quite different from that of DM and BPH + DM rats. Although both dyslipidemic profiles were very alike, yet the DM patients usually show more severe hyperlipidemic manifestations than the BPH (Fig. 4a-b). Literature has indicated that metabolic syndrome-associated dyslipidemia to be the major determinants of prostatic inflammation [25] and overgrowth [1]. Amazingly, EX seemed to have further elevated the TG level in BPH to 140.4 ± 17.4 mg/dL, yet still falling within the normal range (26–145 mg/dL) (Fig. 4b).

According to Nandeesha et al. [26], in human T2DM the levels, total cholesterol, and LDL-cholesterol were significantly higher and HDL-cholesterol was significantly lower in BPH cases as compared to controls. Hammarsten et al. also indicated that there was a larger prostate gland in men with obesity ($p < 0.0001$), and low HDL-cholesterol levels ($p = 0.0132$) than in men without these conditions [27].

Nonetheless, in this investigation we found these two types of dyslipidemia in fact were totally different from each other (Fig. 4a-b), implicating the pathological etiology is completely discrete from each other between BPH and DM.

EX reduced collagen deposition

BPH is usually implicated in detrusor muscle hypertrophy in the early phases of outflow obstruction and deposition of increasing amounts of extracellular matrix (e.g., collagen) [24, 28]. Moreover, DM also induces stromal remodeling and a thickening in the acinar basement membrane of the prostate, accompanied by an increase and disorganization of its proteoglycans, chondroitin sulfate, and collagen [29], as observed in our BPH- and DM-induced models (Fig. 5c).

The combined effect of DM + BPH + EX is still unclear. Previously, we proved EX to alleviate BPH [7]. In this work, we demonstrated that EX not only apparently alleviated the hyperplastic epithelial and stromal growth, inhibiting collagen deposition in BPH (Fig. 5c), but also reduced the collagen deposition in the DM groups. By contrast, the literature demonstrated that in DM, EX restores the DM-induced specific ultrastructural changes in cardiomyopathy, alleviating these symptoms toward non-DM phenotypes, particularly in the mitochondria and extracellular matrix proteins [30].

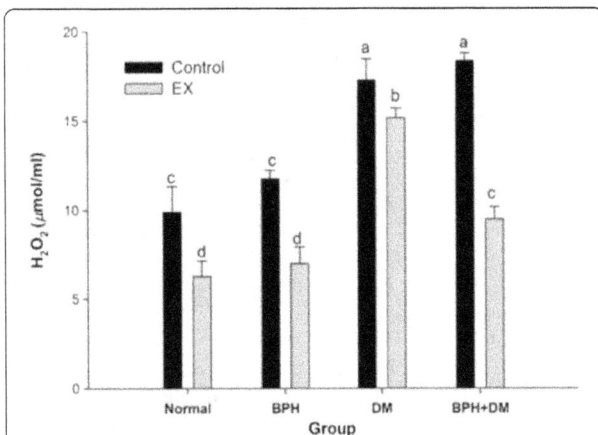

Fig. 8 Levels of serum hydrogen peroxide affected by T1DM, BPH, and exercise intervention. Different symbols indicates statistically different ($p < 0.05$). The different symbols in lower case indicate significantly different from each other. The symbol 'a' denotes the highest data, 'b' the next, and so on

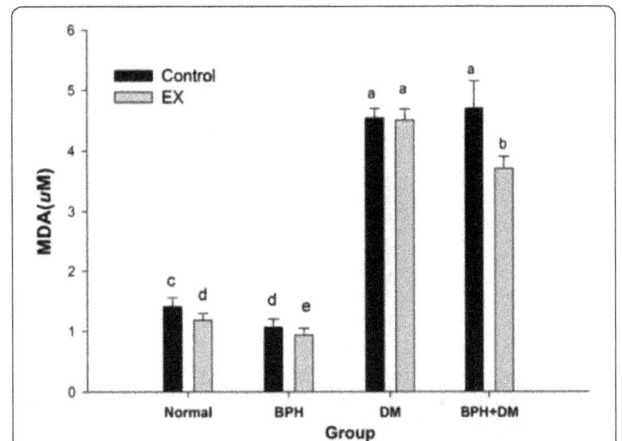

Fig. 9 Levels of serum TBARs affected by T1DM, BPH, and exercise intervention. Different symbols indicates statistically different ($p < 0.05$). The different symbols in lower case indicate significantly different from each other. The symbol 'a' denotes the highest data, 'b' the next, and so on

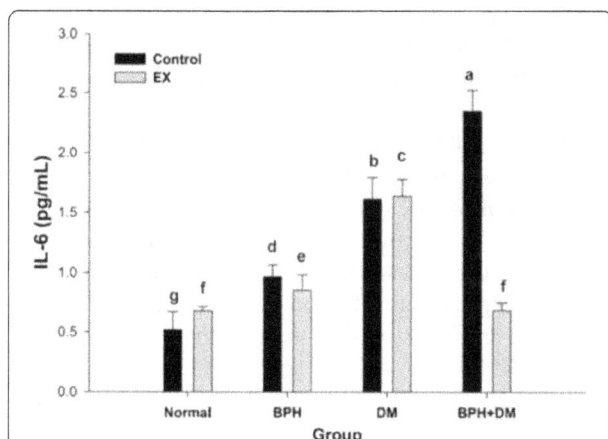

Fig. 10 Levels of prostatic IL-6 affected by T1DM, BPH, and exercise intervention. Different symbols indicates statistically different ($p < 0.05$). The different symbols in lower case indicate significantly different from each other. The symbol 'a' denotes the highest data, 'b' the next, and so on

In the DM and BPH + DM groups, EX substantially decreased the blood glucose and increased the insulin levels

Almeida et al. [31] pointed that body adiposity and glucose homeostasis improved with chronic physical exercise in Wistar male rat model. In addition, total insulin content was reduced in group acute trained, insulin secretion stimulated by glucose was reduced in trained groups (the aerobic trained and the acute trained) [31]. According to Almeida et al. [31], a possible modulating action on insulin secretion is probably related to the association of chronic adaptation with an acute response on cholinergic activity in

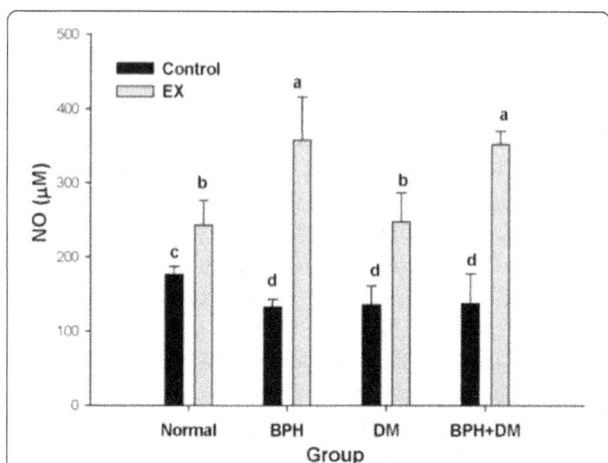

Fig. 11 Serum nitric oxide affected by T1DM, BPH, and exercise intervention. The different symbols in lower case in the figure indicate significantly different from different groups ($p < 0.05$). The symbol 'a' denotes the highest data, 'b' the next, and so on

pancreatic islets. Speculatively, the elevation of IGF and TG and variation of prostate weight by EX could be also dependent on such a phenomenon.

Literature has warranted also that blood glucose concentration is associated with the risk of prostate enlargement. Diabetic patients were more than twice as likely to have prostate enlargement compared with men without DM [13]. Patients with MetS exhibit a high annual prostate growth rate [21–23]. BPH patients with MetS exhibit substantially higher serum glucose levels than do BPH patients without MetS [32]. In subjects with MetS, the fasting glucose levels are usually remaining at higher levels than the normal. Documented data revealed that prostate size correlates positively with the fasting glucose level (r =0.186, $p = 0.007$), but not with BMI, testosterone, insulin level, or insulin resistance (each $p > 0.05$) [30]. Upon multiple adjusted linear regression analysis, prostate size correlated with PSA ($p < 0.01$) and increased fasting glucose levels ($p =0.023$) [33]. Worth noting, Kim et al. also indicated that in non-DM BPH patients with normal testosterone levels, fasting glucose level is an independent risk factor for prostate hyperplasia [33].

In addition, Nandeesha et al. indicated that insulin level in human was significantly associated with prostate size, in human BPH cases. And more importantly in T2DM patients, insulin has been shown to be an independent risk factor in the development of BPH [26].

Previously, Hammarsten et al. had indicated that there was a larger prostate gland in men with non-insulin-dependent diabetes mellitus (NIDDM) ($p = 0.0058$) and high insulin levels ($p < 0.0001$) than in men without these conditions [27].

Taken together, evidently, different animal model (rats vs. human) and different etiological events (Type 1 vs Type 2 DM) could reveal different pathological and biochemical outcomes. We showed in this Type 1 rat model for BPH alone EX did not affect the insilin level, but in case of BPH + DM, the insulin level was substantially reduced in the BPH + DM rats, and EX was seen to slighly ameliorate the insulin level (Fig. 6b), suggesting that although insulin is an independent risk factor in the development of BPH, EX could more or less modulate the pathological (cholinergic adaptation, [31]) condition associated with BPH + T1DM (Fig. 6b).

Moreover, EX seemed to have alleviated the testosterone level in BPH alone group to reach a level higher than the normal (Fig. 7a) (which could be due to the testosterone therapy), while the fasting glucose levels all maintained at extremely high levels (Fig. 6a), implicating the risk to aggravate BPH in the T1DM rats.

EX upregulated the IGF and alleviated the MetS

The IGF-1, although highly suppressed in the normal control, was substantially upregulated by EX in the BPH, DM, and BPH + DM groups (Fig. 6c).

The IGF, another mitogen, and an antiapoptotic agent, binds to the insulin receptor/IGF receptor, and stimulates prostate growth [2]. IGFBP-3 seems to be a mulifunctional protein, which can potentate or inhibit IGF activity [34]. Increased IGF levels and IGF binding proteins (IGFBPs) in prostate tissue and blood are associated with an increased BPH risk, because they regulate the levels of circulating androgen and growth hormone [2].

Regarding the volume variation of the total prostate (TP) volume or transitional zone (TZ) volume, literature has demonstrated that higher PSA ($p < 0.001$), larger waist circumference ($p < 0.001$) and higher IGFBP-3 expression levels ($p = 0.024$) are independently associated with higher TZ volume [34].

The increase of IGF in prostate cancer has been widely studied. But little has been reported on the possible role of IGF in BPH [35]. However, reduced modulatory IGF binding protein levels do seem to be associated with increased BPH risk [35].

Could this be the cause that IGF was decreased in BPH model (Fig. 6c) compared to the control? We really still are not very clear about this.

EX alleviated the BPH and BPH + DM by suppressing the DHT levels, conversely, EX alleviated DM by upregulating androgens

Recently, we demonstrated that EX alleviated BPH [7]. Biochemically, BPH is considered to be an imbalance between androgen and estrogen [36], an overexpression of stromal and epithelial growth factors, cytokines, and steroid hormones [37, 38]. In the BPH groups, the levels of testosterone, 5α-reductase, DHT, and AR were all substantially upregulated (Fig. 7a-e), resulting in substantially increased PSA levels (Fig. 7f), a phenomenon being consistent with the manifestations usually seen in the clinical treatment of BPH. EX alleviated the BPH and BPH + DM by suppressing the DHT levels (Fig. 7c). Subnormal testosterone levels inhibited regular prostate proliferation and differentiation [39].

The biological significance of enzyme like "5-α-reductase" definitely is far different from that of the 'androgen receptor protein'. 5-α-Reductase is responsible for the transformation of testosterone into DHT, the latter activates the translocation of cytosolic AR into the nucleus. In order to differentiate these two biochemical functions, we performed the Western blotting of 5-α-reductase (Fig. 7b), and alternatively, we adopted immunohistochemical (IHC) stain to examine the nuclear translocation of AR (Fig. 7d).

At this stage, we purposely utilized the IHC stain to observe the AR with the goal not only aiming at its quantities, but also its in vivo distribution site. As can be expected, after homogenized the cytosolic and the nuclear AR's would be homogeneously mixed together, and at this stage, even though you could identify a tremendous amount of AR by Western blot, you still could not differentiate the activated AR and its localization into nuclei. On the other hand, we skipped the ER, because ER in reality is not involved in such a biochemical transformation and translocation mechanism.

In the DM group, AR was substantially downregulated (Fig. 6d and e), which was in agreement with Gorbachinsky and Liu and Wang [33, 40]. Literature indicated that the prostatic cytosolic AR content was negatively correlated with the plasma glucose levels [41]. We showed EX alleviated DM by upregulating androgens and AR (Fig. 7d), and EX increased the testosterone levels in the DM + EX group (Fig. 7a)

EX alters the sex hormones and their receptors associated with the balance between apoptosis and cell proliferation in the ventral prostate [41]. EX increased the plasma corticosteroid, DHT, and testosterone levels in the DM groups (Fig. 7a-c), and possibly via these mechanism prevented the apoptosis of glandular epithelium [42] and protected the prostate from MetS-induced prostate hypoxia, fibrosis, and inflammation [43].

The manifestations exhibited by the BPH + DM groups could become even more complicated. No substantial differences in the testosterone levels between the BPH + DM control and the BPH + DM + EX were observed. To compare, the 5α-reductase was upregulated in BPH + DM (Fig. 6b), while the level of DHT was downregulated (Fig. 7c), which implicates the lowering of PSA as shown in Fig. 5f. As contrast, in the BPH group only, EX downregulated 5α-reductase (Fig. 7b) and consequently, DHT was substantially downregulated (Fig. 6c), leading to the lowering of PSA level (Fig. 7f).

Interestingly, EX seemed to exhibit a biphasic action model between BPH and DM. In the BPH only, EX suppressed the serum level of testosterone, 5α-reductase and DHT (Fig. 7a-c). In the DM patients EX elevated T, 5α-reductase and DHT (Fig. 7a-c). While in BPH + DM, although EX stimulated the activity of 5α-reductase, however EX suppressed the DHT without affecting the testosterone level (Fig. 7a-c).

As well known, high zinc level tends to inhibit the activity of 5α-reductase [44]. The middle socioeconomic DM patients exhibited lower serum zinc levels (1.05–4.8 mg/dL in males and 1.7–3.5 mg/mL in females) than the normal non-diabetic population [45]. As contrast, no significant decrease in plasma zinc between BPH and normal controls [46]. Thus in the BPH patients, the production of DHT via the action of 5α-reductase could be merely via the plasma substrate testosterone level controlled kinetics (Fig. 7a-c). Nonetheless, in BPH complicated with DM, the plasma zinc level may play a very important role [45]. As seen, the activity of 5α-reductase was de-repressed in the DM and BPH + DM controls compared to the normal subjects (Fig. 7b). Furthermore, EX tends to accelerate sweating rate. Some endurance runners had significantly lower serum zinc concentrations (<11.5 μmol/L) than did men who were not participating in chronic exercise [47]. Such tremendous zinc loss by sweating could cause further lowering of serum zinc level, resulting in highly de-repressed 5α-reductase (Fig. 7b, c).

EX effectively alleviated the oxidative stress in BPH + DM by suppressing the serum TBARS and H_2O_2

TBARS level was significantly increased in type 2 DM with the duration of disease and development of complications [48]. Similarly we showed the serum TBARs level was highly raised in both the T1DM and the BPH + DM rats (Fig. 9). MetS raised the oxidative stress expressed as H_2O_2 and MDA despite in T1DM or T2DM [49]. BPH is always associated with oxidative stress [50]. DM more severely raised the serum TBARs and H_2O_2 levels (Figs. 8, 9). We demonstrated that EX ineffectively suppressed the serum TBARs level in T1DM (Fig. 9). Consistent with this, Laaksonen and Sen reported that the increased plasma TBARS in the diabetic men both at rest and after exercise [51]. As contrast, EX effectively suppressed the serum TBARs level in the BPH + DM when compared to the BPH + DM control (Fig. 9). To compare, EX effectively inhibited the production of serum H_2O_2 levels in both the DM and BPH + DM groups (Fig. 8). The strongly negative association between plasma TBARS and VO_2 max suggests that good physical fitness may have a protective role against oxidative stress [52]. Results implicated that the oxidative stress associated with DM was more likely related to the lipid peroxidation, whereas that in BPH was more likely due to the elevation of serum H_2O_2 level.

EX effectively alleviated the inflammation in BPH + DM by suppressing the prostate IL-6

Although in BPH, interleukin-6 (IL-6) was localized predominantly in basal cells of epithelia, IL-6 receptor was expressed in benign prostatic tissue in both epithelial and stromal cells [51], no IL-6 expression was detected in stromal cells on immunohistochemistry [53]. IL-6 is a pleiotropic cytokine that interacts with its receptor in prostate cells, thus regulating proliferative response and differentiation in prostates. The consequences of increased IL-6 expression could play a role as a mediator of acute phase reaction and as a pleiotrophic cytokine influencing antigen specific immune responses and

inflammation, as well as a growth factor for prostate epithelial cells [54]. We showed prostatic IL-6 was raised in BPH control, while EX only slightly yet significantly suppressed its level (Fig. 10). as contrast, IL-6 was substantially raised in the DM and BPH + DM controls, in these two groups EX was seen effectively suppressed the elevation of IL-6. In particular, the level of IL-6 in BPH + DM was effectively alleviated to a level as that of control, underlying the promising effect of EX for amelioration of the inflammatory manifestation of BPH + DM, but to a lesser extent for the DM.

Considerable production of NO ameliorated BPH, DM, and BPH + DM

EX highly stimulated the serum NO production (Fig. 11). Pathologically speaking, BPH is always characterized by hypoxia and chronic inflammation [19]. NO plays a crucial role in the autonomic innervations of all compartments of prostatic tissues. In obstructive BPH, the nitrinergic innervation is reduced compared to that in a normal prostate tissue [55], resulting in an enhancement of vasodilatation and blood flow, a promising strategy for treating BPH.

To date, interest in the NO pathway as a potential pharmacological target to treat male LUTS is increasing. Thus, given a potential role of the NO-pathway in the prostate and LUT, enhancing NO production can be a promising strategy to control the smooth muscle function in the human prostate [56].

To emphasize, metabolic syndrome (MetS) is a complex, highly prevalent disorder and a worldwide epidemic. In T2DM, central obesity, insulin resistance, dyslipidemia, and hypertension are the main components of MetS [57]. As contrast, T1DM is insulin-dependent. In our experiment, Streptozotocin induces insulitis and subsequent degeneration of the Langerhans islets beta cells, so the model was a mimic of diabetes type 1 as evidenced by the lowered level of insulin, which in fact was very similarly to the patients affected by DM type 1. While DM type 2 patients, as consequence of insulin resistance, usually show normal or higher level of insulin. Consequently our findings have elicited limitations to the extension of these biochemical findings in a human setting of patients, mostly affected by DM type 2.

Despite T2DM our T1DM, there is growing evidence of the association of MetS with the initiation and clinical progression of BPH and PCa, molecular mechanisms and effects on treatment efficacy remain unclear [57].

Conclusion

EX can alleviate BPH, DM, and BPH + DM. EX provokes androgen remodeling and the specific expression of NO which may play an essential role in enhancing the effect of EX. Data from the peer-reviewed literature suggest an association of MetS with BPH and Pca in humans, although the evidence for a causal relationship remains missing. MetS, including TDM and T2DM, should be considered a new domain in basic and clinical research in patients with prostatic disorders. Further research is required to better understand the role of MetS in BPH and PCa. Even so, clinical urologists need to be cognizant of the effect that MetS has on urologic diseases, as well as on overall patient health. It is of certain that this model in reality has raised some unexpected results that could be haphazard and the consequence due to the small sample size and the complicate model rather than a real biological effect of BPH and/or DM and/or EX. Hence a further research is required to better understand the effects of EX on the oxidative inflammatory pathway.

Abbreviations
5αRd: 5α-reductase; AR: Androgen receptor; BPH: Benign prostatic hyperplasia; BG: Blood glucose; BSA: Bovine serum albumin; ECL: Enhanced chemiluminescence; CHOL: Cholesterol; DM: Diabetes Mellitus; DAB: Diaminobenzidine; DHT: Dihydrotestosterone; EX: Exercise; HDL: High-density lipoprotein; IGFBPs: IGF-binding proteins; IGF: Insulin-like growth factor; IL-6: Interleukin-6; ip: intraperitoneal; LDL: Low-density lipoprotein; LUTS: Low urinary tract symptoms; MetS: Metabolic syndrome; NO: Nitric Oxide; PSA: Prostatic-specific antigen; STZ: Streptozotocin; Ts: Testosterone; TG: Triglyceride; TNF-α: Tumor necrosis factor-α; T2DM: Type 2 DM; T1DM: Type-1 diabetes mellitus; WSLD: Western sample loading dye.

Competing interests
The authors declare that they have no competing interests.

Authors' contributions
KCC, SYS and CCP contributed to this work by designing the study, obtaining data, performing the statistical analysis, writing the manuscript and interpreted the data. CLH and KHS participated in the conception and design of the study and acquisition of data. RYP and YTL participated in the conception and design of the study and interpretation of the data and reviewed and edited the manuscript. All authors read and approved the final manuscript.

Acknowledgments
The authors want to show their gratitude to the financial supports issued by Grant no. MOST103-2313-B-038-002-MY3 from the Ministry Of Science and Technology and Grant no. 104CM-TMU-08 from Chi-Mei Medical Center and no. SJMRP-10303 from St. Joseph's Hospital.
We also want to show our thanks to the technical assistance of Ms Hui-Fong Yeo.

Author details
[1]Department of Urology, Shuang Ho Hospital, Taipei Medical University, 291 Zhongzheng Rd.,, Zhonghe, Taipei 23561, Taiwan. [2]Department of Urology, School of Medicine, College of Medicine, Taipei Medical University, 250 Wu-Shing St., Taipei 11031, Taiwan. [3]The Ph. D. Program for Translational Medicine, College of Medical Science and Technology, Taipei Medical University, Taipei, Taiwan. [4]Department of Urology, St. Joseph's Hospital, 74, Sinsheng Road, Huwei County, Yunlin Hsien 632, Taiwan. [5]Research Institute of Biotechnology, Hungkuang University, 34 Chung-Chie Rd., Shalu County, Taichung Hsien 43302, Taiwan. [6]Graduate Institute of Biotechnology, Changhua University of Education, 1 Jin-De Rd., Changhua 50007, Taiwan. [7]Division of Urology, Department of Surgery, Chi-Mei Medical Center, 901 Chung Hwa Road, Yung Kang City, Tainan 701, Taiwan. [8]Graduate Institute of Clinical Medicine, College of Medicine, Taipei Medical University, 250 Wu-Shing St., Xin-Yi District, Taipei 110, Taiwan.

References
1. Gacci M, Vignozzi L, Sebastianelli A, Salvi M, Giannessi C, De Nunzio C, et al. Metabolic syndrome and lower urinary tract symptoms: the role of inflammation. Prostate Cancer Prostatic Dis. 2013;16:101–6.
2. Wang Z, Olumi AF. Diabetes, growth hormone-insulin-like growth factor pathways and association to benign prostatic hyperplasia. Differentiation. 2011;82:261–71.
3. Zinman B, Ruderman N, Campaigne BN, Devlin JT, Schneider SH. Physical activity/exercise and Diabetes Mellitus. Diabetes care. 2003;26 Suppl 1:S73–7.
4. Sarma AV, Kellogg PJ. Diabetes and benign prostatic hyperplasia: emerging clinical connections. Curr Urol Rep. 2009;10:267–75.
5. de Lemos ET, Oliveira J, Pinheiro JP, Reis F. Regular Physical Exercise as a Strategy to improve antioxidant and anti-Inflammatory status: Benefits in type 2 diabetes mellitus. Oxidative Med and Cellu Longevity. 2012;741545:1–15.
6. Charnow JA. Exercise May Lower BPH, LUTS Risk. April 07, 2008, Renal & Urology News. (http://www.renalandurologynews.com/exercise-may-lower-bph-luts-risk/article/108726/#).
7. Peng CC, Liu JH, Chang CH, Chung JY, Chen KC, Chou KY, et al. Action mechanism of Ginkgo biloba leaf extract intervened by exercise therapy in treatment of benign prostate hyperplasia. Evid Based Complement Alternat Med. 2013;408734:1–12.
8. Sea J, Poon KS, McVary KT. Review of exercise and the risk of benign prostatic hyperplasia. Phys Sports med. 2009;37:75–83.
9. Williams PT. Effects of running distance and performance on incident benign prostatic hyperplasia. Med Sci Sports Exerc. 2008;40:1733–9.
10. Ronald JS, Glen PK, David HW, Carmen C-S, Russell DW. Physical Activity/Exercise and Type 2 Diabetes: A consensus statement from the American Diabetes Association. Diabetes Care. 2006;29:1433–8.
11. Bird SR, Hawley JA. Exercise and type 2 diabetes: new prescription for an old problem. Maturitas. 2012;72:311–6.
12. Stamatiou K, Lardas M, Kostakos E, Koutsonasios V, Michail E. The impact of diabetes type 2 in the pathogenesis of benign prostatic hyperplasia: a review. Adv Urol. 2009;818965:1–3.
13. Parsons JK, Carter HB, Partin AW, Windham BG, Metter EJ, Ferrucci L, et al. Metabolic factors associated with benign prostatic hyperplasia. J Clin Endocrinol Metab. 2006;91(7):2562–68.
14. Berger AP, Deibl M, Leonhartsberger N, Bektic J, Horninger W, Fritsche G, et al. Vascular damage as a risk factor for benign prostatic hyperplasia and erectile dysfunction. BJU Int. 2005;96(7):1073–8.
15. Timms BG, Hofkamp LE. Prostate development and growth in benign prostatic hyperplasia. Differentiation. 2011;82:173–83.
16. Untergasser G, Madersbacher S, Berger P. Benign prostatic hyperplasia: age-related tissue-remodeling. Exp Gerontol. 2005;40:121–8.
17. Ikeda K, Wada Y, Foster Jr HE, Wang Z, Weiss RM, Latifpour J. Experimental diabetes-induced regression of the rat prostate is associated with an increased expression of transforming growth factor-beta. J Urol. 2000;164:180–5.
18. Porto EM, Dos Santos SA, Ribeiro LM, Lacorte LM, Rinaldi JC, Justulin Jr LA, et al. Lobe variation effects of experimental diabetes and insulin replacement on rat prostate. Microsc Res Tech. 2011;74:1040–8.
19. Bostanci Y, Kazzazi A, Momtahen S, Laze J, Djavan B. Correlation between benign prostatic hyperplasia and inflammation. Curr Opin Urol. 2013;23:5–10.
20. Zhang XH, Filippi S, Morelli A, Vignozzi L, Luconi M, Donati S, et al. Testosterone restores diabetes-induced erectile dysfunction and sildenafil responsiveness in two distinct animal models of chemical diabetes. J Sex Med. 2006;3(2):253–64.
21. Ochiai A, Fritsche HA, Babaian RJ. Influence of anthropometric measurements, age, and prostate volume on prostate-specific antigen levels in men with a low risk of prostate cancer. Urol. 2005;66:819–23.
22. Ozden C, Ozdal OL, Urgancioglu G, Koyuncu H, Gokkaya S, Memis A. The correlation between metabolic syndrome and prostatic growth in patients with benign prostatic hyperplasia. Eur Urol. 2007;51:199–203.
23. Parsons JK, Carter HB, Partin AW, Windham BG, Metter EJ, Ferrucci L, et al. Metabolic factors associated with benign prostatic hyperplasia. J Clin Endocrinol Metab. 2006;91:2562–8.

24. Belotto MF, Magdalon J, Rodrigues HG, Vinolo MA, Curi R, Pithon-Curi TC, et al. Moderate exercise improves leukocyte function and decreases inflammation in diabetes. Clin Exp Immunol. 2010;162:237–43.

25. Vignozzi L, Gacci M, Cellai I, Santi R, Corona G, Morelli A, et al. Fat boosts, while androgen receptor activation counteracts, BPH-associated prostate inflammation. Prostate. 2013;73:789–800.

26. Nandeesha H, Koner BC, Dorairajan LN, Sen SK. Hyperinsulinemia and dyslipidemia in non-diabetic benign prostatic hyperplasia. Clin Chim Acta. 2006;370(1-2):89–93.

27. Hammarsten J, Högstedt B, Holthuis N, Mellström D. Components of the metabolic syndrome-risk factors for the development of benign prostatic hyperplasia. Prostate Cancer Prostatic Dis. 1998;1(3):157–62.

28. Schauer IG, Rowley DR. The functional role of reactive stroma in benign prostatic hyperplasia. Differentiation. 2011;82:200–10.

29. Ribeiro DL, Taboga SR, Góes RM. Diabetes induces stromal remodelling and increase in chondroitin sulphate proteoglycans of the rat ventral prostate. Int J Exp Pathol. 2009;90:400–11.

30. Searls YM, Smirnova IV, Fegley BR, Stehno-Bittel L. Exercise attenuates diabetes-induced ultrastructural changes in rat cardiac tissue. Med Sci Sports Exerc. 2004;36:1863–70.

31. Almeida FN, Proença AR, Chimin P, Marçal AC, Bessa-Lima F, Carvalho CR. Physical exercise and pancreatic islets: acute and chronic actions on insulin secretion. Islets. 2012;4(4):296–301.

32. Liu SH, Wang ZS. Study on the expression of androgen receptor in testis, epididymis and prostate of adult rats with diabetes. Zhonghua Nan Ke Xue. 2005;11:891–4.

33. Kim WT, Yun SJ, Choi YD, Kim GY, Moon SK, Choi YH, et al. Prostate size correlates with fasting blood glucose in non-diabetic benign prostatic hyperplasia patients with normal testosterone levels. J Korean Med Sci. 2011;26:1214–18.

34. Protopsaltis I, Ploumidis A, Sergentanis TN, Constantoulakis P, Tzirogiannis K, Kyprianidou C, et al. Linking pre-diabetes with benign prostate hyperplasia. IGFBP-3: a conductor of benign prostate hyperplasia development orchestra? PLoS One. 2013;8(12):e81411.

35. Roberts RO, Jacobson DJ, Girman CJ, Rhodes T, Klee GG, Lieber MM, et al. Insulin-like growth factor I, insulin-like growth factor binding protein 3, and urologic measures of benign prostatic hyperplasia. Am J Epidemiol. 2003;157(9):784–91.

36. Ho CK, Habib FK. Estrogen and androgen signaling in the pathogenesis of BPH. Nat Rev Urol. 2011;8:29–41.

37. Sciarra A, Mariotti G, Salciccia S, Autran Gomez A, Monti S, Toscano V, et al. Prostate growth and inflammation. J Steroid Biochem Mol Biol. 2008;108:254–60.

38. Lucia MS, Lambert JR. Growth factors in benign prostatic hyperplasia: basic science implications. Curr Urol Rep. 2008;9:272–8.

39. Sudha S, Sankar BR, Valli G, Govindarajulu P, Balasubramanian K. Streptozotocin-diabetes impairs prolactin binding to Leydig cells in prepubertal and pubertal rats. Horm Metab Res. 1999;31:583–6.

40. Gorbachinsky I, Akpinar H, Assimos DG. Metabolic Syndrome and Urologic Diseases. Rev Urol. 2010;12:e157–80.

41. Teixeira GR, Fávaro WJ, Pinheiro PF, Chuffa LG, Amorim JP, Mendes LO, et al. Physical exercise on the rat ventral prostate: steroid hormone receptors, apoptosis and cell proliferation. Scand J Med Sci Sports. 2012;22:e86–92.

42. Timms BG, Chandler JA. Ultrastructural and analytical studies on the prostate of castrated rats. Prostate. 1983;4:37–55.

43. Vignozzi L, Morelli A, Sarchielli E, Comeglio P, Filippi S, Cellai I, et al. Testosterone protects from metabolic syndrome-associated prostate inflammation: an experimental study in rabbit. J Endocrinol. 2012;212:71–84.

44. Stamatiadis D, Bulteau-Portois MC, Mowszowicz I. Inhibition of 5 alpha-reductase activity in human skin by zinc and azelaic acid. The Brit J Dermat. 1988;119(5):627–32.

45. Yahya H, Yahya KM, Saqib A. Minerals and type 2 diabetes mellitus –level of zinc, magnesium and chromium in diabetic and non diabetic population. J Univer Med & Dent College. 2011;2:34–8.

46. Christudoss P, Selvakumar R, Fleming JJ, Gopalakrishnan G. Zinc status of patients with benign prostatic hyperplasia and prostate carcinoma. Indian J Urol. 2011;27(1):14–8.

47. Dressendorfer RA, Sockolov R. Hypozincemia in runners. Phys Sports Med. 1980;8:97–100.

48. Sundaram RK, Bhaskar A, Vijayalingam S, Viswanathan M, Mohan R, et al. Antioxidant status and lipid peroxidation in type II diabetes mellitus with and without complications. Clin Sci. 1996;90:255–60.

49. Wierusz-Wysocka B, Wysocki H, Byks H, Zozulińska D, Wykretowicz A, Kaźmierczak M. Metabolic control quality and free radical activity in diabetic patients. Diabetes Res Clin Practice. 1995;27:193–7.

50. Aryal M, Pandeya A, Gautam N, Baral N, Lamsal M, Majhi S, et al. Oxidative stress in benign prostate hyperplasia. Nepal Med Coll J. 2007;9:222–4.

51. Laaksonen DE, Sen CK. Exercise and Oxidative Stress in Diabetes Mellitus. In: Sen CK, Packer L, Hanninen O, editors. Handbook of Oxidants and Antioxidants in Exercise. Amsterdam: Elsevier; 2000. p. 1105–36.

52. Atalay M, Laaksonen DE. Diabetes, oxidative stress and physical exercise. J Sports Sci Med. 2002;1:1–14.

53. Hobisch A, Rogatsch H, Hittmair A, Fuchs D, Bartsch Jr G, Klocker H, et al. Immunohistochemical localization of interleukin-6 and its receptor in benign, premalignant and malignant prostate tissue. J Pathol. 2000;191:239–44.

54. Okamoto M, Lee C, Oyasu R. Interleukin-6 as a paracrine and autocrine growth factor in human prostatic carcinoma cells in vitro. Cancer Res. 1997;57:141–6.

55. Bloch W, Klotz T, Loch C, Schmidt G, Engelmann U, Addicks K. Distribution of nitric oxide synthase implies a regulation of circulation, smooth muscle tone, and secretory function in the human prostate by nitric oxide. Prostate. 1997;33:1–8.

56. Kedia GT, Uckert S, Jonas U, Kuczyk MA, Burchardt M. The nitric oxide pathway in the human prostate: clinical implications in men with lower urinary tract symptoms. World J Urol. 2008;26:603–9.

57. De Nunzio C, Aronson W, Freedland SJ, Giovannucci E, Parsons JK. The correlation between metabolic syndrome and prostatic diseases. Eur Urol. 2012;61(3):560–70.

6

New medical treatments for lower urinary tract symptoms due to benign prostatic hyperplasia and future perspectives

Simone Albisinni[1]*[ID], Ibrahim Biaou[1], Quentin Marcelis[1], Fouad Aoun[1], Cosimo De Nunzio[2] and Thierry Roumeguère[1]

Abstract

Background: Lower Urinary Tract Symptoms (LUTS) in men are a common clinical problem in urology and have been historically strictly linked to benign prostatic hyperplasia (BPH), which may lead to bladder outlet obstruction (BOO). New molecules have been approved and have entered the urologists' armamentarium, targeting new signaling pathways and tackling specific aspects of LUTS. Objective of this review is to summarize the evidence regarding the new medical therapies currently available for male non-neurogenic LUTS, including superselective α1-antagonists, PDE-5 inhibitors, anticholinergic drugs and intraprostatic onabotulinum toxin injections.

Methods: The National Library of Medicine Database was searched for relevant articles published between January 2006 and December 2015, including the combination of "BPH", "LUTS", "medical" and "new". Each article's title, abstract and text were reviewed for their appropriateness and their relevance. One hundred forty eight articles were reviewed.

Results: Of the 148 articles reviewed, 92 were excluded. Silodosin may be considered a valid alternative to non-selective α1-antagonists, especially in the older patients where blood pressure alterations may determine major clinical problems and ejaculatory alterations may be not truly bothersome. Tadalafil 5 mg causes a significant decrease of IPSS score with an amelioration of patients' QoL, although with no significant increase in Q_{max}. Antimuscarinic drugs are effective on storage symptoms but should be used with caution in patients with elevated post-void residual. Intraprostatic injections of botulinum toxin are well-tolerated and effective, with a low rate of adverse events; however profound ameliorations were seen also in the sham arms of RCTs evaluating intraprostatic injections.

Conclusion: New drugs have been approved in the last years in the medical treatment of BPH-related LUTS. Practicing urologists should be familair with their pharmacodynamics and pharmacokinetics.

Keywords: Benign prostatic hyperplasia, Medical treatment, Prostate

Background

Lower Urinary Tract Symptoms (LUTS) in men are a common clinical problem in urology, and have been historically strictly linked to benign prostatic hyperplasia (BPH). These are classified into storage, voiding and post micturition symptoms [1]. However, BPH does not describe symptoms, but is instead a

histologic diagnosis, characterized by a micronodular hyperplasia evolving into a macroscopic nodular enlargement, which in turn may determine bladder outlet obstruction (BOO). Although BOO as a consequence of BPH may be responsible for a part of male LUTS, studies have found that the prostate is not the only actor in the complex play of male LUTS. The bladder and it's articulated neuronal control has been found to be another main character in this plot [2]. To support this theory, also women suffer from storage LUTS, with overactive bladder

---
* Correspondence: albisinni.simone@gmail.com
[1]Urology Department, Erasme Hospital, Université Libre de Bruxelles, Route de Lennik 808, B-1070 Brussels, Belgium
Full list of author information is available at the end of the article

(OAB) being the most frequent cause. Moreover, although voiding LUTS are the most common symptoms in BPH, storage are the most bothersome with great impact on the patients' quality of life (QoL) [3]. As such, today it is insufficient and inappropriate to consider the prostate as the only therapeutic target in the management of LUTS in men, even when BOO is present. Rather, the entire lower urinary tract, from the afferent sensory nerves to the urethra, must be seen as a whole and in this direction research is moving [4].

Historically, the standard medical treatment for LUTS in men with BPH included α1-antagonists, 5α-reductase inhibitors and phytotherapy. These agents remain indeed today the mainstay of BPH treatment. Nonetheless, albeit full dose treatment, some patients remain symptomatic or may experience BPH progression, defined as the onset of acute urinary retention (AUR), urinary infection (UI) or the need of BPH-related surgery [5]. In addition, the drugs routinely used in the management of LUTS carry potential adverse effects (AE), which in turn may be the cause of non-compliance of patients [6]. Therefore, research is progressing in order to expand and optimize medical strategies in the management of BPH-related LUTS. Selective α1-antagonists, phosphodiesterase 5 (PDE5) inhibitors, and anticholinergics have been tested and have entered our armamentarium for the management of male LUTS. These agents, their pharmacodynamics, pharmacokinetics and AEs should be well known to the practicing urologist. Furthermore, our knowledge of bladder and prostatic molecular anatomy is constantly growing, and in parallel new biomolecular targets are being identified and explored as new candidates in BPH management. Objective of this systematic review is to summarize the evidence regarding the new medical therapies currently available for BPH-related LUTS, and to give an overview on current research and agents which may enter our everyday clinical practice in the close future.

Methods

The National Library of Medicine Database was searched for relevant articles published between January 2006 and December 2015. A wide search was performed including the combination of following words: "BPH", "LUTS", "medical" "new". Although recent articles were prioritized, manuscripts with relevant historical findings were referenced if necessary. Publications in English language were preferred, though if necessary data was extrapolated even from manuscripts in other languages. Evidence was not limited to human data; results from animal and in vitro experiments were also included in the review. Helsinki declaration principles were respected and informed consent was obtained. Each article's title, abstract and text were reviewed for their appropriateness and their relevance. The initial list of selected papers was enriched by individual suggestions of the authors of the present review. Overall, 148 articles were reviewed. Of these, 92 were excluded after screening by the authors, leaving 56 articles eligible for the review (Fig. 1).

Results and Discussion
Selective α1-antagonists

α1-receptors are highly concentrated along the urinary and ejaculatory tracts [7], and non-selective α1-antagonists, alfuzosin, doxazosin, terazosin and tamsulosine are today the first line medical treatment in men with moderate to severe symptoms of BPH [8]. There are three main subtypes of α1-receptors expressed in the human organism: $α1_A$, $α1_B$ and $α1_D$-receptors. These are all composed of seven transmembrane domains and are coupled with G proteins, and their stimulation results in the activation of phospholipase C with consequent increase in intracellular Ca^{2+}, which in turn stimulates contraction in smooth muscular cells [7]. While $α1_B$-receptors are typically found in vascular tissue, where they mediate arterial contraction, $α1_A$ and $α1_D$ are more specific of the lower urinary tract [7]. Kojima et al. explored the expression of these two subtypes in the transitional zone of 28 prostatic tissue of men affected by BPH, and found that 43 % were $α1_A$ dominant, whereas 57 % $α1_D$dominant [9]. These receptors are found also in the human detrusor muscle and in the spinal cord, although the role of these localizations in the pathology of LUTS remains controversial. Moreover, in a rat model, α1-receptors stimulation determined an increase in bladder vascular resistance, with doxazosin determining an increase in bladder blood flow [10].

Non-selective α1-antagonists act on the dynamic component of BPH, counteracting smooth muscle contraction in the prostate, which is augmented in BPH, with a consequent increase in urinary flow, reduction of LUTS and improvement in QoL [11, 12]. A recent metanalysis has demonstrated the reduction of bladder outlet obstruction index of −30.45 for silodosin, effect which was higher than all other available α1-antagonists [13]. However, due to their concurrent action on $α1_B$-receptors, their use is associated with vascular AE, notably orthostatic hypotension, headaches and dizziness [8].

Silodosin is the most recently developed, highly selective antagonist of $α1_A$-receptors. Its selectivity towards $α1_A$-receptor blockade was reported to be 38 times higher than tamsulosin [13]. It has been shown that in vitro silodosin possesses an elevated $α1_A/α1_B$ binding ratio of 162/1 [14], and in vivo experiments have demonstrated its higher affinity for the urinary tract compared

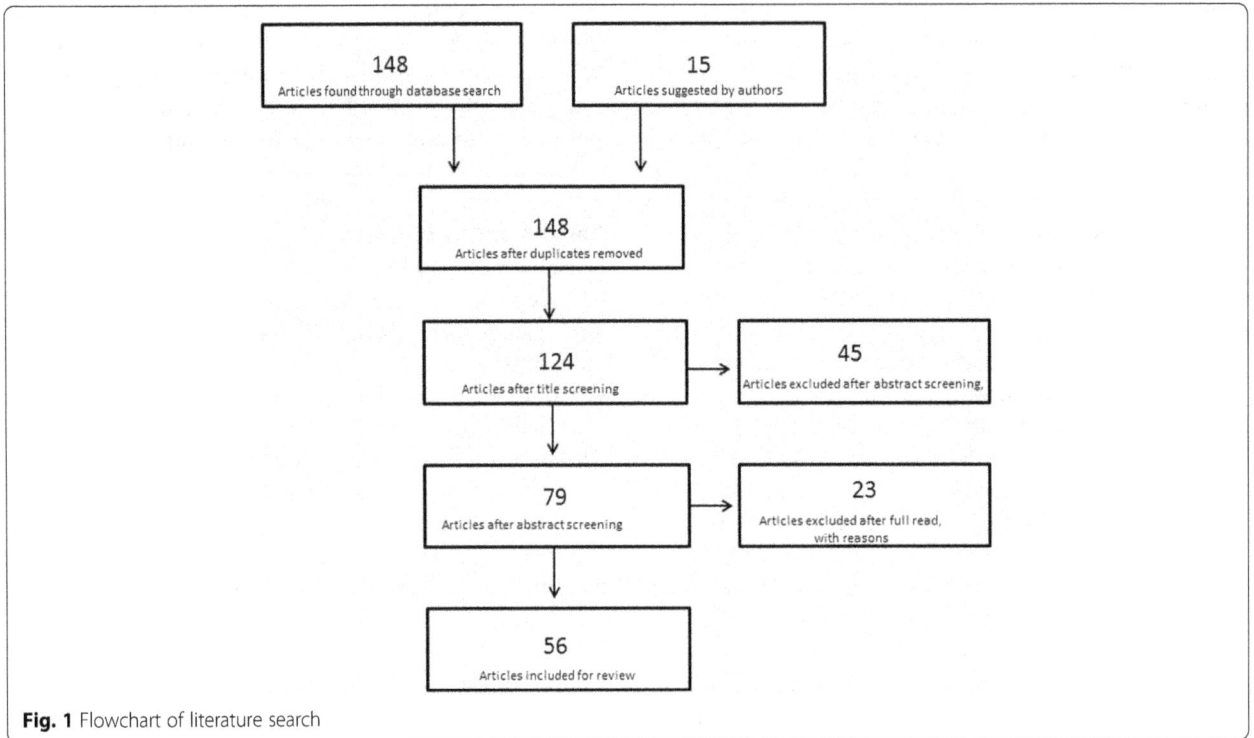

Fig. 1 Flowchart of literature search

to the vascular system [15]. Kobayashi et al. demonstrated that in dogs, while tamsulosin inhibits intraurethral pressure in a dose dependent manner with a concurrent reduction of blood pressure (especially in old dogs), silodosin determines similar effects on intraurethral pressures without altering blood pressure [16]. The recommended dosage is 8 mg once –daily, which has been found to be non-inferior to 4 mg twice-daily in a double-blind randomized controlled trial (RCT) [17]. After administration, Silodosin is quickly absorbed and has a bioavailability of 32 % at 8 mg/day (therapeutic dose) [18]. Tmax is reached in 2.6 h and half life of the drug is 13.3 h. The drug is then eliminated via fecal (55 %) and renal (45 %) route [18].

On this pharmacologic basis, silodosin has been tested in order to evaluate its non-inferior effect on BPH, while minimizing peripheral vasodilatation and cardiovascular effects which may be cause of falls and fractures, especially in the elderly [19]. Chapple et al. have explored the efficacy of silodosin in a prospective, placebo controlled trial [20]. Nine hundred ninety five European men were randomized to receive either 8 mg silodosin, 0,4 mg tamsulosin or placebo on a daily basis for 12 weeks. The authors found a significant improvement of voiding and storage LUTS after treatment with silodosin compared to placebo (Δ IPSS: 2.3, 95%CI 1.4-3.2, $p < 0.001$)*, similar to that of tamsulosin, with a significant amelioration of patients' QoL. Furthermore, silodosin determined a reduction of nycturia (Change from baseline silodosin vs

placebo: -0.9 vs-0.7, $p = 0.013$), effect which was non-significant ($p = 0.095$) for tamsulosin vs placebo. Silodosin also caused an increase in urinary flow of 3.77 ml/s, though this was not significantly higher compared to placebo ($p = 0.089$). Kawabe et al. reported results of a RCT which included 457 Japanese men treated by silodosin, tamsulosin or placebo, and found a significant decrease in total IPSS in the silodosin arm compared to placebo [21]. Similarly, Marks et al. found that 8 mg daily silodosin caused a significant reduction of both storage and voiding LUTS compared to placebo (Δ total 1.9, $p < 0.0001$; Δ storage 0.5, $p = 0.0002$; Δ voiding 1.4 $p < 0.0001$) [22]. Finally, it appears that Silodosin may decrease nycturia, especially in patients >65 years old in which desmopressin therapy may be problematic: in a pooled analysis of three RCTs, Eisenhardt et al. found that silodosin, compared to placebo, determined a significant nicturia improvement (53.4 vs. 42.8 %, $p < 0.0001$) [23], making it an interesting drug in the elderly population.

Most studies reported that truly silodosin determines less peripheral vascular AE compared to non-selective α1-antagonists, as it does not determine significant effects on supine or orthotopic blood pressure [20, 24]. However, silodosin caused in most trials a higher rate of anejaculation compared to non-selective α1-antagonists or tamsulosin, with rates between 14.2 and 20.9 %: this has been hypothesized to be a consequence of its selectivity for $\alpha1_A$-receptors, which are highly expressed along the vas deferens, with a consequent reduction of their contractility [20]. In 30 young sexually active patients, Bozkurt et al. have found impaired ejaculation in 27/30 men, with significant enlargement of seminal vesicles [24]. A long-term analysis following 104 men for 6 years found a quite high discontinuation of silodosin (75 %), mostly due to progression of disease and need for surgery or to unknown causes; only 9/78 stopped treatment due to side effects [25].

As such, silodosin may be considered a valid alternative to non-selective α1-antagonists, especially in the older patients where blood pressure alterations may determine major clinical problems and ejaculatory alterations may be not truly bothersome.

Phosphodiesterase 5 Inhibitors

In addition to adrenergic fibers, key actors in micturition are the nonadrenergic-noncholinergic fibers. This neural system is implicated in the release and increase of nitric oxide (NO), a cardinal molecule for intracellular signaling which causes an increase of cyclic guanosine monophosphate (cGMP), consequently catabolized by the enzyme PDE. After its fundamental discovery in the cavernous tissue and the development of PDE5 inhibitors in the treatment of erectile dysfunction (ED), researchers have demonstrated the presence of PDE-5 isoenzymes all along the lower urinary tract: they are in fact expressed in the detrusor, the prostate, the urethra and in pelvic vessels [26]. Here PDE-5 inhibition determines intracellular cGMP increase, which in turn may promote micturition via different though yet unclear mechanisms of action [27]. First, cGMP phosphorylates and inactivates a protein kinase G (ρ-kinase) to promote smooth muscle cells relaxation [28]. In addition, this ρ-kinase stimulates endothelin-1, which is a potent vasoconstrictor which can mediate muscle contraction [28]. Therefore, PDE-5 inhibition, via a cGMP increase, reduces ρ-kinase activity and thus increases relaxation in the lower urinary tract. Additionally, PDE inhibition enhances smooth muscle cell relaxation increasing NO activity as observed in the bladder neck, where nitrergic innervation is prominent [26], in the prostate, were PDE inhibition determines a dose-dependent tissue relaxation [29], and in urethral tissue [30]. Finally, PDE-5 inhibition leads to increased perfusion of pelvic organs with the hypothesis that pelvic atherosclerosis with consequent ischaemia may have a role in male LUTS [31], the vasodilatation and increased end-organ perfusion determined by PDE-5 inhibitors on blood vessels may be beneficial for LUTS. Of note, Bertolotto et al. demonstrated increased prostatic perfusion on contrast-enhanced ultrasound after administration of tadalafil 20 mg [32]. Moreover, soluble cGMP plays a key role in the NO-mediated inhibition of leukocyte rolling, and PDE5 inhibition may reduce atherosclerotic damage and overall inflammation

by reducing leukocyte recruitment. Tadalafil was shown to attenuate in vitro the expression of the inflammatory cytokines TNF-α and IL-1βin pulmonary arteries [33] and of TNF-α and IL-8 in endothelial cells [34]. Finally, cGMP modulates afferent nerve fibers from the bladder and urethra, and PDE inhibitors may decrease the sensation of bladder filling, thus reducing urgency [26, 35]. In this context Minagawa et al. found that tadalafil significantly decreased afferent activity from the bladder in response to bladder filling in a rat model [35] and Behr-Roussel et al. reported a reduction of afferent signaling in rats with spinal cord injury in response to bladder filling after treatment with vardenafil [36].

Randomized, placebo-controlled clinical trials have demonstrated that daily treatment with 5 mg tadalafil improves safely BPH-related LUTS [37–39]. McVary et al. found that tadalafil determined a decrease of total IPSS of −3.8 compared to −1.7 with placebo after 12 weeks of treatment ($p < 0.0001$) [37]. QoL also significantly improved (−0.7 vs −0.3, $p = 0.008$), while no significant differences were observed for peak urinary flow (Q_{max}). Roehrborn et al. confirmed these findings, and noted in their trial that the dose of tadalafil with the best risk-benefit profile was 5 mg, determining a reduction of IPSS of −4.87 vs −2.27 with placebo ($p < 0.001$) [38]. Similarly, also QoL was significantly improved with tadalafil 5 mg. On post hoc analysis, the authors found that although tadalafil caused a numerically superior increase in Q_{max} compared to placebo, this increase was nonsignificant [40]. Oelke et al. reported an amelioration of total IPSS after 12 weeks of tadalafil 5 mg (Δ IPSS vs placebo: −2.1, $p = 0.001$) and of QoL (−0.3, $p = 0.022$) [39]. Moreover, these investigators described a significant increase in Q_{max}: +2.4 ml/s (tadalafil) vs +1.2 ml/s (placebo), $p = 0.009$: although this result is not consistent with those previously reported [41], it must be kept in mind that Q_{max} is intra individually variable and influenced by age, sexual activity and baseline Q_{max} severity [40]. In a meta-analysis, Gacci et al. synthesized that tadalafil determines a significant −2.85 decrease in overall IPSS compared to placebo and a significant −1.85 decrease in association with α1-inhibitors compared to α1-inhibitors alone [42]. Clearly, tadalafil also significantly improves erectile function with a net increase of the International Index of Erectile Function. Indeed, a point of controversy is whether the amelioration of IPSS and QoL, which are subjective measurements, is a direct consequence of tadalafil's pharmacologic effect on the lower urinary tract or if the results observed are confounded by the fact that the patients, having an improved potency, are more sexually active and thus more satisfied. It appears however that the amelioration seen in IPSS and QoL is observed both in potent and impotent patients [43] and pooled data analyses determined that the LUTS amelioration was largely

(92.5 %) determined by a direct effect of the drug [44]. Tadalafil is also being tested in combination therapy with tamsulosin [45] or finasteride [46], demonstrating a more pronounced amelioration of LUTS and ED symptoms in the combination arms. Concerning AE, the vast majority of manuscripts reported mild to moderate grade AE (dyspepsia and flushing), with a low rate (2–4 %) of discontinuation of the therapy secondary to AE [42, 47].

In conclusion, tadalafil 5 mg is an effective and well tolerated treatment for BPH-related LUTS, and is of cardinal importance when treating patients with concomitant ED. Tadalafil causes a significant decrease of IPSS score with an amelioration of patients' QoL, although with no significant increase in Q_{max}.

Great caution is advised when prescribing iPDE5. As a consequence of systemic vasodilation, reduced venous blood flow to the heart may trigger cardiac failure in patients with preexisting cardiac insufficiency [42]. As such, before prescribing iPDE5, the clinician must always exclude signs of cardiac insufficiency as dyspnea, lower extremity oedema, chest pain. Moreover, for the same pharmacologic reasons, concomitant treatment with nitroderivates is an absolute contraindication to iPDE5 utilisation [8].

Antimuscarinics

Two main subtypes of muscarinic receptor (MR) are expressed in the lower urinary tract: M2 and M3 receptors. Their proportions in detrusor membranes are respectively evaluated at 71 % and 22 % [48]. While M3 are mainly responsible for detrusor contraction in both healthy and pathologic conditions, M2 are predominant in the urothelium and may be associated with pathologic changes in the bladder [49]. It has been commonly and reasonably thought that the main mechanism of action of antimuscarinics in the treatment of LUTS is mediated by a reduction of detrusor contractility. Specimens from patients with bladder overactivity are consistently denervated, and as such it has been hypothesized that possible denervation supersensibility to acetylcholine may be crucial in OAB physiopathology [50]. However MR are also present in the urothelium and are here involved in urothelial sensory function. The urothelium in fact releases multiple signal molecules, including acetylcholine, which activate unmyelinated afferent C-fibers present in the suburothelial layer of the bladder wall, and this release of acetylcholine is increased by bladder overstretching . This, associated to the denervation supersensitivity of the detrusor to acetylcholine, may induce disorganized contraction of small muscular units in the detrusor, generating pathologic afferent signals which in turn may determine urgency symptoms [51].

Antimuscarinics have been prevalently used in female patients with OAB: however today it is clear that in men

with BPH, storage symptoms are partially caused by the bladder, with urodynamically proven OAB being a common cause [52]. As such antimuscarinic therapy has emerged as a new option in male LUTS management [8]. Chun-Hou Liao et al. have studied the predictors of therapeutic success with a first line antimuscarinic treatment in BPH men with predominant storage symptoms. In their 197 patients group, receiving tolterodine in monotherapy, higher baseline IPSS, higher baseline Qmax and lower prostate volume were each associated with a better response [53]. Treatment with antimuscarinics alone is still felt as dangerous in patients with BOO by many urologists, due to the possible increased risk of AUR. Abrams et al. reported that in men with mild to moderate BOO, the antimuscarinic tolterodine 2 mg twice daily for 12 weeks caused a significant increase in post void residual (PVR) urine compared to placebo (49 ml vs 16 ml): however, rates of AUR (3 %) and Q_{max} were equal across both groups [54]. This is probably a consequence of the action of antimuscarinics on the storage phase of micturition and not on voiding, as there is little evidence that these agents, at the therapeutic recommended doses, determine a significant reduction of voiding contraction [55]. Nonetheless, in daily clinical practice, the majority of patients is already under treatment with an α1-antagonist, and present with persisting storage symptoms. In this context, several trials have explored the efficacy and safety of the addition of an antimuscarinic to the α1-antagonist in these patients [56–58]. The TIMES study included 879 men with symptoms of BPH and OAB [56]. Patients were randomized to receive either tolterodine 4 mg ER + tamsuloin, one of the two drugs alone or placebo. After 12 weeks, in the combination arm the patients reported significant decrease in urgency incontinence episodes (−0.88 vs −0.31, $p = 0.005$), frequency (−2.54 vs −1.41, $p < 0.001$) and an amelioration of QoL. Although higher than for placebo and for tamsulosin alone, the rate of AUR was low for the combination (0.4 %) and the tolterodine arm alone (0.5 %). MacDiarmid et al. reported significant amelioration of both storage and voiding symptoms ($p = 0.006$) in men affected by BPH treated with tamsulosin + oxybutinin 10 mg, with a non-significant increase in PVR in treated patients compared to placebo [57]. Similarly, in the VICTOR study, 398 men were randomized to receive tamsulosin plus either solifenacin 5 mg or placebo. In the solifenacin group, patients showed a significant reduction of urgency episodes (−2.18 vs −1.10, $p = 0.001$) but a non-significant reduction of frequency (−1.05 vs −0.67, $p = 0.135$) [58]. In most trials the most frequent AE associated with antimuscarinics is xerostomia [56, 57]. Increase in PVR urine, though statistically significant in many studies, frequently did not determine a significant increase in the risk of AUR requiring catheterization [56, 57]. However, as recommended by current EAU guidelines, antimuscarinics are therefore medications which can be prescribed in men with BPH with residual storage symptoms after treatment with α1-antagonists. Before to start a treatment with an antimuscarinic, BPH patients should be monitored for PVR and then closely followed [8]. Some authors have been questioning the compliance to bi-therapy, considering the fact that the common chronic combination of antimuscarinics and αl-antagonists could be a burden for the patients. Barkin et al. reported a retrospective analysis based on patients prescriptions reimbursement data. They concluded that patients treated in combination therapy showed an improved persistence over a year period, compared to those on αl-antagonists monotherapy [59].

Concerning anticholinergic drugs, great care is necessary when prescribing these drugs in the elderly, as cognitive deterioration may be a serious consequence and one must bear in mind that 16 % of patients >70 years show some form of cognitive impairment [60]. Indeed, encephalic cholinergic activity, and in particular M1 and M2 receptors which represent over 60 % of the brains cholinergic receptors, are vital in cognitive function [61]. The only antimuscarinic which was accorded a beneficial safety profile in the elderly is Fesoterodine, as this drug was studied specifically in the ageing population [62–64]. In the SOFIA trial 581 patients >65, of which 33 % were >75 years old and frequently on polypharmacy, completed a 3 month double-blind randomized trial of Fesoterodine versus placebo [62]. At 12 weeks, patients in the treatment arm demonstrated reduced urgency (–3.8 episodes), pollakiuria and nycturia (–0.55 episodes) (all $p < 0.001$) compared to placeebo. Fesoterodine determined a similar rate of adverse events compared to placebo (39.8 % vs 36.1 %), mostly mild xerostomia. Of note, no clinically relevant changes in cognitive function (evaluated through the mini-mental status examination) were observed throughout the study in both arms. This may be attributed to the high affinity of Fesoterodine for the M3 receptor and its inability to pass the blood–brain barrier [65]. In any case, great care is advised with anticholinergic drugs and a high level of suspiciousness in case of cognitive deterioration while receiving treatment.

Intraprostatic agents
In addition to classic oral therapy, medical agents may be injected directly in the prostate [66]. This is a promising minimally invasive approach in patients who are unresponsive to medical treatment, who experience debilitating AE or who are poor candidates for surgery. The rationale for this therapy is the ability of some agents to determine prostatic involution and promote apoptosis, thus shrinking prostatic volume and

ameliorating LUTS [66]. In addition, these agents may modulate prostatic afferent nerves, reducing nociception and improving BPH-related symptoms. However, it must be remembered that profound ameliorations were seen also in the sham arms of RCTs evaluating intraprostatic injections [67]: as such, the results of such trials must always be redimensioned and relativized to the sham-control arm, rather than considering the absolute results.

Ethanol has been explored as agent for intraprostatic administration, with favorable results. Investigators found a significant reduction of IPSS and an amelioration of Q_{max} and QoL [68, 69]. However results are seldom durable, and patients frequently require re-treatment, which has been reported necessary in over 40 % of patients [70]. Intraprostatic botulinum toxin injection is a very promising and is being throughout fully explored. This neurotoxin exists in seven different subtypes, and the most widely used has been Onabotulinum toxin A. Though yet unclear, it has been hypothesized that this may enhance prostatic apoptosis, downregulate α-receptors and modulate afferent signaling in the prostate [71]. Investigators have reported positive and significant improvement of LUTS in men with BPH treated by Onabotulinum toxin injection [72]. Generally, doses between 100U and 300U have been used during most trials but Arnouk et al. reported similar functional and safety results after injection of 100U and 200U [73]. To date the largest trial testing botulinum in BPH was recently published by Marberger et al. in a phase II placebo-controlled trial, enrolling 380 men [74]. Patients were randomized to receive 100U, 200U or 300U Onabotulinum toxin A or 0.9 % saline, and were followed for 72 weeks. The investigators found a meaningful improvement of BPH parameters after botulinum injection, including IPSS (Δ IPSS: 5.6 to 6.6, according to dose), $Q_{max}(\Delta = 2.0$ to 2.4 ml/s, according to dose) and QoL. However, a pronounced placebo effect was observed, with patients in the control arm experiencing a similar symptom amelioration, yielding non-significant differences in outcomes across the treatment and control arm. Overall, intraprostatic injections of botulinum toxin are well-tolerated, with a low rate of AE mainly associated with the administration of the drug (2 % prostatitis) [74] and not the compound itself. Moreover, no sexual AEs are reported, with full conservation of sexual potency [75].

Future perspectives in the medical treatment of BPH
Research in the field of BPH therapy is continuously progressing. As our molecular understanding of bladder, prostatic, urethral anatomy and pathophysiology advances, so do the experimental studies and clinical trials exploring new drugs in this domain. In particular

there is growing interest in the role of inflammation, the vitamin D receptor signaling pathway and the activity of β_3-receptors in BPH-mediated LUTS.

Inflammation has been associated with BPH pathogenesis and progression, with multiple cytokines and inflammatory cells responsible for the increased risk of BPH determined by prostatic inflammation [76]. The COX pathway leads to the production of free radicals and consequent oxidative stress: as such, a possible therapeutic effect of non-steroidal anti-inflammatory drugs has been hypothesized [77, 78]. Di Silverio et al. found that the combination of finasteride and a COX-2 inhibitor, rofecoxib 25 mg/die, caused a significant improvement in IPSS score ($p = 0.0001$) and of Q_{max} ($p = 0.03$) compared to finasteride alone [77]. Moreover flavocoxid, an inhibitor of COX and 5-lipoxygenase enzymes, reduced prostate weight, increased the expression of Bax and caspase-9 mRNA (pro-apoptotic) and decreased that of Bcl-2 (anti-apoptotic) in mice with induced BPH [78]. Although COX inhibitors could have a future role in the management of BPH, clinical evidence is still lacking and their application in BPH must be considered experimental.

The vitamin D receptor (VDR) signaling pathway could be associated with BPH and LUTS [79, 80]. Investigators have found that VDR agonists, notably elocalcitol, a synthetic derivative of vitamin D3 that regulates cell proliferation and apoptosis may inhibit the androgen-dependent and androgen-independentprostatic cell proliferation [81]. It can also reduce IL-8 secretion by inflammatory cells in the prostate by targeting the NF-kB pathway [80]. Elocalcitol modulates bladder contractility by inhibiting the calcium-sensitizing RhoA/ROCK with a potential interest in storage symptoms control [82]. In a phase II RCT, Colli et al. treated 57 men with prostate volumes ≥40 ml with elocalcitol for 12 weeks, finding a significant reduction of prostate growth compared to placebo (-2.90 vs $+4.32$, $p < 0.0001$) [79]. However until now in humans, elocalcitol was demonstrated with a very good safety profile but only exhibited limited efficacy on LUTS in patients with BPH and overactive bladder. Recent data in animals reported the interest of association of elicalcitol with tolterodine [83]. Clinical experimentation is continuing to evaluate its potential role in LUTS due to BPH and OAB management.

In the bladder the predominant form of β-adrenoceptor is the β3-receptor subtype. Its activation is associated with increased bladder capacity without change in micturition pressure, residual volume, or voiding contraction [84]. Mirabegron is a β3-receptor agonist that has been successfully tested in male and female patients suffering from OAB without BOO [85, 86] and is now being evaluated also in men with associated BOO. Nitti et al. in a randomized, double-blind, phase II study, treated 200 men affected by BOO with mirabegron 50, 100 mg or placebo.

Mirabegron 50 mg was effective in reducing urgency and frequency, without impairing Q_{max} and with a non-significant increase in PVR urine [87]. Otsuki et al. studied the response to mirabegron 50 mg in two groups of patient, newly diagnosed OAB and BPH related OAB unresponsive to antimuscarinics [88]. They showed a significant improvement of OAB Symptom Score and IPSS –QOL index, voiding symptoms with no significant difference on post-void residual, supporting the use of Mirabegron in second line after failure of antimuscarinics. A recent randomized controlled trial tested the add-on of Mirabegron 50 mg to 0.2 mg tamsulosine compared to tamsulosine alone, with a significant benefit on urgency, daytime frequency and quality of life index after 2 months of therapy [89]. Although the increase in post-void residual urine volume was significantly greater in the add-on group, AUR was observed only in one man. The results of these trials suggest that Mirabegron may be effective in reducing storage LUTS and safe in patients affected by BOO.

Ion channel transient receptor potential subtype melastatin 8 (TRPM8) is an important factor in the mechanism of detection of bladder filling, whose activation can activate the initiation of micturition. Ito et al. described their activity in a rat model, finding [90] that administration of the TRPM8 antagonist RQ-00203078 significantly increased bladder capacity and voided volume. Moreover, the activation of TRPM8 is enhanced by cold temperatures, as found by Uvin et al. [91], demonstrating the known empirical finding that cold temperatures worsen urgency. Although these findings represent important steps in the understanding of the physiology of micturition, their clinical relevance to date remains limited: TRPM8 antagonists (PF-05105679) have been tested in phase 1 trials, however given the generalized expression of these receptors, significant side effects were recorded including hypothermia [92], thus limiting their possible clinical application.

PRX302 is a PSA-activated bacterial protoxin which has the ability to bind to cellular membranes, where it creates transmembrane channels with consequent lytic cell death. After intriguing results in animal models where intraprostatic injection of PRX302 caused extensive, organ-confined prostatic shrinkage [93], this molecule has been tested in humans with favorable preliminary results. In a phase II trial, 18 men received intraprostatic injections of PRX302 [94]. After one year there was an average change from baseline IPPS of -9.7 and of $+2.8$ ml/s inQ_{max}. Moreover, 12/18 (67 %) patients showed a ≥20 % reduction inprostate volume at day 90. Of note, no patient experienced sexual AEs. Clearly, though these results appear very encouraging, the small sample size limits their interpretation and PRX302 is still considered experimental.

NX-1207 is another protein for intraprostatic injection currently under evaluation in preliminary studies. This molecule promotes focal apoptosis, with significant reductions of prostate volumes in animal models [95]. Human phase II studies found that intraprostatic injection of NX-1207 determined a reduction of AUA Symptom Score, maintained during 6 months follow-up, with no significant AE [95]. Two phase III trials are underway and their results are awaited to better analyze the true potential of this drug in BPH management.

Conclusions

Today, BPH should not be considered a strictly prostatic disease, as it has been demonstrated that the entire lower urinary tract is involved in a complex pathophysiology. New medical treatments are available and the right drugs should be prescribed t the correct patients. Silodosin has similar efficacy compared to tamsulosin, with a lower risk of cardiovascular AE, making it a good choice for older patients requiring α1-antagonists. Tadalafil improves BPH symptoms in men with and without ED, and could be considered especially when ED and BPH coexist. Antimuscarinics are effective on residual storage symptoms after α1-antagonist therapy and appears to be safe even in men with moderate BOO, though these patients should be strictly monitored with regular PVR measurements. Intraprostatic injections of onabotulinum toxin A are a promising minimally invasive option for LUTS management, although their true efficacy is still object of evaluation. Finally, research in the field of BPH medical treatment is actively progressing, with new agents as elocalcitol and mirabegron being tested. Future basic research and prospective clinical trials must continue in order to increase our pharmacologic armamentarium for men suffering from LUTS, in order to reduce BPH progression, improve QoL and decrease AEs.

Abbreviations

AE: Adverse effects; AUR: Acute urinary retention; BOO: Bladder outlet obstruction; BPH: Benign prostatic hyperplasia; cGMP: Cyclic guanosine monophosphate; ED: Erectile dysfonction; IPSS: International prostatic symptom score; LUTS: Lower urinary tract symtoms; NO: Nitric oxide; OAB: Overactive bladder; PDE5: Phosphodiesterase 5; QoL: Quality of Life; UI: Urinary infection

Acknowledgements

None.

Funding

No funding was obtained for the present study.

Authors' contributions
Study concept and design: SA, CDN, TR. Acquisition of data: SA, IB, QM, FA. Analysis and interpretation of data: SA, FA, CDN, TR. Drafting of the manuscript: SA, IB, QM, FA. Critical revision of the manuscript for important intellectual content: FA, CDN, TR. All authors read and approved the final manuscript.

Competing interest
The authors declare that they have no competing interests.

Author details
[1]Urology Department, Erasme Hospital, Université Libre de Bruxelles, Route de Lennik 808, B-1070 Brussels, Belgium. [2]Department of Urology, Ospedale Sant'Andrea, University "La Sapienza", Roma, Italy.

References

1. Abrams P, Cardozo L, Fall M, Griffiths D, Rosier P, Ulmsten U, et al. The standardisation of terminology of lower urinary tract function: report from the Standardisation Sub-committee of the International Continence Society. Am J Obstet Gynecol. 2002;187:116–26.
2. Chapple CR, Roehrborn CG. A shifted paradigm for the further understanding, evaluation, and treatment of lower urinary tract symptoms in men: focus on the bladder. Eur Urol. 2006;49:651–8.
3. Peters TJ, Donovan JL, Kay HE, Abrams P, de la Rosette JJ, Porru D, et al. The International Continence Society "Benign Prostatic Hyperplasia" Study: the botherosomeness of urinary symptoms. J Urol. 1997;157:885–9.
4. Soler R, Andersson K-E, Chancellor MB, Chapple CR, de Groat WC, Drake MJ, et al. Future direction in pharmacotherapy for non-neurogenic male lower urinary tract symptoms. Eur Urol. 2013;64:610–21.
5. Andriole GL, Bostwick DG, Brawley OW, Gomella LG, Marberger M, Montorsi F, et al. Effect of dutasteride on the risk of prostate cancer. N Engl J Med. 2010;362:1192–202.
6. Masumori N, Hashimoto J, Itoh N, Tsukamoto T, Group TSMUNS. Short-term efficacy and long-term compliance/treatment failure of the alpha1 blocker naftopidil for patients with lower urinary tract symptoms suggestive of benign prostatic hyperplasia. Scand J Urol Nephrol. 2007;41:422–9.
7. Michel MC, Vrydag W. Alpha1-, alpha2- and beta-adrenoceptors in the urinary bladder, urethra and prostate. Br J Pharmacol. 2006;147 Suppl 2: S88–119.
8. Oelke M, Bachmann A, Descazeaud A, Emberton M, Gravas S, Michel MC, et al. EAU guidelines on the treatment and follow-up of non-neurogenic male lower urinary tract symptoms including benign prostatic obstruction. Eur Urol. 2013;64:118–40.
9. Kojima Y, Kubota Y, Sasaki S, Hayashi Y, Kohri K. Translational pharmacology in aging men with benign prostatic hyperplasia: molecular and clinical approaches to alpha1-adrenoceptors. Curr Aging Sci. 2009;2:223–39.
10. Das AK, Leggett RE, Whitbeck C, Eagen G, Levin RM. Effect of doxazosin on rat urinary bladder function after partial outlet obstruction. Neurourol Urodyn. 2002;21:160–6.
11. Yamanishi T, Mizuno T, Tatsumiya K, Watanabe M, Kamai T, Yoshida K-I. Urodynamic effects of silodosin, a new alpha 1A-adrenoceptor selective antagonist, for the treatment of benign prostatic hyperplasia. Neurourol Urodyn. 2010;29:558–62.
12. Matsukawa Y, Gotoh M, Komatsu T, Funahashi Y, Sassa N, Hattori R. Efficacy of silodosin for relieving benign prostatic obstruction: prospective pressure flow study. J Urol. 2009;182:2831–5.
13. Rossi M, Roumeguère T. Silodosin in the treatment of benign prostatic hyperplasia. Drug Des Devel Ther. 2010;4:291–7.
14. Tatemichi S, Kobayashi K, Maezawa A, Kobayashi M, Yamazaki Y, Shibata N. Alpha1-adrenoceptor subtype selectivity and organ specificity of silodosin (KMD-3213). Yakugaku Zasshi. 2006;126(Spec no):209–16.
15. Akiyama K, Noto H, Nishizawa O, Sugaya K, Yamagishi R, Kitazawa M, et al. Effect of KMD-3213, an alpha1A-adrenoceptor antagonist, on the prostatic urethral pressure and blood pressure in male decerebrate dogs. Int J Urol Off J Jpn Urol Assoc. 2001;8:177–83.

16. Kobayashi S, Tomiyama Y, Tatemichi S, Hoyano Y, Kobayashi M, Yamazaki Y. Effects of silodosin and tamsulosin on the urethra and cardiovascular system in young and old dogs with benign prostatic hyperplasia. Eur J Pharmacol. 2009;613:135–40.

17. Choo M-S, Song M, Kim JH, Lee K-S, Kim JC, Kim SW, et al. Safety and efficacy of 8-mg once-daily vs 4-mg twice-daily silodosin in patients with lower urinary tract symptoms suggestive of benign prostatic hyperplasia (SILVER Study): a 12-week, double-blind, randomized, parallel, multicenter study. Urology. 2014;83:875–81.

18. Keating GM. Silodosin: a review of its use in the treatment of the signs and symptoms of benign prostatic hyperplasia. Drugs. 2015;75:207–17.

19. Welk B, McArthur E, Fraser L-A, Hayward J, Dixon S, Hwang YJ, et al. The risk of fall and fracture with the initiation of a prostate-selective α antagonist: a population based cohort study. BMJ. 2015;351:h5398.

20. Chapple CR, Montorsi F, Tammela TLJ, Wirth M, Koldewijn E, Fernández Fernández E, et al. Silodosin therapy for lower urinary tract symptoms in men with suspected benign prostatic hyperplasia: results of an international, randomized, double-blind, placebo- and active-controlled clinical trial performed in Europe. Eur Urol. 2011;59:342–52.

21. Kawabe K, Yoshida M, Homma Y, Silodosin Clinical Study Group. Silodosin, a new alpha1A-adrenoceptor-selective antagonist for treating benign prostatic hyperplasia: results of a phase III randomized, placebo-controlled, double-blind study in Japanese men. BJU Int. 2006;98:1019–24.

22. Marks LS, Gittelman MC, Hill LA, Volinn W, Hoel G. Rapid efficacy of the highly selective alpha1A-adrenoceptor antagonist silodosin in men with signs and symptoms of benign prostatic hyperplasia: pooled results of 2 phase 3 studies. J Urol. 2009;181:2634–40.

23. Eisenhardt A, Schneider T, Cruz F, Oelke M. Consistent and significant improvement of nighttime voiding frequency (nocturia) with silodosin in men with LUTS suggestive of BPH: pooled analysis of three randomized, placebo-controlled, double-blind phase III studies. World J Urol. 2014;32:1119–25.

24. Bozkurt O, Demir O, Sen V, Esen A. Silodosin causes impaired ejaculation and enlargement of seminal vesicles in sexually active men treated for lower urinary tract symptoms suggestive of benign prostatic hyperplasia. Urology. 2015;85:1085–9.

25. Yamanishi T, Kaga K, Fuse M, Shibata C, Kamai T, Uchiyama T. Six-year follow up of silodosin monotherapy for the treatment of lower urinary tract symptoms suggestive of benign prostatic hyperplasia: What are the factors for continuation or withdrawal? Int J Urol Off J Jpn Urol Assoc. 2015;22:1143–8.

26. Giuliano F, Ückert S, Maggi M, Birder L, Kissel J, Viktrup L. The mechanism of action of phosphodiesterase type 5 inhibitors in the treatment of lower urinary tract symptoms related to benign prostatic hyperplasia. Eur Urol. 2013;63:506–16.

27. Roumeguere T, Aoun F, Marcelis Q. Minimally invasive devices for treating lower urinary tract symptoms in benign prostate hyperplasia: technology update. Res Rep Urol. 2015;7:125.

28. Rees RW, Foxwell NA, Ralph DJ, Kell PD, Moncada S, Cellek S. Y-27632, a Rho-kinase inhibitor, inhibits proliferation and adrenergic contraction of prostatic smooth muscle cells. J Urol. 2003;170:2517–22.

29. Ückert S, Sormes M, Kedia G, Scheller F, Knapp WH, Jonas U, et al. Effects of phosphodiesterase inhibitors on tension induced by norepinephrine and accumulation of cyclic nucleotides in isolated human prostatic tissue. Urology. 2008;71:526–30.

30. Lee JG, Moon DG, Kang SH, Cho DY, Park HS, Bae JH. Relaxation effect of phosphodiesterase-5 inhibitor on the animal bladder and prostatic urethra: in vitro and in vivo study. Urol Int. 2010;84:231–5.

31. Azadzoi KM, Babayan RK, Kozlowski R, Siroky MB. Chronic ischemia increases prostatic smooth muscle contraction in the rabbit. J Urol. 2003;170:659–63.

32. Bertolotto M, Trincia E, Zappetti R, Bernich R, Savoca G, Cova MA. Effect of Tadalafil on prostate haemodynamics: preliminary evaluation with contrast-enhanced US. Radiol Med (Torino). 2009;114:1106–14.

33. Tsai BM, Turrentine MW, Sheridan BC, Wang M, Fiore AC, Brown JW, et al. Differential effects of phosphodiesterase-5 inhibitors on hypoxic pulmonary vasoconstriction and pulmonary artery cytokine expression. Ann Thorac Surg. 2006;81:272–8.

34. Roumeguère T, Zouaoui Boudjeltia K, Babar S, Nuyens V, Rousseau A, Van Antwerpen P, et al. Effects of phosphodiesterase inhibitors on the inflammatory response of endothelial cells stimulated by myeloperoxidase-modified low-density lipoprotein or tumor necrosis factor alpha. Eur Urol. 2010;57:522–8.

35. Minagawa T, Aizawa N, Igawa Y, Wyndaele J-J. Inhibitory effects of phosphodiesterase 5 inhibitor, tadalafil, on mechanosensitive bladder

36. Behr-Roussel D, Oger S, Caisey S, Sandner P, Bernabé J, Alexandre L, et al. Vardenafil decreases bladder afferent nerve activity in unanesthetized, decerebrate, spinal cord-injured rats. Eur Urol. 2011;59:272–9.

37. McVary KT, Roehrborn CG, Kaminetsky JC, Auerbach SM, Wachs B, Young JM, et al. Tadalafil relieves lower urinary tract symptoms secondary to benign prostatic hyperplasia. J Urol. 2007;177:1401–7.

38. Roehrborn CG, McVary KT, Elion-Mboussa A, Viktrup L. Tadalafil administered once daily for lower urinary tract symptoms secondary to benign prostatic hyperplasia: a dose finding study. J Urol. 2008;180:1228–34.

39. Oelke M, Giuliano F, Mirone V, Xu L, Cox D, Viktrup L. Monotherapy with tadalafil or tamsulosin similarly improved lower urinary tract symptoms suggestive of benign prostatic hyperplasia in an international, randomised, parallel, placebo-controlled clinical trial. Eur Urol. 2012;61:917–25.

40. Roehrborn CG, Kaminetsky JC, Auerbach SM, Montelongo RM, Elion-Mboussa A, Viktrup L. Changes in peak urinary flow and voiding efficiency in men with signs and symptoms of benign prostatic hyperplasia during once daily tadalafil treatment. BJU Int. 2010;105:502–7.

41. Laydner HK, Oliveira P, Oliveira CRA, Makarawo TP, Andrade WS, Tannus M, et al. Phosphodiesterase 5 inhibitors for lower urinary tract symptoms secondary to benign prostatic hyperplasia: a systematic review. BJU Int. 2011;107:1104–9.

42. Gacci M, Corona G, Salvi M, Vignozzi L, McVary KT, Kaplan SA, et al. A systematic review and meta-analysis on the use of phosphodiesterase 5 inhibitors alone or in combination with α-blockers for lower urinary tract symptoms due to benign prostatic hyperplasia. Eur Urol. 2012;61:994–1003.

43. Broderick GA, Brock GB, Roehrborn CG, Watts SD, Elion-Mboussa A, Viktrup L. Effects of tadalafil on lower urinary tract symptoms secondary to benign prostatic hyperplasia in men with or without erectile dysfunction. Urology. 2010;75:1452–8.

44. Brock GB, McVary KT, Roehrborn CG, Watts S, Ni X, Viktrup L, et al. Direct effects of tadalafil on lower urinary tract symptoms versus indirect effects mediated through erectile dysfunction symptom improvement: integrated data analyses from 4 placebo controlled clinical studies. J Urol. 2014;191:405–11.

45. Singh DV, Mete UK, Mandal AK, Singh SK. A comparative randomized prospective study to evaluate efficacy and safety of combination of tamsulosin and tadalafil vs. tamsulosin or tadalafil alone in patients with lower urinary tract symptoms due to benign prostatic hyperplasia. J Sex Med. 2014;11:187–96.

46. Glina S, Roehrborn CG, Esen A, Plekhanov A, Sorsaburu S, Henneges C, et al. Sexual function in men with lower urinary tract symptoms and prostatic enlargement secondary to benign prostatic hyperplasia: results of a 6-month, randomized, double-blind, placebo-controlled study of tadalafil coadministered with finasteride. J Sex Med. 2015;12:129–38.

47. Donatucci CF, Brock GB, Goldfischer ER, Pommerville PJ, Elion-Mboussa A, Kissel JD, et al. Tadalafil administered once daily for lower urinary tract symptoms secondary to benign prostatic hyperplasia: a 1-year, open-label extension study. BJU Int. 2011;107:1110–6.

48. Mansfield KJ, Liu L, Mitchelson FJ, Moore KH, Millard RJ, Burcher E. Muscarinic receptor subtypes in human bladder detrusor and mucosa, studied by radioligand binding and quantitative competitive RT-PCR: changes in ageing. Br J Pharmacol. 2005;144:1089–99.

49. Mukerji G, Yiangou Y, Grogono J, Underwood J, Agarwal SK, Khullar V, et al. Localization of M2 and M3 muscarinic receptors in human bladder disorders and their clinical correlations. J Urol. 2006;176:367–73.

50. Yoshida M, Inadome A, Maeda Y, Satoji Y, Masunaga K, Sugiyama Y, et al. Non-neuronal cholinergic system in human bladder urothelium. Urology. 2006;67:425–30.

51. Drake MJ, Harvey IJ, Gillespie JI, Van Duyl WA. Localized contractions in the normal human bladder and in urinary urgency. BJU Int. 2005;95:1002–5.

52. Lee JY, Kim HW, Lee SJ, Koh JS, Suh HJ, Chancellor MB. Comparison of doxazosin with or without tolterodine in men with symptomatic bladder outlet obstruction and an overactive bladder. BJU Int. 2004;94:817–20.

53. Liao C-H, Kuo Y-C, Kuo H-C. Predictors of successful first-line antimuscarinic monotherapy in men with enlarged prostate and predominant storage symptoms. Urology. 2013;81:1030–3.

54. Abrams P, Kaplan S, De Koning Gans HJ, Millard R. Safety and tolerability of tolterodine for the treatment of overactive bladder in men with bladder outlet obstruction. J Urol. 2006;175:999–1004. discussion 1004.

55. Andersson K-E. Antimuscarinics for treatment of overactive bladder. Lancet Neurol. 2004;3:46–53.

56. Kaplan SA, Roehrborn CG, Rovner ES, Carlsson M, Bavendam T, Guan Z. Tolterodine and tamsulosin for treatment of men with lower urinary tract symptoms and overactive bladder: a randomized controlled trial. JAMA. 2006;296:2319–28.

57. MacDiarmid SA, Peters KM, Chen A, Armstrong RB, Orman C, Aquilina JW, et al. Efficacy and safety of extended-release oxybutynin in combination with tamsulosin for treatment of lower urinary tract symptoms in men: randomized, double-blind, placebo-controlled study. Mayo Clin Proc. 2008;83:1002–10.

58. Kaplan SA, McCammon K, Fincher R, Fakhoury A, He W. Safety and tolerability of solifenacin add-on therapy to alpha-blocker treated men with residual urgency and frequency. J Urol. 2009;182:2825–30.

59. Barkin J, Diles D, Franks B, Berner T. Alpha blocker monotherapy versus combination therapy with antimuscarinics in men with persistent LUTS refractory to alpha-adrenergic treatment: patterns of persistence. Can J Urol. 2015;22:7914–23.

60. Petersen RC, Roberts RO, Knopman DS, Geda YE, Cha RH, Pankratz VS, et al. Prevalence of mild cognitive impairment is higher in men. The Mayo Clinic Study of Aging. Neurology. 2010;75:889–97.

61. Jiang S, Li Y, Zhang C, Zhao Y, Bu G, Xu H, et al. M1 muscarinic acetylcholine receptor in Alzheimer's disease. Neurosci Bull. 2014;30:295–307.

62. Wagg A, Khullar V, Marschall-Kehrel D, Michel MC, Oelke M, Darekar A, et al. Flexible-dose fesoterodine in elderly adults with overactive bladder: results of the randomized, double-blind, placebo-controlled study of fesoterodine in an aging population trial. J Am Geriatr Soc. 2013;61:185–93.

63. DuBeau CE, Kraus SR, Griebling TL, Newman DK, Wyman JF, Johnson TM, et al. Effect of fesoterodine in vulnerable elderly subjects with urgency incontinence: a double-blind, placebo controlled trial. J Urol. 2014;191:395–404.

64. Sand PK, Heesakkers J, Kraus SR, Carlsson M, Guan Z, Berriman S. Long-term safety, tolerability and efficacy of fesoterodine in subjects with overactive bladder symptoms stratified by age: pooled analysis of two open-label extension studies. Drugs Aging. 2012;29:119–31.

65. Chancellor MB, Staskin DR, Kay GG, Sandage BW, Oefelein MG, Tsao JW. Blood–brain barrier permeation and efflux exclusion of anticholinergics used in the treatment of overactive bladder. Drugs Aging. 2012;29:259–73.

66. Andersson K-E. Treatment of lower urinary tract symptoms: agents for intraprostatic injection. Scand J Urol. 2013;47:83–90.

67. Welliver C, Kottwitz M, Feustel P, McVary K. Clinically and statistically significant changes seen in sham surgery arms of randomized, controlled benign prostatic hyperplasia surgery trials. J Urol. 2015;194:1682–7.

68. El-Husseiny T, Buchholz N. Transurethral ethanol ablation of the prostate for symptomatic benign prostatic hyperplasia: long-term follow-up. J Endourol Endourol Soc. 2011;25:477–80.

69. Grise P, Plante M, Palmer J, Martinez-Sagarra J, Hernandez C, Schettini M, et al. Evaluation of the transurethral ethanol ablation of the prostate (TEAP) for symptomatic benign prostatic hyperplasia (BPH): a European multi-center evaluation. Eur Urol. 2004;46:496–501. discussion 501–2.

70. Goya N, Ishikawa N, Ito F, Kobayashi C, Tomizawa Y, Toma H. Transurethral ethanol injection therapy for prostatic hyperplasia: 3-year results. J Urol. 2004;172:1017–20.

71. Chuang Y-C, Huang C-C, Kang H-Y, Chiang P-H, Demiguel F, Yoshimura N, et al. Novel action of botulinum toxin on the stromal and epithelial components of the prostate gland. J Urol. 2006;175:1158–63.

72. Crawford ED, Hirst K, Kusek JW, Donnell RF, Kaplan SA, McVary KT, et al. Effects of 100 and 300 units of onabotulinum toxin a on lower urinary tract symptoms of benign prostatic hyperplasia: a phase II randomized clinical trial. J Urol. 2011;186:965–70.

73. Arnouk R, Suzuki Bellucci CH, Benatuil Stull R, de Bessa J, Malave CA, Mendes Gome C. Botulinum neurotoxin type A for the treatment of benign prostatic hyperplasia: randomized study comparing two doses. Sci World J. 2012;2012:463574.

74. Marberger M, Chartier-Kastler E, Egerdie B, Lee K-S, Grosse J, Bugarin D, et al. A randomized double-blind placebo-controlled phase 2 dose-ranging study of OnabotulinumtoxinA in men with benign prostatic hyperplasia. Eur Urol. 2013;63:496–503.

75. Silva J, Pinto R, Carvalho T, Botelho F, Silva P, Silva C, et al. Intraprostatic botulinum toxin type A administration: evaluation of the effects on sexual function. BJU Int. 2011;107:1950–4.

76. De Nunzio C, Kramer G, Marberger M, Montironi R, Nelson W, Schröder F, et al. The controversial relationship between benign prostatic hyperplasia and prostate cancer: the role of inflammation. Eur Urol. 2011;60:106–17.

77. Di Silverio F, Bosman C, Salvatori M, Albanesi L, Proietti Pannunzi L, Ciccariello M, et al. Combination therapy with rofecoxib and finasteride in the treatment of men with lower urinary tract symptoms (LUTS) and benign prostatic hyperplasia (BPH). Eur Urol. 2005;47:72–8. discussion 78–9.

78. Altavilla D, Minutoli L, Polito F, Irrera N, Arena S, Magno C, et al. Effects of flavocoxid, a dual inhibitor of COX and 5-lipoxygenase enzymes, on benign prostatic hyperplasia. Br J Pharmacol. 2012;167:95–108.

79. Colli E, Rigatti P, Montorsi F, Artibani W, Petta S, Mondaini N, et al. BXL628, a novel vitamin D3 analog arrests prostate growth in patients with benign prostatic hyperplasia: a randomized clinical trial. Eur Urol. 2006;49:82–6.

80. Penna G, Fibbi B, Amuchastegui S, Corsiero E, Laverny G, Silvestrini E, et al. The vitamin D receptor agonist elocalcitol inhibits IL-8-dependent benign prostatic hyperplasia stromal cell proliferation and inflammatory response by targeting the RhoA/Rho kinase and NF-kappaB pathways. Prostate. 2009;69:480–93.

81. Crescioli C, Ferruzzi P, Caporali A, Scaltriti M, Bettuzzi S, Mancina R, et al. Inhibition of prostate cell growth by BXL-628, a calcitriol analogue selected for a phase II clinical trial in patients with benign prostate hyperplasia. Eur J Endocrinol Eur Fed Endocr Soc. 2004;150:591–603.

82. Adorini L, Penna G, Amuchastegui S, Cossetti C, Aquilano F, Mariani R, et al. Inhibition of prostate growth and inflammation by the vitamin D receptor agonist BXL-628 (elocalcitol). J Steroid Biochem Mol Biol. 2007;103:689–93.

83. Streng T, Andersson K-E, Hedlund P, Gratzke C, Baroni E, D'Ambrosio D, et al. Effects on bladder function of combining elocalcitol and tolterodine in rats with outflow obstruction. BJU Int. 2012;110:E125–31.

84. Tyagi P, Tyagi V. Mirabegron, a β₃-adrenoceptor agonist for the potential treatment of urinary frequency, urinary incontinence or urgency associated with overactive bladder. IDrugs Investig Drugs J. 2010;13:713–22.

85. Herschorn S, Barkin J, Castro-Diaz D, Frankel JM, Espuna-Pons M, Gousse AE, et al. A phase III, randomized, double-blind, parallel-group, placebo-controlled, multicentre study to assess the efficacy and safety of the β₃ adrenoceptor agonist, mirabegron, in patients with symptoms of overactive bladder. Urology. 2013;82:313–20.

86. Nitti VW, Khullar V, van Kerrebroeck P, Herschorn S, Cambronero J, Angulo JC, et al. Mirabegron for the treatment of overactive bladder: a prespecified pooled efficacy analysis and pooled safety analysis of three randomised, double-blind, placebo-controlled, phase III studies. Int J Clin Pract. 2013;67:619–32.

87. Nitti VW, Rosenberg S, Mitcheson DH, He W, Fakhoury A, Martin NE. Urodynamics and safety of the β₃-adrenoceptor agonist mirabegron in males with lower urinary tract symptoms and bladder outlet obstruction. J Urol. 2013;190:1320–7.

88. Otsuki H, Kosaka T, Nakamura K, Mishima J, Kuwahara Y, Tsukamoto T. β3-Adrenoceptor agonist mirabegron is effective for overactive bladder that is unresponsive to antimuscarinic treatment or is related to benign prostatic hyperplasia in men. Int Urol Nephrol. 2013;45:53–60.

89. Ichihara K, Masumori N, Fukuta F, Tsukamoto T, Iwasawa A, Tanaka Y. A randomized controlled study of the efficacy of tamsulosin monotherapy and its combination with mirabegron for overactive bladder induced by benign prostatic obstruction. J Urol. 2015;193:921–6.

90. Ito H, Aizawa N, Sugiyama R, Watanabe S, Takahashi N, Tajimi M, et al. Functional role of the transient receptor potential melastatin 8 (TRPM8) ion channel in the urinary bladder assessed by conscious cystometry and ex vivo measurements of single-unit mechanosensitive bladder afferent activities in the rat. BJU Int. 2016;117:484–94.

91. Uvin P, Franken J, Pinto S, Rietjens R, Grammet L, Deruyver Y, et al. Essential role of transient receptor potential M8 (TRPM8) in a model of acute cold-induced urinary urgency. Eur Urol. 2015;68:655–61.

92. Winchester WJ, Gore K, Glatt S, Petit W, Gardiner JC, Conlon K, et al. Inhibition of TRPM8 channels reduces pain in the cold pressor test in humans. J Pharmacol Exp Ther. 2014;351:259–69.

93. Williams SA, Merchant RF, Garrett-Mayer E, Isaacs JT, Buckley JT, Denmeade SR. A prostate-specific antigen-activated channel-forming toxin as therapy for prostatic disease. J Natl Cancer Inst. 2007;99:376–85.

94. Denmeade SR, Egerdie B, Steinhoff G, Merchant R, Abi-Habib R, Pommerville P. Phase 1 and 2 studies demonstrate the safety and efficacy of intraprostatic injection of PRX302 for the targeted treatment of lower urinary tract symptoms secondary to benign prostatic hyperplasia. Eur Urol. 2011;59:747–54.

95. Shore N. NX-1207: a novel investigational drug for the treatment of benign prostatic hyperplasia. Expert Opin Investig Drugs. 2010;19:305–10.

7

Rates of prostate surgery and acute urinary retention for benign prostatic hyperplasia in men treated with dutasteride or finasteride

Josephina G. Kuiper[1*], Irene D. Bezemer[1], Maurice T. Driessen[2], Averyan Vasylyev[3], Claus G. Roehrborn[4], Fernie J. A. Penning-van Beest[1] and Ron M. C. Herings[1]

Abstract

Background: Previous studies have suggested a greater benefit for various outcomes in men diagnosed with benign prostatic hyperplasia (BPH) who are treated with dutasteride than for men treated with finasteride. This study investigates whether the rates of BPH-related prostate surgery and acute urinary retention (AUR) differ between dutasteride and finasteride users in the Netherlands.

Methods: From the PHARMO Database Network, men aged ≥50 years with a dispensing of dutasteride or finasteride with or without concomitant alpha-blocker treatment between March 1, 2003 and December 31, 2011 were selected. The incidence of BPH-related prostate surgery and AUR was determined during dutasteride or finasteride treatment and stratified by type of initial BPH-treatment (5-ARI monotherapy or combination with alpha-blocker) and prescriber (general practitioner (GP) or urologist). Comparison of the incidence of BPH-related prostate surgery and AUR between the treatment groups was done by Cox proportional hazard regression.

Results: 11,822 dutasteride users and 5,781 finasteride users were identified. Most users started treatment in combination with an alpha-blocker. Overall, dutasteride users had a lower risk of BPH-related prostate surgery was lower among dutasteride users than finasteride users (HR: 0.75; 95 % CI: 0.56–0.99). This lower risk among dutasteride users was also seen when stratifying by monotherapy or combination therapy (HR: 0.73; 95 % CI: 0.54–0.98 for monotherapy and HR: 0.85; 95 % CI: 0.74–0.97 for combination therapy). However, the association was only present among men treated by urologists. For AUR the rates were low and no statistical significant difference was observed between dutasteride and finasteride users.

Conclusions: The risk of undergoing BPH-related prostate surgery was lower among men using dutasteride compared to men using finasteride. The association was observed for monotherapy as well as combination therapy, however, only among men who received their prescription from a urologist.

Keywords: Benign prostatic hyperplasia, Prostate surgery, Acute urinary retention, 5-alpha reductase inhibitors, Alpha-blocker

Abbreviations: 5-ARIs, 5-alpha reductase inhibitors; ATC, Anatomical therapeutic chemical; AUR, Acute urinary retention; BPH, Benign prostatic hyperplasia; CDS, Chronic disease score; CI, Confidence interval; DHT, Dihydrotestosterone; GP, General practitioner; HR, Hazard ratio; ICPC, International Classification of Primary Care; IPSS, International Prostate Symptom Score; IQR, Interquartile range; LUTS, Lower urinary tract symptoms; MPR, Medication possession rate; PSA, Prostate-specific antigen; PY, Person-years; SD, Standard deviation; WHO, World Health Organization

* Correspondence: josine.kuiper@pharmo.nl
[1]PHARMO Institute for Drug Outcomes Research, van Deventerlaan 30-40, 3528 AE Utrecht, Netherlands
Full list of author information is available at the end of the article

Background

Benign prostatic hyperplasia (BPH) affects 32–52 % of men aged 51–60 years and 77–99 % of men ≥81 years of age [1, 2]. Lower urinary tract symptoms (LUTS), such as poor stream and hesitancy, are common in patients with BPH. Progression of BPH may result in acute urinary retention (AUR) and need for surgical procedures that (partially) remove the prostate [3]. In order to relief BPH related symptoms, alpha-adrenoreceptor antagonists ("alpha-blockers") can be used. Previous studies suggests that the combination of alpha-blockers and 5-alpha reductase inhibitors (5-ARIs) can be beneficial in the treatment of BPH associated with LUTS [4]. The greatest efficacy for this combination treatment was shown in patients with a large prostate size, a prostate-specific antigen (PSA) value of > 1.5 ng/ml, and with moderate to severe symptoms based on the International Prostate Symptom Score (IPSS). They experienced significant symptom relief and a decreased risk of AUR and surgery compared to patients treated with monotherapy [5]. Dihydrotestosterone (DHT), a metabolite of testosterone is the main mediator of prostate growth. As a class, 5-ARIs aimed to reduce the size of the prostate by blocking the activity of 5-alpha reductase enzymes in converting testosterone to DHT [6, 7]. The currently available 5-ARI agents in the United States and European market (dutasteride and finasteride), have been shown to reduce prostate volume by 20–30 % [8]. Long-term use of 5-ARI agents results in symptomatic improvements and reduction of the risk for AUR and prostate surgery [6, 9, 10]. Dutasteride blocks the type 1 as well as type 2 5-alpha reductase isoenzymes whereas finasteride blocks only the type 2 isoenzyme. Suppression of serum DHT has been shown to be more than 90 % by dutasteride and 70 % by finasteride [7].

In retrospective studies, the efficacy of finasteride and dutasteride has been compared for AUR and BPH-related surgeries showing significantly lower rates of AUR and BPH-related surgeries among dutasteride treated patients as compared with finasteride treated patients [11]. In another study, patients treated with dutasteride were less likely to experience AUR and prostate surgery than patients treated with finasteride [12]. A previous study conducted in Italy showed that the incidence of BPH-related hospitalization was lower among patients treated with dutasteride compared to patients treated with finasteride [13].

The purpose of this study was to compare the rates of BPH-related prostate surgery and AUR between dutasteride and finasteride alone or in combination with an alpha-blocker in the Dutch setting.

Methods

Data source

Data were obtained from the PHARMO Database Network in the Netherlands. This population-based network of healthcare databases combines data from different healthcare settings. Data sources are linked on a patient level through validated algorithms. The longitudinal nature of the PHARMO Database Network system enables to follow-up more than 4 million (25 %) residents of a well-defined population in the Netherlands for an average of ten years. For this study the Hospitalisation Database, the Out-patient Pharmacy Database and the General Practitioner (GP) Database were used. The Hospitalisation Database comprises hospital admissions from the Dutch Hospital Data Foundation [14], i.e., admissions for more than 24 h and admissions for less than 24 h for which a bed is required. The records include information about discharge diagnoses, procedures, and hospital admission and discharge dates. Diagnoses are coded according to the International Classification of Diseases [15] and procedures are coded according to the Dutch Classification of Procedures [16]. The Out-patient Pharmacy Database comprises GP or specialist prescribed healthcare products dispensed by the out-patient pharmacy. The dispensing records include information about type of medicine, dispensing date, strength, dosage regimen, quantity, route of administration, and prescriber specialty. Drug dispensings are coded according to the World Health Organization (WHO) Anatomical Therapeutic Chemical (ATC) Classification System. The GP Database comprises data from electronic patient records registered by GPs. The records include information on diagnoses and symptoms, laboratory test results, referrals to specialists and healthcare product/drug prescriptions. Diagnoses and symptoms are coded according to the International Classification of Primary Care (ICPC) [17]. The prescription records include information on type of product, date, strength, dosage regimen, quantity and route of administration. Drug prescriptions are coded according to the WHO ATC Classification System (WHO Anatomical Therapeutic Chemical Classification System) [18].

Study population

From the Out-patient Pharmacy Database, men aged 50 years or older who were treated with dutasteride or finasteride between March 1, 2003 and December 31, 2011 were selected for inclusion in this study. The date of the first dispensing was designated as cohort entry date. Men were classified as either receiving 5-ARI monotherapy or 5-ARI in combination with an alpha-blocker at cohort entry date. 5-ARI in combination with an alpha-blocker was defined as continuous use of an alpha-blocker at cohort entry date or starting an alpha-blocker within 7 days of cohort entry date. The alpha-blocker and 5-ARI could be used as separate preparations or as combination pill. From the selected population, we excluded 1) men using 1 mg finasteride tablets (as these were indicated for the treatment of alopecia), and 2) men who had a hospitalization for prostate surgery, urinary retention, prostate cancer or bladder cancer before cohort entry date. To be able to define comorbidities in recent history and the risk of BPH-related prostate surgery, users were required to have continuous enrollment in the PHARMO Database Network of at least 12 months before and 12 months after the index date. All men were followed from cohort entry until moving out of the PHARMO catchment region, death, or end of the study period (December 31, 2011), whichever occurred first.

Type of treatment

Dispensings of dutasteride, finasteride and alpha-blocker at cohort entry date and during follow-up were converted into treatment episodes of uninterrupted use. For each drug dispensing the duration of use was calculated by dividing the number of units dispensed by the number of units to be used per day, as defined in the dispensing records. In case of an interruption between two dispensings, use was considered uninterrupted if the duration of this gap was less than half the period of the given dispensing, or seven days, whichever is greater, according to the method of Catalan [19]. Episodes of uninterrupted use were constructed on the level of 5-ARI (dutasteride and finasteride episodes) and on the level of total BPH treatment (dutasteride monotherapy, finasteride monotherapy, dutasteride combination therapy or finasteride combination therapy). The first episode of 5-ARI treatment ended at the dispensing date of the alternative 5-ARI. The first episode of BPH treatment ended when the dutasteride or finasteride episode ended, when the alpha-blocker episode ended (for men on combined therapy) or when an alpha-blocker was dispensed (for men on monotherapy). Adherence with 5-ARI treatment during the first episode of BPH treatment was reflected by the medication possession rate (MPR), defined as the total number of days of 5-ARI treatment, divided by the duration of episode.

Study endpoint

The primary endpoints in the current study were the rate of BPH-related prostate surgery and AUR during treatment with dutasteride compared to finasteride. BPH-related prostate surgery was defined by surgical procedures on the prostate during hospitalization with a primary or secondary discharge diagnosis of BPH (either coded as benign neoplasm or hyperplasia) and no diagnosis of prostate cancer. AUR was defined as a hospital admission with a primary or secondary discharge diagnosis of urinary retention.

BPH-related prostate surgery and AUR were determined during the first episode of 5-ARI treatment. Sensitivity analyses were performed by adding a washout period of 6 months after discontinuation of 5-ARI treatment to the observation period, and by limiting the observation period to the first episode of BPH treatment, i.e. ending observation upon addition (for initial monotherapy) or discontinuation (for initial combination therapy) of alpha-blocker therapy.

Data analysis

Incidence rates of BPH-related prostate surgery and AUR were calculated by dividing the number of men with the event under investigation by the person-time at risk of the event under investigation in the population. Rates were stratified by concomitant use of alpha-blocker (mono- or combination therapy). As the setting of care is an indicator of severity of disease and may as well be related to surgery rates, results were also stratified by initial prescriber (GP or urologist). Hazard ratios (HR) and confidence intervals (CI) for comparison between the treatment groups were calculated using Cox proportional hazards regression adjusting for confounders. Potential confounders were age, chronic disease score (CDS), prescriber, adherence with 5-ARI treatment (medication possession rate (MPR)), history of bladder/kidney stones, urological care, haematuria, PSA, duration of alpha-blocker use, hypertension, hypercholesterolemia, diabetes type I, diabetes type II, Parkinson's disease, multiple sclerosis, number of hospital admissions, number of drug dispensings (of any drug), and number of GP visits. Potential covariates that were associated with the outcome at an alpha of 5 % (univariate $p < 0.05$) and also were associated with choice of 5-ARI (t-test $p < 0.05$ for continuous variables and chi-square $p < 0.05$ for categorical variables) were included in the multivariate model if they changed the association between treatment and outcome by at least 5 %. All HRs were adjusted for geographic location to account for potential missing outcomes in combination with local prescriber preference.

All data were analysed using SAS programs organized within SAS Enterprise Guide version 4.3 (SAS Institute Inc., Cary, NC, USA) and conducted under Windows using SAS version 9.2.

Results

Patient characteristics

A total of 11,822 men treated with dutasteride (8,675 men (73 %) on combination therapy) and 5,781 men treated with finasteride (3,517 men (61 %) on combination therapy) between March 1, 2003 and December 31, 2011 were included in the analysis (Table 1). Most men on combination therapy were already using an alpha-blocker when they started 5-ARI (68 % of the dutasteride users and 75 % of the finasteride users). The mean age among the different cohorts was approximately 70 years. The initial

Table 1 General characteristics of men with BPH using finasteride or dutasteride

	Dutasteride		Finasteride	
	monotherapy	& alpha-blocker	monotherapy	& alpha-blocker
	$N = 3,147$	$N = 8,675$	$N = 2,264$	$N = 3,517$
	n (%)	n (%)	n (%)	n (%)
Age at cohort entry				
50–54 years	150 (5)	330 (4)	172 (8)	148 (4)
55–59 years	320 (10)	860 (10)	255 (11)	371 (11)
60–64 years	468 (15)	1,541 (18)	341 (15)	577 (16)
65–79 years	1,659 (53)	4,681 (54)	1,101 (49)	1,847 (53)
80–84 years	330 (10)	848 (10)	246 (11)	378 (11)
85–89 years	169 (5)	348 (4)	101 (4)	151 (4)
≥ 90	51 (2)	67 (1)	48 (2)	45 (1)
Mean (±SD)	70 ± 10	70 ± 9	69 ± 10	70 ± 9
Prescriber of first 5-ARI				
Urologist	1,705 (54)	5,053 (58)	653 (29)	1,412 (40)
GP	1,063 (34)	2,242 (26)	1,275 (56)	1,546 (44)
Other	379 (12)	1,380 (16)	336 (15)	559 (16)
Prior use of urological care				
Yes	2,055 (65)	6,164 (71)	943 (42)	1,946 (55)
History of bladder or kidney stones				
Yes	50 (2)	148 (2)	16 (1)	48 (1)
Comorbidities				
Hypertension	1,653 (53)	4,444 (51)	1,116 (49)	1,771 (50)
Hypercholesterolemia	1,060 (34)	2,948 (34)	662 (29)	1,094 (31)
Diabetes type I	42 (1)	113 (1)	50 (2)	73 (2)
Diabetes type II	322 (10)	930 (11)	209 (9)	372 (11)
Parkinson's disease	42 (1)	148 (2)	41 (2)	50 (1)
Multiple sclerosis	1 (<0.5)	1 (<0.5)	0 (0)	2 (<0.5)
Chronic disease score				
0–3	1,402 (45)	3,987 (46)	1,137 (50)	1,634 (46)
4–7	939 (30)	2,516 (29)	619 (27)	1,017 (29)
≥ 8	806 (26)	2,172 (25)	508 (22)	866 (25)
Mean (±SD)	5 ± 4	5 ± 4	4 ± 4	5 ± 4
Adherence (MPR 5-ARI) (%)				
Mean (±SD)	84 ± 13	85 ± 13	81 ± 14	84 ± 13
Database follow-up after cohort entry date				
≥ 1 year	2,264 (100)	3,517 (100)	3,147 (100)	8,675 (100)
≥ 2 years	1,906 (84)	2,975 (85)	2,361 (75)	6,395 (74)
≥ 3 years	1,596 (70)	2,463 (70)	1,700 (54)	4,526 (52)
≥ 4 years	1,291 (57)	1,991 (57)	1,115 (35)	2,972 (34)
≥ 5 years	970 (43)	1,490 (42)	618 (20)	1,715 (20)

SD standard deviation, *IQR* interquartile range, *MPR* medication possession rate

prescriber of the first dutasteride dispensing was a urologist (57 %), while the first finasteride dispensing was primarily issued by the GP (49 %). The proportion of men that had received prior urological care was higher among dutasteride users than among finasteride users. The duration of the first 5-ARI treatment episode was on average

17 months for men receiving monotherapy of either finasteride or dutasteride. For men on combination therapy, the duration of the first 5-ARI treatment episode was on average 20 months for men on finasteride combination therapy and 18 months for men on dutasteride combination therapy.

Incidence of outcomes

The incidence of BPH-related prostate surgery among men using finasteride ranged from 12 per 1,000 person-years among those using monotherapy prescribed by a GP to 472 per 1,000 person-years among those using combination therapy prescribed by a urologist (Table 2). For men using dutasteride this was 10 per 1,000 person-years among those using monotherapy prescribed by a GP to 248 per 1,000 person-years among those using combination therapy prescribed by a urologist. A transurethral resection of the prostate (TURP) was most common in all cohorts (data not shown).

Figure 1 shows the proportion of men free of BPH-related prostate surgery over time, stratified by type of initial BPH treatment and prescriber. Overall, dutasteride users had a lower risk of BPH-related prostate surgery than finasteride users. The crude HR was 0.83 (95 % CI: 0.62–1.10), however when adjusted for geographic location, cohort (mono- or combination therapy), adherence with 5-ARI treatment, prescriber, chronic disease score and number of GP visits the HR was 0.75 (95 % CI: 0.56–0.99). The strongest confounder was the initial prescriber. This lower risk was seen for men on monotherapy (adjusted HR: 0.73; 95 % CI: 0.54–0.98) as well as

combination therapy (adjusted HR: 0.85; 95 % CI: 0.74–0.97) (Table 2). This association, however, was only present among men with a first dispensing from a urologist (HR: 0.77; 95 % CI: 0.46–1.30 for men on monotherapy and HR: 0.62; 95 % CI: 0.50–0.78 for combination therapy), while there was no difference in the risk of BPH-related prostate surgery among men with a first dispensing from a GP. In a sensitivity analysis, BPH-related prostate surgery was determined during total BPH treatment (censoring upon changes in alpha-blocker use) and in another sensitivity analysis during 5-ARI treatment (regardless of alpha-blocker use) with a wash-out period of 6 months after discontinuation. The difference in incidence of BPH-related prostate surgery between mono- and combination therapy remained, but the association with type of 5-ARI was less clear.

Only 1 % of the finasteride or dutasteride users were admitted for AUR during the first 5-ARI treatment episode. The incidence rates were 6 per 1,000 person-years for men on dutasteride monotherapy, 5 per 1,000 person-years for men on finasteride monotherapy, 9 per 1,000 person-years for men on dutasteride combination therapy and 5 per 1,000 person-years for men on finasteride combination therapy. Due to the low number of men admitted for AUR, no HR could be calculated.

Discussion

To our knowledge, this is the first population-based study to report the incidence of BPH-related prostate surgery and AUR among men using dutasteride or finasteride in the Netherlands. Disease severity was

Table 2 Hazard ratios of BPH-related prostate surgery among men with BPH using finasteride or dutasteride

	Finasteride			Dutasteride			Dutasteride vs finasteride	
	Men with BPH-related surgery n (%)[f]	PY at risk	Incidence per 1,000 PY (95 % CI)	Men with BPH-related surgery n (%)[f]	PY at risk	Incidence per 1,000 PY (95 % CI)	Hazard ratio	
							Crude (95 % CI)[a]	Adjusted (95 % CI)
Overall							0.83 (0.62–1.10)	0.75 (0.56–0.99)[b]
Monotherapy	86 (4)	3,132	28 (22–34)	108 (3)	4,356	25 (20–30)	0.85 (0.64–1.13)	0.73 (0.54–0.98)[c]
Combination therapy	317 (9)	5,646	56 (50–63)	767 (9)	12,685	61 (56–65)	0.91 (0.80–1.04)	0.85 (0.74–0.97)[c]
Prescriber: GP								
Monotherapy	14 (1)	1,201	12 (6–20)	9 (1)	915	10 (5–19)	0.91 (0.39–2.13)	–[g]
Combination therapy	44 (4)	1,710	26 (19–35)	74 (4)	2389	31 (24–39)	1.07 (0.74–1.56)	1.10 (0.76–1.60)[d]
Prescriber: Urologist								
Monotherapy	26 (11)	142	183 (120–268)	45 (7)	433	104 (76–139)	0.56 (0.35–0.92)	0.77 (0.46–1.30)[d]
Combination therapy	105 (24)	223	472 (386–571)	272 (16)	1097	248 (219–279)	0.53 (0.42–0.66)	0.62 (0.50–0.78)[e]

PY person-years, *CI* confidence interval, *GP* general practitioner; [a]Adjusted for geographic location; [b]Adjusted for geographic location, cohort (mono- or combination therapy), adherence with 5-ARI treatment, prescriber, chronic disease score and number of GP visits; [c]Adjusted for geographic location, adherence with 5-ARI treatment, prescriber and number of GP visits; [d]Adjusted for geographic location and adherence with 5-ARI treatment; [e]Adjusted for geographic location, adherence with 5-ARI treatment and number of drug dispensings; [f]percentage of patients with an event in the specific group; [g]None of the covariates were associated with BPH-related prostate surgery or 5-ARI treatment

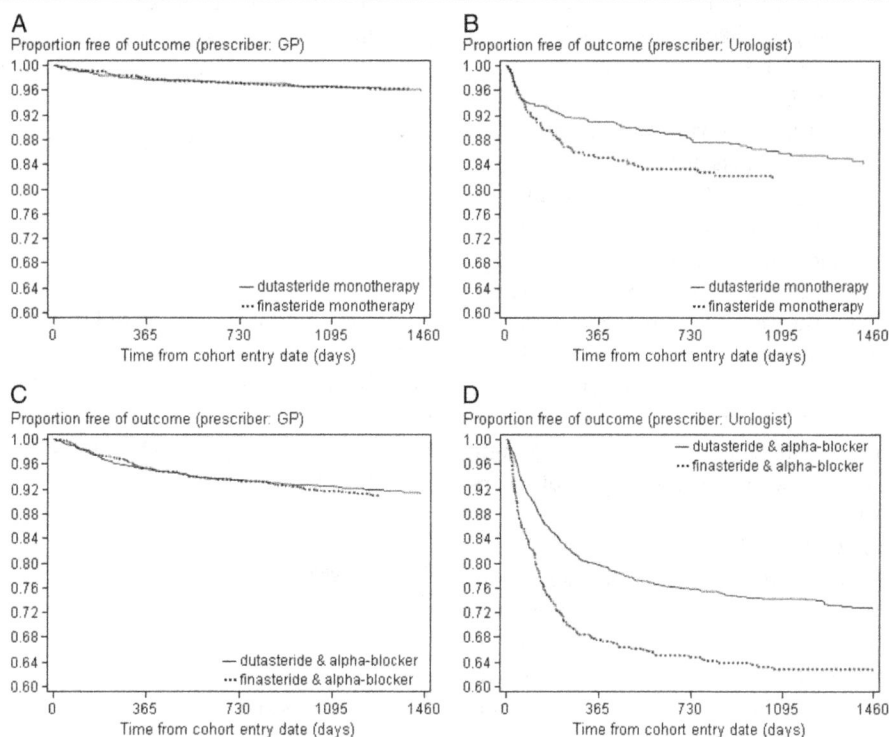

Fig. 1 Kaplan-Meier survival curve showing the proportion of men free of BPH-related prostate surgery, stratified by type of initial BPH treatment and prescriber. **a**) dutasteride or finasteride monotherapy prescribed by GP, **b**) dutasteride or finasteride monotherapy prescribed by urologist, **c**) dutasteride or finasteride & alpha-blocker prescribed by GP, **d**) dutasteride or finasteride & alpha-blocker prescribed by urologist

accounted for by stratifying the results by type of therapy (mono- or combination with alpha-blocker) and prescriber (GP or urologist) in the absence of information on symptom severity, flow rate parameter, serum PSA or prostate size. In line with previous retrospective studies it was confirmed that the risk of BPH-related prostate surgery was lower among men using dutasteride compared to men using finasteride. The association was observed with either mono- or alpha-blocker combination therapy, however only among men who received their prescription from a urologist. Both dutasteride and finasteride blocks the type 2 5-alpha reductase enzymes and converts testosterone into DHT, which makes them both effective treatments for BPH [6, 7]. Dutasteride also blocks the type 1 5-alpha reductase enzymes which may suggest the possibility of improved outcomes with this treatment. Furthermore, dutasteride has a longer half-life compared to finasteride (approximately 4 weeks vs 6 h), which also might lead to better efficacy with dutasteride [6, 20].

The incidence of BPH-related prostate surgery was higher among men on combination therapy, which may reflect the treatment choices based on perceived severity of the condition. Furthermore, the incidence of BPH-related prostate surgery was higher in men treated by urologists compared to those treated by GPs. This

difference may be explained by the fact that the choice for surgery takes place in secondary care. According to Dutch guidelines, watchful waiting is advised for patients without complications and with mild symptoms and/complaints [21]. This is mainly based on the finding that the effectiveness of both drug and invasive treatment in these patients is limited, especially if it is weighed against the potential side effects or complications. Patients with severe symptoms who do not benefit enough from lifestyle changes should be treated with an alpha-blocker according to Dutch guidelines. When results of alpha-blocker treatment are unsatisfactory after 6 weeks, the medication should be stopped and the patients should be referred to a specialist to discuss the possibilities of invasive procedures. Treatment with a 5-alpha reductase inhibitor (finasteride or dutasteride) is an appropriate option for patients with moderate to severe complaints and a prostate volume >30–40 ml. If a fast reduction of complaints is desired, a 5-alpha reductase inhibitor can be given (temporarily) in combination with an alpha-blocker. When other possible causes of BPH are suspected, for example prostate cancer, the primary care guidelines refer the patient to a specialist for additional examination [21]. Furthermore, when the symptoms are severe and surgical treatment is the only option, the patient will be directly referred to a specialist.

Urologists have the choice to recommend surgical treatment and conduct the surgery themselves. This is not the case for GPs, who have to refer patients when a BPH-related prostate surgery is needed. As a result, BPH patients in primary care are less severe and patients have less room for improvement. This was also shown in a study performed among four GP practices in the Netherlands. In this study, it was shown that 30 % of the BPH patients were immediately referred to the urologist. For the majority of the patients, the main reason for referral was the nature and the severity of the micturition, a suspicious rectal toucher or requested by the patient [22].

Until the early 90s, the choice of therapy in patients with BPH consisted of either watchful waiting or surgical treatment. In the last 15 years, many new therapies were introduced of which alpha-blockers and 5-ARI are most common.

Extending the follow-up with 6 months after discontinuation of 5-ARI affected the incidence rates only marginally. Applying a more strict definition of treatment, i.e. not only continuous 5-ARI treatment but also no change in alpha-blocker therapy, resulted in a more pronounced difference in rates between mono- and combination therapy, but the difference between dutasteride and finasteride users did not change.

Finasteride became available on the European market in 1992, while dutasteride became available in 2002. As new drugs are usually first given to a selected group of patients, mostly the more severe, this may create a bias in favor of older products and thus a confounded comparison of the risks of BPH-related prostate surgery between dutasteride and finasteride. In order to assess this potential introduction bias, a sensitivity analysis was performed excluding men starting with 5-ARI between 2003 and 2006. However, excluding those years did not change the comparison of risk of BPH-related prostate surgery between dutasteride and finasteride. Therefore, introduction bias seems unlikely. Furthermore, for this study, data up to and including 2011 was used. As in more recent years no substantial changes occurred with respect to the management and treatment of BPH, major changes in the association between type of 5-ARI and BPH-related prostate surgery are not likely.

Consistent with the current results, a previous study showed that dutasteride was associated with a lower risk of BPH-related surgery (HR 0.75; 95 % CI: 0.58–0.98) [13]. However, whether the patients in this study were on monotherapy or combination therapy was not specified. In another study among men aged ≥50 years, no significant difference in surgery rates was found between patients using dutasteride or finasteride [12].

AUR was a relatively infrequent event in this study, occurring in only 1 % of the men using finasteride or dutasteride. AUR was probably underreported in this study because the database did not capture emergency department visits. In a previous study among patients aged 50 years or older diagnosed with BPH, the rate of AUR after 5 to 12 months was significantly lower in the dutasteride group compared with the finasteride group (5.3 % vs 8.3 %) [12].

Conclusions

In conclusion, the risk of BPH-related prostate surgery was lower among men using dutasteride than among men using finasteride. This association was present among men treated with 5-ARI monotherapy as well as men treated with 5-ARI combination therapy. The difference in surgery rates was limited to BPH patients treated in secondary care.

Acknowledgements
None.

Funding
This work was supported by a grant from GlaxoSmithKline.

Authors' contribution
JGK protocol development, data management, data analysis, manuscript writing. IDB protocol development, data management, data analysis, manuscript writing. MTD protocol development, interpretation of data, manuscript editing. AV interpretation of data, manuscript editing. CGR interpretation of data, manuscript editing. FJAPB protocol development, interpretation of data, manuscript editing. RMCH protocol development, interpretation of data, manuscript editing. All authors read and approved the final manuscript.

Competing interest
JG Kuiper, ID Bezemer, FJA Penning-van Beest and RMC Herings are employees from the PHARMO Institute for Drug Outcomes Research. This independent research institute performs financially supported studies for government and related healthcare authorities and several pharmaceutical companies.
A Vasylyev is an employee of GSK and receives stock/stock options in GSK.
MT Driessen is an employee of GSK and receives stock/stock options in GSK.
CG Roehrborn is a professor in Urology and has been a consultant to GSK in the area of LUTS and BPH.

Ethics approval and consent to participate
Each research project request is assessed by PHARMO's Governance & Ethics Board. The research request should be in accordance with the agreed terms of use of datasets from the various healthcare providers in the PHARMO Database Network. This study was approved by the Governance & Ethics Board and supported by a grant from GlaxoSmithKline.

Author details
[1]PHARMO Institute for Drug Outcomes Research, van Deventerlaan 30-40, 3528 AE Utrecht, Netherlands. [2]GlaxoSmithKline, 980 Great West Road, TW8 9 GS, Brentford, London, UK. [3]GlaxoSmithKline, 980 Great West RdBrentford, London, UK. [4]Department of Urology, University of Texas Southwestern Medical Center, 5323 Harry Hines Bldv, TX 75390 Dallas, TX, USA.

References

1. Roehrborn CG, Rosen RC. Medical therapy options for aging men with benign prostatic hyperplasia: focus on alfuzosin 10 mg once daily. Clin Interv Aging. 2008;3:511–24.
2. Berry SJ, Coffey DS, Walsh PC, Ewing LL. The development of human benign prostatic hyperplasia with age. J Urol. 1984;132:474–9.
3. Fitzpatrick JM. The natural history of benign prostatic hyperplasia. BJU Int. 2006;97 Suppl 2:3–6. discussion 21-22.
4. Roehrborn CG, Oyarzabal Perez I, Roos EP, Calomfirescu N, Brotherton B, Wang F, Palacios JM, Vasylyev A, Manyak MJ. Efficacy and safety of a fixed-dose combination of dutasteride and tamsulosin treatment (Duodart((R))) compared with watchful waiting with initiation of tamsulosin therapy if symptoms do not improve, both provided with lifestyle advice, in the management of treatment-naive men with moderately symptomatic benign prostatic hyperplasia: 2-year CONDUCT study results. BJU Int. 2015; 116:450–59.
5. Roehrborn CG, Siami P, Barkin J, Damiao R, Major-Walker K, Nandy I, Morrill BB, Gagnier RP, Montorsi F, Comb ATSG. The effects of combination therapy with dutasteride and tamsulosin on clinical outcomes in men with symptomatic benign prostatic hyperplasia: 4-year results from the CombAT study. Eur Urol. 2010;57:123–31.
6. Roehrborn CG, Boyle P, Nickel JC, Hoefner K, Andriole G. Efficacy and safety of a dual inhibitor of 5-alpha-reductase types 1 and 2 (dutasteride) in men with benign prostatic hyperplasia. Urology. 2002;60:434–41.
7. Clark RV, Hermann DJ, Cunningham GR, Wilson TH, Morrill BB, Hobbs S. Marked suppression of dihydrotestosterone in men with benign prostatic hyperplasia by dutasteride, a dual 5alpha-reductase inhibitor. J Clin Endocrinol Metab. 2004;89:2179–84.
8. Nickel JC, Gilling P, Tammela TL, Morrill B, Wilson TH, Rittmaster RS. Comparison of dutasteride and finasteride for treating benign prostatic hyperplasia: the Enlarged Prostate International Comparator Study (EPICS). BJU Int. 2011;108:388–94.
9. McConnell JD, Bruskewitz R, Walsh P, Andriole G, Lieber M, Holtgrewe HL, Albertsen P, Roehrborn CG, Nickel JC, Wang DZ, Finasteride Long-Term Efficacy and Safety Study Group, et al. The effect of finasteride on the risk of acute urinary retention and the need for surgical treatment among men with benign prostatic hyperplasia. N Engl J Med. 1998;338:557–63.
10. Debruyne F, Barkin J, van Erps P, Reis M, Tammela TL, Roehrborn C. Efficacy and safety of long-term treatment with the dual 5 alpha-reductase inhibitor dutasteride in men with symptomatic benign prostatic hyperplasia. Eur Urol. 2004;46:488–94. discussion 495.
11. Fenter TC, Davis EA, Shah MB, Lin PJ. Dutasteride vs finasteride: assessment of differences in acute urinary retention rates and surgical risk outcomes in an elderly population aged > or =65 years. Am J Manag Care. 2008;14:S154–159.
12. Issa MM, Runken MC, Grogg AL, Shah MB. A large retrospective analysis of acute urinary retention and prostate-related surgery in BPH patients treated with 5-alpha reductase inhibitors: dutasteride versus finasteride. Am J Manag Care. 2007;13 Suppl 1:S10–16.
13. Cindolo L, Fanizza C, Romero M, Pirozzi L, Autorino R, Berardinelli F, Schips L. The effects of dutasteride and finasteride on BPH-related hospitalization, surgery and prostate cancer diagnosis: a record-linkage analysis. World J Urol. 2013;31:665–71.
14. Foundation DHD: www.dutchhospitaldata.nl. Accessed 14 June 2016.
15. WHO International Classification of Diseases. [www.who.int]. Accessed 14 June 2016.
16. Dutch Classification of Procedures. [www.dhd.nl]. Accessed 14 June 2016.
17. Care ICoP: https://www.nhg.org/themas/artikelen/icpc. Accessed 25 Aug 2016.
18. WHO Anatomical Therapeutic Chemical Classification System. [www.whocc. no]. Accessed 14 June 2016.
19. Catalan V, Lelorier J. Predictors of long-term persistence on statins in a subsidized clinical population. Value in Health. 2000;3:417–26.
20. Wurzel R, Ray P, Major-Walker K, Shannon J, Rittmaster R. The effect of dutasteride on intraprostatic dihydrotestosterone concentrations in men with benign prostatic hyperplasia. Prostate Cancer Prostatic Dis. 2007;10:149–54.
21. Urologie NV. Richtlijn Diagnostiek en behandeling van LUTS/BPH. 2006.
22. Dijstelbloem DALA, Schouten MA, Lagro-Janssen ALM. Benigne prostaathyperplasie in vierhuisartsenpraktijken. Vóórkomen, beleid en beloop. Huisarts Wet. 2003;46(3):133–37.

8

Quantitative volumetric imaging of normal, neoplastic and hyperplastic mouse prostate using ultrasound

Shalini Singh[1,4], Chunliu Pan[1,4], Ronald Wood[2,3], Chiuan-Ren Yeh[3], Shuyuan Yeh[1,3], Kai Sha[1,4], John J. Krolewski[1,4] and Kent L. Nastiuk[1,4*]

Abstract

Background: Genetically engineered mouse models are essential to the investigation of the molecular mechanisms underlying human prostate pathology and the effects of therapy on the diseased prostate. Serial *in vivo* volumetric imaging expands the scope and accuracy of experimental investigations of models of normal prostate physiology, benign prostatic hyperplasia and prostate cancer, which are otherwise limited by the anatomy of the mouse prostate. Moreover, accurate imaging of hyperplastic and tumorigenic prostates is now recognized as essential to rigorous pre-clinical trials of new therapies. Bioluminescent imaging has been widely used to determine prostate tumor size, but is semi-quantitative at best. Magnetic resonance imaging can determine prostate volume very accurately, but is expensive and has low throughput. We therefore sought to develop and implement a high throughput, low cost, and accurate serial imaging protocol for the mouse prostate.

Methods: We developed a high frequency ultrasound imaging technique employing 3D reconstruction that allows rapid and precise assessment of mouse prostate volume. Wild-type mouse prostates were examined ($n = 4$) for reproducible baseline imaging, and treatment effects on volume were compared, and blinded data analyzed for intra- and inter-operator assessments of reproducibility by correlation and for Bland-Altman analysis. Examples of benign prostatic hyperplasia mouse model prostate ($n = 2$) and mouse prostate implantation of orthotopic human prostate cancer tumor and its growth ($n = 6$) are also demonstrated.

Results: Serial measurement volume of the mouse prostate revealed that high frequency ultrasound was very precise. Following endocrine manipulation, regression and regrowth of the prostate could be monitored with very low intra- and interobserver variability. This technique was also valuable to monitor the development of prostate growth in a model of benign prostatic hyperplasia. Additionally, we demonstrate accurate ultrasound image-guided implantation of orthotopic tumor xenografts and monitoring of subsequent tumor growth from ~10 to ~750 mm^3 volume.

Discussion: High frequency ultrasound imaging allows precise determination of normal, neoplastic and hyperplastic mouse prostate. Low cost and small image size allows incorporation of this imaging modality inside clean animal facilities, and thereby imaging of immunocompromised models. 3D reconstruction for volume determination is easily mastered, and both small and large relative changes in volume are accurately visualized. Ultrasound imaging does not rely on penetration of exogenous imaging agents, and so may therefore better measure poorly vascularized or necrotic diseased tissue, relative to bioluminescent imaging (IVIS).

(Continued on next page)

* Correspondence: kent.nastiuk@roswellpark.org
[1]Departments of Pathology and Laboratory Medicine, University of Rochester School of Medicine and Dentistry, Rochester, NY, USA
[4]Current address: Department of Cancer Genetics, Roswell Park Cancer Institute, Buffalo 14263NY, USA
Full list of author information is available at the end of the article

(Continued from previous page)

Conclusions: Our method is precise and reproducible with very low inter- and intra-observer variability. Because it is non-invasive, mouse models of prostatic disease states can be imaged serially, reducing inter-animal variability, and enhancing the power to detect small volume changes following therapeutic intervention.

Keywords: Prostate cancer, BPH, Mouse model, IVIS, 3D volume

Background

Prostate cancer (PrCa) is the most prevalent non-cutaneous cancer and second leading cause of cancer mortality in men [1]. Despite effective therapy for localized disease, treatment of recurrent and metastatic PrCa is problematic and therefore the focus of intense investigation. Mouse models have proven valuable for studying human disease, including prostate cancer, because of their short breeding cycles and manageable costs, but particularly because of the ease of genetic manipulation compared to larger animals. Mice are also useful as immunocompromised hosts for xenografts of human prostate cancers [2, 3]. Genetically engineered mouse models have been particularly informative in revealing the molecular and cellular mechanisms underlying prostate tumor biology, and to evaluate new therapeutic inventions [4]. Although fewer models are available, benign prostatic hyperplasia can also be genetically engineered in mice, which may be useful in developing therapies for this highly prevalent disease [5].

US Food and Drug Administration approval rates for drugs has been declining since 1990 and oncology drug development has been particularly inefficient [6]. Only about one in twenty drugs entering phase I human clinical trials for cancer are eventually approved and among those that progress to phase III trials, only about 30 % are eventually approved [6]. A major cause of this failure is lack of efficacy in human trials, rather than safety issues. Specifically, the apparent efficacy in murine models is frequently not replicable in human trials [7, 8]. To enhance reproducibility, and ultimately the translation of pre-clinical trial success into human clinical trials, it has been proposed that all pre-clinical trials include randomization of tumor bearing animals to treatment groups; blinding to those treating, and subsequently evaluating, endpoints; a pre-determined statistical analysis protocol; and treatment designs that are adequately powered to test the null hypotheses [9, 10]. Accurate volumetric imaging serves an important role in executing such rigorous preclinical trials by ensuring that all animals undergoing randomization to treatment groups have tumors of similar size. This is particularly important in models where tumor formation does not occur in 100 % of mice or where there is significant variation in the rate of tumor formation [11]. In addition, live animal imaging of tumor volume provides an accurate assessment of tumor response kinetics, controlled for animal-to-animal variation, since each animal serves as its own control [12]. The alternatives – serially sacrificing

groups of animals at intermediate time points, or simply measuring tumor size at the end of the trial – are less informative or require many more animals, compromising the statistical power of the preclinical study design [13].

While rodent and human prostates are functionally equivalent, the mouse prostate is small (~25 mm^3), multi-lobular (ventral, dorsal, lateral and anterior), and interdigitated with surrounding genitourinary organs. Many reports have monitored prostate tumor growth and regression using optical imaging (fluorescence or luciferase reporters). However, tumors must be engineered to express a reporter gene and quantitation is very problematic [14, 15], particularly for longitudinal imaging [16, 17]. Optical imaging is both higher throughput and lower in cost than other modalities, but has relatively poor anatomic resolution [18]. We have previously described a quantitative and reproducible anatomical imaging approach, utilizing high-field magnetic resonance imaging with chemical shift suppression (MRI-CHESS) [19, 20] to measure murine prostate volumes changes resulting from a variety of manipulations in mouse models. Since MRI instrumentation is costly and not widely available, we sought to develop a 3D-ultrasound imaging protocol to precisely measure very small changes in the volume of the mouse prostate, in living animals.

High-frequency ultrasound imaging of the mouse prostate has many advantages: it is low cost and high throughput, enables 3D reconstruction for precise volume determination, and allows real-time imaging to facilitate surgical manipulations [21]. Here, we describe the use of high-resolution *in vivo* ultrasound imaging for quantitative analysis of prostate volume. Monitoring changes in the prostate of normal mice, we demonstrate that this ultrasound technique can precisely detect sub-cubic millimeter changes in volume following hormonal manipulations that result in regression and regrowth of the normal prostate. We then apply this technique to two distinct prostate disease models: growth of the prostate in a prolactin-driven benign prostatic hyperplasia model [22], and growth of human prostate cancer orthotopic xenografts implanted in the anterior lobe of the mouse prostate [23].

Methods

Animals

All animal studies were approved by the University of Rochester institutional animal use committee (UCAR #2012-030) and conducted according to the guidelines of the local committee on animal resources, as well as all relevant national guidelines. Six to nine month old male C57/BL6 mice, and 12–14 week old male nude mice, used as orthotopic xenograft hosts, were purchased from Charles River Labs. Probasin-driven prolactin (Pb-PRL) transgenic mice were provided by John Kindbloom [22] and backcrossed into an FVB background [24]. All mice were housed individually and provided food and water *ad libitum*. Endocrine perturbation was as described previously [19]. Briefly, animals were anesthetized via intra-peritoneal Ketamine (87 mg/kg) and Xylazine (13 mg/kg) injection and then surgically castrated via scrotal incision. Testes were removed, and blood vessels and vas deferens ligated. The incision was closed with wound clips. Three days following castration clips were removed to allow ultrasound imaging. Fourteen days following castration, 5 mg/kg 5alpha-androstan-17beta-ol-3-one (dihydrotestosterone, DHT, Sigma) in corn oil was injected sub-cutaneously daily.

High-resolution ultrasound image acquisition and analysis

Each mouse was imaged with a high-resolution ultrasound system (Vevo770 high resolution imaging system, VisualSonics, Toronto, Ontario, Canada) using the highest resolution scan head (either 710 or 704b) that was able to image the entire prostate or tumor. The 704b scan head probe is driven by a linear motor with a center frequency of 40 MHz and provides a 40 μm axial and 80 μm lateral resolution at a focal depth of 6 mm, affording a 14.5 μm field of view. The corresponding values for the 710 scan head are 25 MHz, 70 μm × 140 μm, and 20.8 μm, respectively. Mice were anesthetized in a chamber using 3 % isoflurane and then fixed in the transverse position on a heated imaging platform (Vevo Integrated Rail System III, VisualSonics) with a nose cone for maintenance of anesthesia using 2 % isoflurane. Animals were monitored for heart rate and respiratory cycle using surface electrodes. The abdomens of the mice were depilated using a commercial calcium thioglycolate product ("Nair"), and ultrasound gel (Aquasonic 100, Parker Laboratories, Fairfield, NJ) was applied to the abdomen. The location of the anterior, dorsal and ventral prostate lobes was identified by mechanically adjusting the position of the ultrasound transducer, with the bladder and urethra as landmarks. Images of 585 sections of each ultrasound series were acquired at a resolution of 1600 × 1200 pixels using the VisualSonics software. Following acquisition, images were imported into Amira software (Visualization Sciences Group, Burlington MA), for 3D mouse prostate volume reconstruction. The images were set to 8-bit gray scale and the contrast enhanced using Amira. Anatomic boundaries of the prostate lobes were manually outlined in parallel slices. Based on these areas, the volume was subsequently computed with Amira. Slice alignment, segmentation and generation of surface meshes were also performed with Amira.

Volume, in cubic millimeters, or mean volumes, accompanied by standard error of the mean (SEM) if multiple equivalent imaging sessions were analyzed, are presented. In the reproducibility study, the coefficient(s) of variation (CV) was calculated as the appropriate standard deviation divided by the mean, and expressed as a percentage. For all other studies, a single determination is presented.

Cell culture

For orthotopic prostate tumor implantation in nude mice, CWR22Rv1 cells [25] were acquired from American Type Culture Collection (Manassas, VA) and grown in Roswell Park Memorial Institute 1640 (RPMI) medium containing glutamine and antibiotics with 10 % fetal calf serum. Prior to injection, cells were washed with phosphate buffered saline, harvested with trypsin/Ethylenediaminetetraacetic acid solution, and pelleted. Cells were re-suspended in RPMI media and an equal volume of Matrigel (Corning, Bedford, MA) was added.

Image-guided orthotopic prostate tumor establishment

Nude mice were imaged using high-frequency ultrasound, as above, prior to tumor xenografting to establish baseline images. For implantation, image acquisition was performed with the 704b probe using enhanced abdominal visualization in 3D-mode. Physiological status (electrocardiogram, respiration, blood pressure, and body temperature) of the mice was monitored during each image-guided injection. While monitoring these images, a 30-gauge needle on a syringe was positioned with a micro-manipulator into the junction of the two lobes of the anterior prostate. A volume of 10 μL containing 1×10^6 tumor cells in 50 % Matrigel was injected over 20 s. The syringe was then withdrawn, ultrasound gel removed, and mice allowed to recover. Mice were imaged weekly for eight weeks to monitor development of the orthotopic prostate tumor xenografts.

Statistical analysis

Prostate volume was normalized to pre-castration volume for each animal and the mean of group of each time (+/− SEM), relative to pre-castration volume is presented in each data set. Comparison between groups was analyzed by one-way ANOVA with Dunnetts's post-hoc test. Subsets of the data were quantitated independently by two blinded observers to create a Bland-Altman plot [26, 27]. The means of the prostate volumes, generated by two independent observers, were plotted on the horizontal axis, and the differences between the two observers were plotted on the vertical axis. Differences were considered statistically significant for a value of $P < 0.05$.

Results

Ultrasound imaging of WT mouse prostate

Prostates of four normal mature mice were imaged using high frequency ultrasound to assess organ volume. Images of three orthogonal (transverse, coronal and sagittal) planes of the ventral prostate (VP) were acquired and integrated 3D images produced using VisualSonics software. The rodent prostate gland is composed of multiple lobes: ventral, dorsal, lateral and anterior, which are interdigitated into surrounding tissues [28], while in humans the gland is non-lobular (unitary). The mouse VP has a larger epithelial component and therefore a larger volume of luminal prostatic secretions relative to the dorsal-lateral prostate (DLP) lobes, which share ducts and have similar proportions of epithelial and stromal components, and therefore are often considered together. As the VP is most echogenically distinct, segmentation of this lobe is most accurate, and henceforth reported when describing normal prostate volume changes. Image sets for two of these mice, M1 and M2, are illustrated in Fig. 1a. 3D images were imported into Amira visualization software, manually outlining the bladder (yellow) and VP (green) in all three

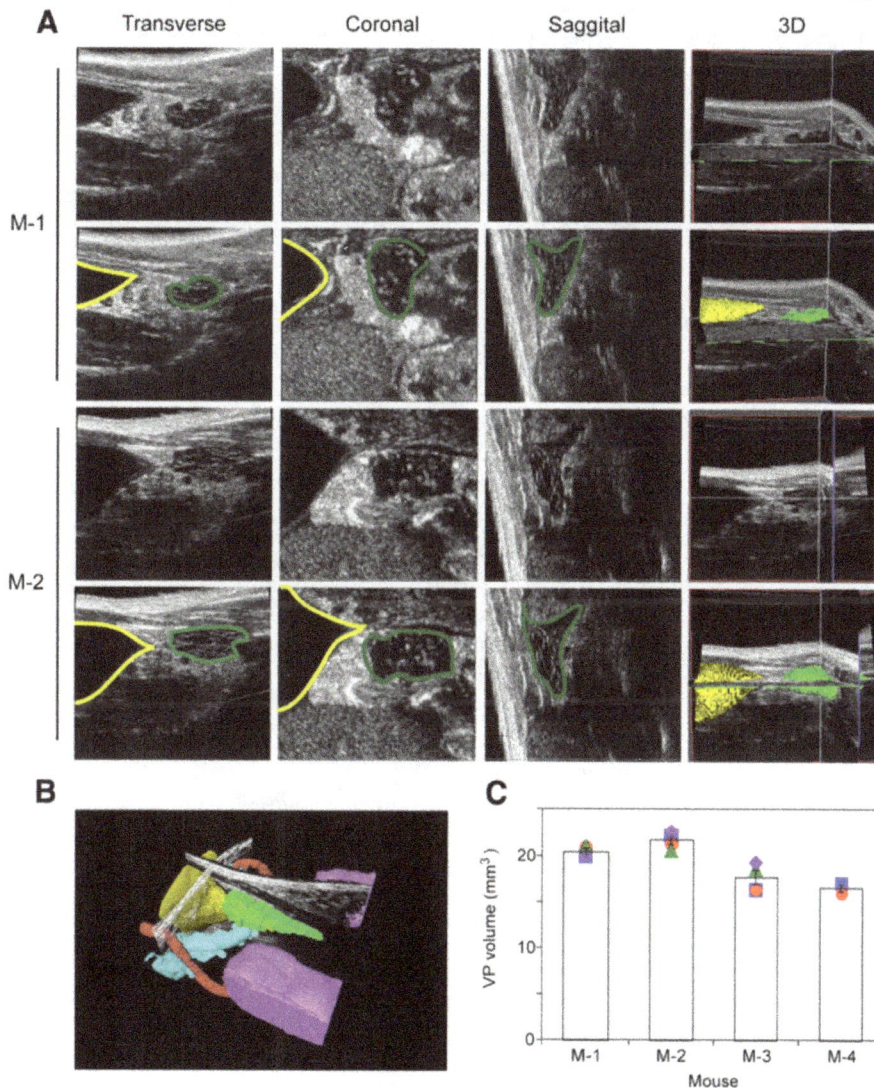

Fig. 1 Ultrasound volume quantitation of mouse ventral prostate is highly reproducible. **a** Upper sets of panels (for mice M-1 and M-2) depict the ultrasound images of the lower genitourinary system resolved into three orthogonal planes (transverse, coronal and sagittal, as indicated) and the corresponding integrated 3D images. The lower set of panels (for mice M-1 and M-2) illustrates the process of segmentation of the relevant anatomic structures (*bladder in yellow, ventral prostate in green*) using the Amira software. **b** Amira generated segmented ultrasound image of the lower genitourinary system from mouse M-1, including bladder (*yellow*), seminal vesicle (*blue*), testes (*purple*), ventral prostate (*green*) and vas deferens (*red*). **c** The ventral prostate volume for each of four mice was repeatedly determined. Each symbol represents an independent determination for a given mouse. Columns denote the mean and error bars the SEM. M-1, M-2 and M-3 were imaged four times, while M-4 was imaged twice.

planes (Fig. 1a, lower set of panels for each mouse). Using the segmentation illustrated in Fig. 1a, Amira was employed to produce 3D reconstructions of these organs, as well as the seminal vesicles and vas deferens (Fig. 1b). To assess the reproducibility of this method for determining the volume of the VP, the same four mice were each imaged four times. Based on the corresponding segmentation and 3D reconstruction, the volumes of the ventral lobes of these mouse prostates were computed using Amira (Fig. 1c). The average VP volume for these mice was 19.03 +/− 3.01 mm^3; (mean +/− SEM, $n = 4$). The intra-mouse variability was quite low (CV% = 5.0 %), suggesting that for a mature mouse a single imaging session is sufficient to determine the baseline prostate volume for further studies that measure organ volume regulation.

Regression of WT prostate volume after castration

Advanced, recurrent, and metastatic prostate cancer is typically controlled using androgen deprivation therapy (ADT) [29]. ADT induces apoptosis of the epithelial cells, resulting in regression of normal and diseased prostate glands as well as disseminated tumor in both patients and the corresponding mouse models [3, 28, 30]. During castration, the VP undergoes greater regression than other lobes due to the relatively higher proportion of epithelial cells [19, 31, 32]. To determine the ability of high frequency 3D ultrasound to monitor prostate regression, four WT mice were surgically castrated and VP volume assessed every 3 or 4 days thereafter by ultrasound imaging. We observed significant reduction of VP volume in all mice from day 4 through day 14 (Fig. 2a). Amira derived volumes indicate that by day 4, the ventral prostate lobes regressed 39 ± 3 %. This progressed to 68 ± 3 % on day 7 and was further reduced to 84 ± 2 and 92 ± 2 % on day 10 and 14, respectively, relative to the corresponding mouse's intact VP volume ($P < 0.001$, Fig. 2b). The normalized CVs (relative to the intact VP volume for each mouse, "intra-mouse CV") were 6.8 %, 5.3 %, 2.2 %, 3.8 % for days 4, 7, 10, and 14, respectively, much smaller than the overall VP volume variance of 12.6 % ("inter-mouse CV") when not normalized to pre-castration volume, as would be the case if one were to examine VP volumes for groups of mice sacrificed serially.

Regrowth of ventral prostate volume in normal mice

The prostate of castrated mice returns to its pre-castrated size following 2 to 3 weeks of androgen supplementation [19, 31]. Two weeks following castration, the four mice depicted in Fig. 2 were supplemented daily with DHT and changes in prostate volume were monitored using high frequency 3D ultrasound imaging.

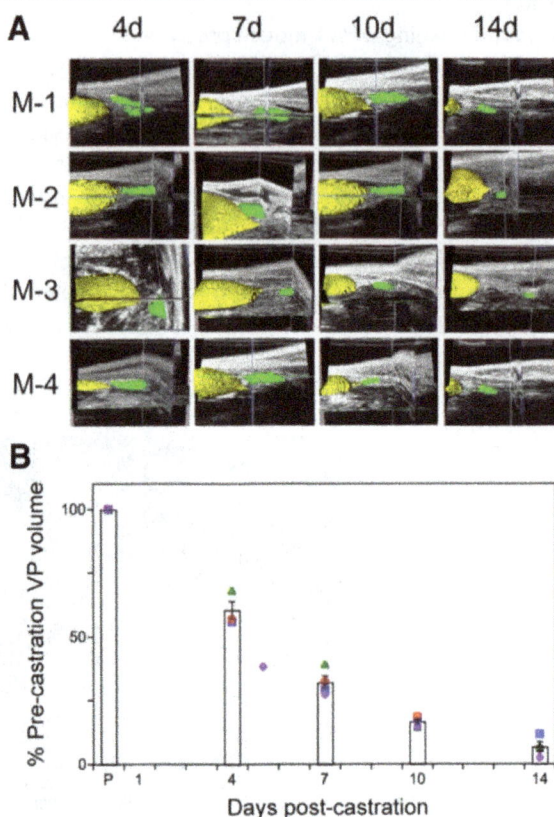

Fig. 2 Castration induced prostate regression monitored by high-resolution 3D ultrasound imaging. Imaging of VP volume in four mice, post-castration. **a** Amira generated 3D volume reconstructions from ultrasound images, for four mice (M-1 through M-4). Segmentation of the bladder (*yellow*) and the ventral prostate (*green*) is illustrated. **b** Plot of ventral prostate volume regression. VP volume was normalized to pre-castration (P) volume for each animal and the mean (columns, ± SEM) of the group at the indicated day, relative to pre-castration volume. Symbols correspond to M-1 (*square*); M-2 (*circle*); M-3 (*diamond*) and M-4 (*triangle*).

Following manual segmentation and 3D reconstruction using Amira software to delineate the bladder (yellow pseudocolored structure in Fig. 3a) and ventral prostate (green structure in Fig. 3a), we calculated the volume of the VP for these mice. There was a steady increase in the ventral prostate volume, from 8 % of the pre-castrated volume at the beginning of DHT treatment, to 36.4 ± 5, 49.57 ± 4, 59 ± 5, and 70 ± 0.5 % on days 2, 4, 6, and 8, respectively. This represents regeneration of two-thirds of the VP volume in eight days (Fig. 3b). The variability of this regeneration appears to be higher at intermediate time points (21.7 % CV at day 2, 16.7 % CV at day 4, 13.6 % CV at day 6) compared to the final measurement (2.4 % CV at day 8), suggesting that this represents underlying biological variability in the rate of regrowth, rather than reflecting inherent variability in our imaging technique.

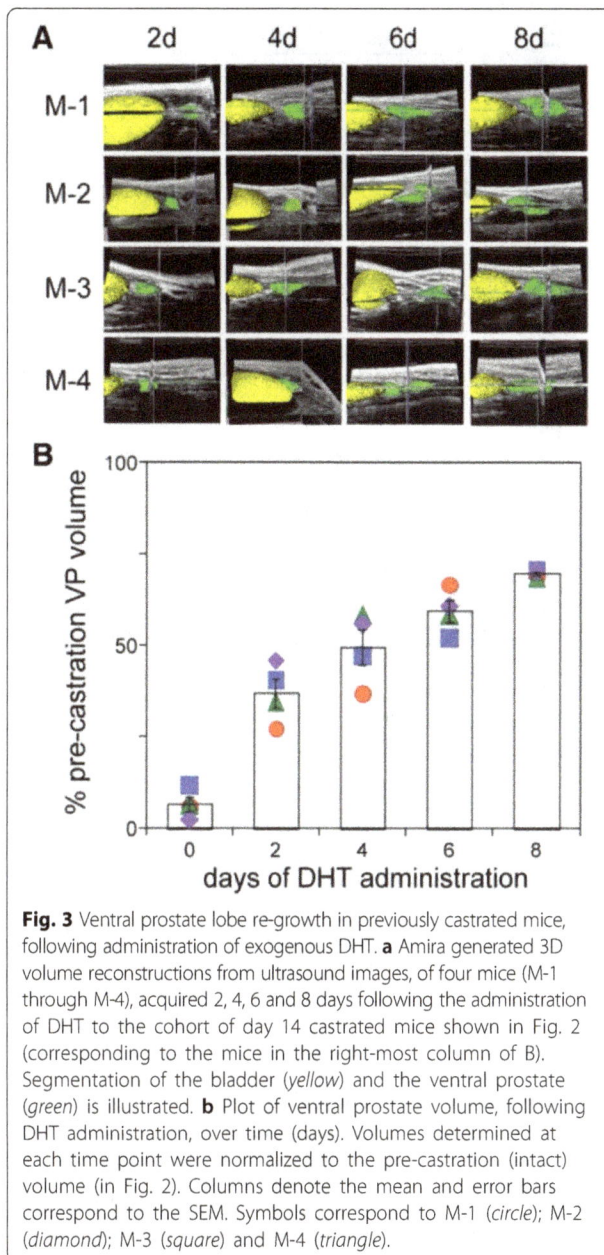

Fig. 3 Ventral prostate lobe re-growth in previously castrated mice, following administration of exogenous DHT. **a** Amira generated 3D volume reconstructions from ultrasound images, of four mice (M-1 through M-4), acquired 2, 4, 6 and 8 days following the administration of DHT to the cohort of day 14 castrated mice shown in Fig. 2 (corresponding to the mice in the right-most column of B). Segmentation of the bladder (*yellow*) and the ventral prostate (*green*) is illustrated. **b** Plot of ventral prostate volume, following DHT administration, over time (days). Volumes determined at each time point were normalized to the pre-castration (intact) volume (in Fig. 2). Columns denote the mean and error bars correspond to the SEM. Symbols correspond to M-1 (*circle*); M-2 (*diamond*); M-3 (*square*) and M-4 (*triangle*).

Intra- and inter-observer variability

To examine the precision of high frequency ultrasound measurement of the mouse VP volume, the images generated in Figs. 2 and 3 were blinded and reanalyzed by the primary reviewer and a secondary reviewer [20, 33–35]. Following segmentation and 3D reconstruction, the volumes were recorded, sent to an honest broker, decoded, and the intraclass correlation coefficients and variability for intra- and inter-observer assessments were calculated [33]. Intra-observer correlation was quite robust, with $r^2 = 0.995$ (Fig. 4a). The mean intra-observer deviation of individual measurements, as measured by Bland-Altman analysis was 0.8 % (Fig. 4b), suggesting

strong confidence in the reproducibility of the high frequency ultrasound 3D reconstruction of the VP volume. In addition, this data was blinded and quantitated by two independent observers and inter-observer agreement analyzed by Bland Altman analysis (Fig. 4c and d). Volume correlation for the VP was $r^2 = 0.945$ (Fig. 4c), and the mean deviation 3.0 % (Fig. 4d). The interclass correlation coefficient for measurements of volume between the first and second examiner also revealed that the intra- and inter-observer variability for regression of the ventral prostate was 2.5 and 6 %, respectively, indicating that differences between the groups of mice were not due to observer bias.

Ultrasound imaging of hyperplastic mouse prostate

The volume of the ventral prostate was monitored during development in a mouse model of benign prostatic hyperplasia using high frequency ultrasound imaging. Pb-PRL transgenic males developed a significant enlargement of the prostate gland, characterized primarily by hyperplasia of the stromal compartment, distended ductal structures, and focal areas of glandular dysplasia [22]. Two Pb-PRL mice were monitored from 16 to 30 weeks of age, and one of these an additional four weeks. Ventral prostate and bladder were manually segmented and boundaries in parallel slices and Amira three-dimensional reconstructions are shown in Fig. 5a. Ultrasound images of the hyperplastic prostates were acquired using the 710 probe for the wider field of view. Computed VP volumes of the Pb-PRL transgenic mice from 16 to 30 weeks (and 34 weeks for mouse B1) are plotted in Fig. 5b. Fortuitously, an animal care issue unrelated to prostate volume required that a single Pb-PRL mouse (not one of the two monitored in Fig. 5) be sacrificed at 28 weeks of age, and so the wet weight of microdissected ventral prostate was then determined to be 80 mg, while 3D reconstruction of high frequency ultrasound of this mouse abdomen, performed on the same day, resulted in a prostate volume of 82 mm³ (data not shown). Prolactin-driven prostate volume increases rapidly from 20 weeks of age, and slows by 30 weeks of age, while continuing to grow slowly thereafter (data not shown). Unfortunately, attempts to microdissect the BPH prostates at later ages proved unsuccessful due to the interdigitated nature of the diseased prostate into the surrounding tissues.

Development of orthotopic xenografts

We used high frequency ultrasound imaging to guide the establishment and monitor the growth of an orthotopic human prostate cancer mouse xenograft model. The genitourinary anatomy of nude mice was imaged by high resolution, high frequency ultrasound (using the VisualSonics 704 probe) and the junction of the anterior

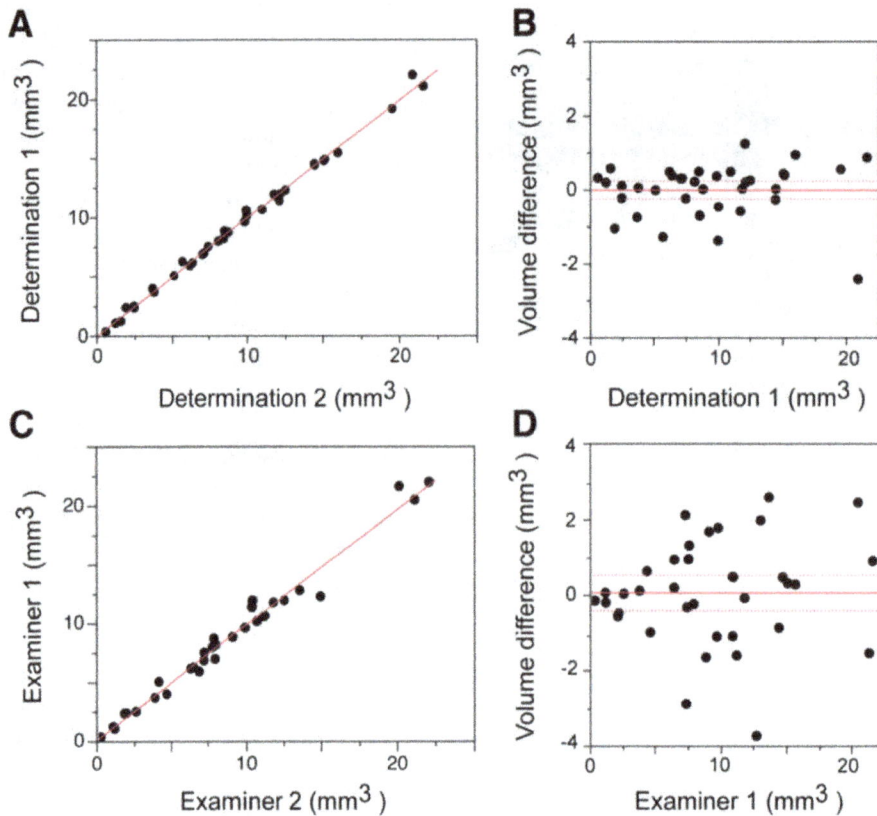

Fig. 4 Intra- and inter-observer variability of volume measurement by ultrasound imaging. Intra-observer variation (**a**, **b**). **a** Linear correlation plot of two independent sets of volume measurements, performed (blinded) by a single observer (data from Figs. 2 and 3 image sets). The correlation coefficient, $r^2 = 0.995$. **b** Bland-Altman plot of the data from (**a**). Dashed lines correspond to the 95 % confidence interval. The mean deviation of individual measurements was 0.8 % ($n = 36$). **c** Inter-observer variation (**c**, **d**). **c** Linear correlation plot of two independent sets of volume determinations, performed (blinded) by two separate examiners (data from Figs. 2 and 3 image sets). The correlation coefficient, $r^2 = 0.945$. **d** Bland-Altman plot of the data from (**c**). Dashed lines correspond to the 95 % confidence interval. The mean deviation of individual measurements was 3.0 % ($n = 32$).

prostate lobes was identified. A syringe needle was then aligned with the junction and advanced into a lobe of the anterior prostate (circled in Fig. 6a) using the needle guide overlay feature of the VisualSonics software that allows for the simultaneous visualization of the needle alignment and injection target on the monitor. CWR22Rv1 cells in matrigel were injected directly into a lobe of the anterior prostate and were visualized post-injection as the hyperechoic signature at the end of the hypoechoic needle displacement track in Fig. 6a (right side). Non-invasive high frequency ultrasound imaging was used to identify the site of origin of the tumor and then to serially monitor growth of the CWR22Rv1xenografts. We observed tumor growth starting at week 3 in one lobe of the anterior prostate (volume approximately 10 mm³; Fig. 6b, "W3" and by the fourth week tumor volume increased rapidly, reaching the field of view limit of the 704 probe to simultaneously visualize the entire tumor volume (approximately 60 mm³; Fig. 6b, "W4"). Tumor growth was further monitored using the 25 MHz frequency 710b probe from week 5 to week 7

post-implantation (Fig. 6b, bottom) or until tumor volume reached 750 mm³, when the xenograft hosts were sacrificed. For the six xenografts in this proof of principle, we observed most xenografts grew at a rate of ~50 mm³ per week, while one xenograft had a much more aggressive growth phenotype (doubling every week, Fig. 6c).

Discussion

Androgens regulate prostate growth and neoplastic phenotype. They promote mitosis and differentiation of rodents prostate ductal epithelium, and further inhibit apoptosis of differentiated cells [36]. Androgen withdrawal, through surgical castration or pharmacological blockade, induces apoptosis of the ductal secretory epithelium, but not the basal epithelium or stromal cells [37]. The small size of the mouse prostate (25 mm³) versus the human prostate (25 cm³) and the difficulty in reproducibly excising the prostate from surrounding tissues makes it challenging to accurately determine prostate volume by weighing or histological analysis at

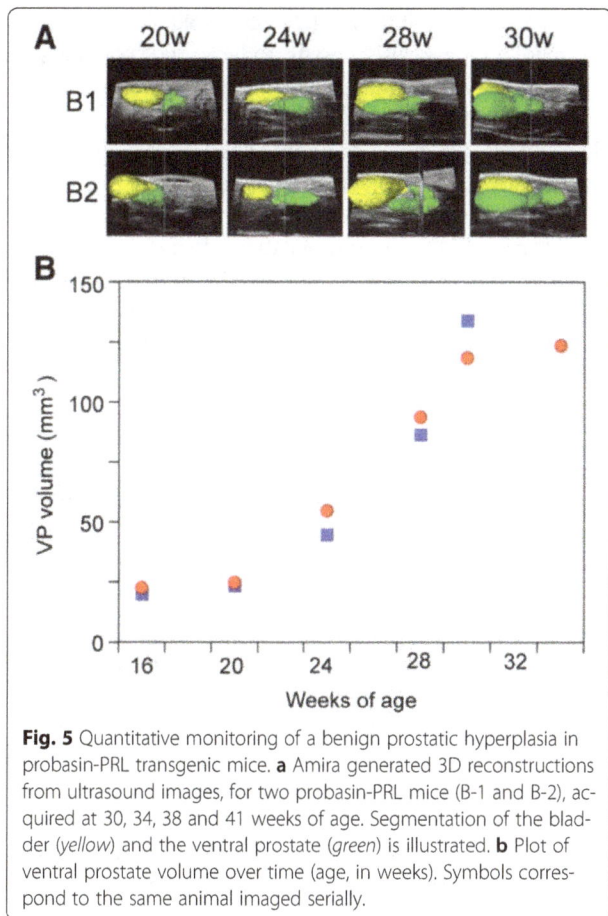

Fig. 5 Quantitative monitoring of a benign prostatic hyperplasia in probasin-PRL transgenic mice. **a** Amira generated 3D reconstructions from ultrasound images, for two probasin-PRL mice (B-1 and B-2), acquired at 30, 34, 38 and 41 weeks of age. Segmentation of the bladder (*yellow*) and the ventral prostate (*green*) is illustrated. **b** Plot of ventral prostate volume over time (age, in weeks). Symbols correspond to the same animal imaged serially.

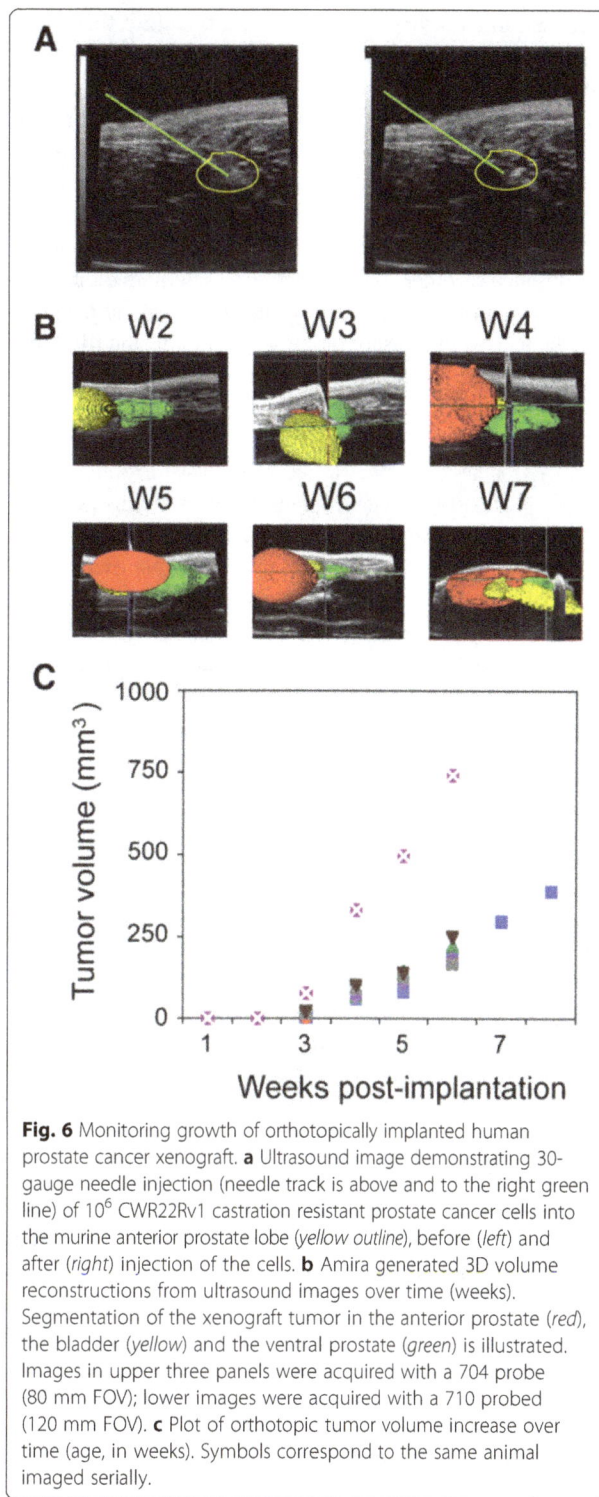

Fig. 6 Monitoring growth of orthotopically implanted human prostate cancer xenograft. **a** Ultrasound image demonstrating 30-gauge needle injection (needle track is above and to the right green line) of 10^6 CWR22Rv1 castration resistant prostate cancer cells into the murine anterior prostate lobe (*yellow outline*), before (*left*) and after (*right*) injection of the cells. **b** Amira generated 3D volume reconstructions from ultrasound images over time (weeks). Segmentation of the xenograft tumor in the anterior prostate (*red*), the bladder (*yellow*) and the ventral prostate (*green*) is illustrated. Images in upper three panels were acquired with a 704 probe (80 mm FOV); lower images were acquired with a 710 probed (120 mm FOV). **c** Plot of orthotopic tumor volume increase over time (age, in weeks). Symbols correspond to the same animal imaged serially.

necropsy [3, 19, 20, 38–40]. Moreover, as noted in the Introduction, restricting analysis to animals at necropsy would require large numbers of animals for longitudinal studies of tumor or BPH response to therapy and is inherently less accurate than repeated volumetric imaging of individual animals over time. Biochemical cancer biomarkers, such as serum PSA for human prostate xenograft volume [11, 41], and serum PSP94 for mouse tumor volume [42], correlate well with tumor volume but are androgen driven, and therefore problematic for monitoring therapies directed at androgen signaling. Thus, there is a need for a relatively rapid and inexpensive, yet quantitative, methodology for imaging the murine prostate.

In 2006, Albanese and colleagues [43] pioneered the use of high field strength MRI to measure prostate volume in mouse tumor models. Subsequently, we developed [19] and utilized [20] a quantitative and reproducible magnetic resonance-based anatomical imaging approach (MRI-CHESS) to quantitate murine prostate volume changes in mouse models. CHESS (chemical shift suppression) allows suppression of MR signal arising artifactually from surrounding peri-prostatic fat, revealing boundaries of the prostatic lobes more accurately, and differentiating the

ventral from the dorsal-lateral lobes. However, since MRI requires costly instrumentation, with high operating costs, and the additional expense of a dedicated operator [44], it is not available to the vast majority of prostate cancer investigators. Moreover, achieving the very high spatial resolution required to accurately determine prostate volumes with

MRI necessitates long scan times, and therefore this methodology is decidedly low throughput. Finally, the significant infrastructure required to support an MRI facility often precludes location within the clean zone of an animal facility, which hampers the ability to image immunocompromised animals (such as xenograft-bearing athymic nude mice) which require a pathogen-free environment.

Given these obstacles to the implementation of MRI, and in the absence of other well-characterized alternative quantitative imaging protocols, optical imaging, employing constitutive luciferase reporters for bioluminescent imaging (BLI), has become the *de facto* technology for monitoring the growth and regression (in response to therapy). However, correlation of BLI intensity with tumor volume is poor ($R^2 = 0.6$-0.8), particularly for larger tumors (>200 mm^3) [44]. Problems arise due to inconsistent luciferin penetration of organs generally [45], and tumor specifically due to vascularity of the hypoxic tumor necrotic core [46], and this may be further exacerbated in a trial of pro-apoptotic therapies. Further, BLI intensity can be reduced by surrounding tissues, such as bladder with variable urine content [16] or incomplete fur removal [44], and thus volume estimates may be unreliable for prostate. Increasing tumor volume also directly reduces the ability of light to escape [14], and this imaging modality may be more properly described as qualitative [15].

While micro-computed tomography is lower cost than MR imaging, it cannot effectively distinguish prostate tumor from surrounding normal tissue [11]. In contrast, ultrasound imaging instrumentation is much more amenable to use in animal core facilities due to both acquisition and operating costs, as well as instrument size. Volume determinations using a micro-transrectal transceiver [41], has been shown to correlate well with volumes determined from the wet weight of dissected orthotopic prostate tumors, but are technically challenging. High frequency ultrasound measurements using the VisualSonics Vevo 770, that employs an external probe, show good correlation ($r^2 = 0.85$) with dissected large autochthonous tumors [11]. Moreover, the relative ease of operation facilitates reasonable through-put, since scan times are on the order of 30 min including preparative anesthesia and depilation. 2D-ultrasound allows in-plane sizing of tumors with a diameter as small as ~3 mm, which is within 10 % of the diameter of mouse prostate, as revealed by histology [35], but single slice imaging is subject to sampling error, few prostate tumor imaging studies report volume changes less than 10 mm^3, and tumors with non-uniform shapes are poorly described by 2D-imaging. 3D-ultrasound for human prostate is a more precise and accurate methodology for determining prostate volume [47, 48]. High resolution 3D-ultrasound computed volumes from 0.5 to 10 mm^3 correlate well with caliper measurements and histology for endometriotic cysts [45], and colorectal xenografts [34]. We therefore sought to exploit the precision of 3D-ultrasound by adapting it to accurately quantitate very

small changes (as little as 3 % of a volume as small as ~10 mm^3) in the mouse prostate under various physiological and pathological conditions. Figs. 1, 2 and 3 demonstrate that our use of the VisualSonics instrumentation and Amira 3D software for reconstruction allows very reproducible measurements of VP volume in intact mice (Fig. 1), mice undergoing castration induced regression (Fig. 2) and mice undergoing DHT supplementation induced re-growth (Fig. 3). In these imaging sessions the VP volumes varied from ~20 mm^3 for intact animals to ~5 mm^3 for regressed animals, emphasizing the high degree of accuracy in measuring very small glands. Because image processing involves operator-dependent segmentation of the raw US images, we performed blinded intra- and inter-operator assessments of reproducibility (Fig. 4) and found excellent agreement (CV ~3 %). We should note that assessment does not require extensive training in mouse anatomy, as individuals who had no prior experience were able to readily master the segmentation protocol within weeks. We also applied our methodology to two pathological animals models: prolactin transgene-driven benign prostatic hyperplasia (Fig. 5) and orthotopic implantation of human prostate cancer xenografts (Fig. 6). In both cases, we were able to detect pathological changes which increased the volumes by as little as 10 % (*c.f.* Fig. 6b, W3). In addition, the small size of the normal anterior prostate host site for implantation leads to variability when injecting tumor cells to establish prostate orthotopic xenografts, impairing reproducibility in the either the microenvironment or mis-location of the implantation and concomitant dissemination of the tumor in the peritoneum [49]. Thus, in contrast to other imaging modalities, which require large volume changes to be appreciated, this methodology reveals the magnitude of morphological changes more typically seen in human pathology, where the volumetric alterations are a small fraction of the original organ volume. Finally, in data not shown here, we have use the same protocol to image tumor formation in PTEN deficient mouse models of human prostate cancer and can similarly detect presumptive tumor which represents less than 10 % of prostate volume.

Conclusions

We have developed an accurate, precise, and reproducible high frequency ultrasound imaging and 3D reconstruction protocol to serially quantitate prostate volume in live mice. This protocol allows determination of normal prostate growth and regression following hormone manipulation (ADT), as well as growth following androgen supplementation, in a model of BPH and in orthotopic prostatic tumor xenograft models. We anticipate that the utility of this technique can be extended to determining the efficacy of novel therapeutics in pre-clinical trials in mouse models of prostate cancer and benign prostatic hyperplasia.

Abbreviations
PrCa: Prostate cancer; MRI-CHESS: Magnetic resonance imaging with chemical shift suppression; Pb-PRL: Probasin-driven prolactin; CV(s): Coefficient(s) of variation; RPMI: Roswell park memorial institute 1640 media; VP: Ventral prostate; DLP: Dorsal-lateral prostate; ADT: Androgen deprivation therapy; SEM: Standard error of the mean; BLI: Bioluminescent imaging.

Competing interests
The author declares that there is no competing interests.

Authors' contributions
SS participated in the design of the study, manipulated and imaged the mice, evaluated the images, and performed the analysis. CP evaluated images. RW optimized imaging parameters and developed 3D reconstruction protocols. C-RY developed xenograft protocols. C-RY and KS manipulated mice. SS and CP drafted the manuscript and figures. RW and SY critically reviewed the manuscript. KLN blinded all data and served as the honest broker. JJK and KLN conceived of the study, participated in its coordination, and finalized the manuscript and figures. All authors read and approved the final manuscript.

Acknowledgements
We thank the University of Rochester Center for Musculo-skeletal Research (directed by Dr. Edward Schwarz, in the Department of Orthopedics) for access to the VisualSonics ultrasound instrumentation. We also thank Jon Kindblom for providing the prolactin transgenic mouse model of benign prostatic hyperplasia used in these studies. Grant sponsor: National Institutes of Health; Grant numbers: CA151753, P30AR061307

Funding
This work was supported by the National Institutes of Health; Grant numbers: CA151753 (JJK),P30AR061307 (University of Rochester Musculoskeletal center). The funders had no role in study design,data collection and analysis, decision to publish, or preparation of the manuscript.

Author details
[1]Departments of Pathology and Laboratory Medicine, University of Rochester School of Medicine and Dentistry, Rochester, NY, USA. [2]Departments of Neurobiology and Anatomy and Obstetrics and Gynecology, University of Rochester School of Medicine and Dentistry, Rochester, NY, USA. [3]Department of Urology, University of Rochester School of Medicine and Dentistry, Rochester, NY, USA. [4]Current address: Department of Cancer Genetics, Roswell Park Cancer Institute, Buffalo 14263NY, USA.

References
1. Siegel R, Ma J, Zou Z, Jemal A. Cancer statistics, 2014. CA Cancer J Clin. 2014;64(1):9–29.
2. Pienta KJ, Abate-Shen C, Agus DB, Attar RM, Chung LW, Greenberg NM, et al. The current state of preclinical prostate cancer animal models. Prostate. 2008;68(6):629–39.
3. Ittmann M, Huang J, Radaelli E, Martin P, Signoretti S, Sullivan R, et al. Animal models of human prostate cancer: the consensus report of the New York meeting of the Mouse Models of Human Cancers Consortium Prostate Pathology Committee. Cancer Res. 2013;73(9):2718–36.
4. Parisotto M, Metzger D. Genetically engineered mouse models of prostate cancer. Mol Oncol. 2013;7(2):190–205.
5. Kindblom J, Dillner K, Ling C, Tornell J, Wennbo H. Progressive prostate hyperplasia in adult prolactin transgenic mice is not dependent on elevated serum androgen levels. Prostate. 2002;53(1):24–33.
6. Hay M, Thomas DW, Craighead JL, Economides C, Rosenthal J. Clinical development success rates for investigational drugs. Nat Biotechnol. 2014;32(1):40–51.
7. Begley CG, Ellis LM. Drug development: Raise standards for preclinical cancer research. Nature. 2012;483(7391):531–3.
8. Collins FS, Tabak LA. NIH plans to enhance reproducibility. Nature. 2014;505:612–3.
9. Landis SC, Amara SG, Asadullah K, Austin CP, Blumenstein R, Bradley EW, et al. A call for transparent reporting to optimize the predictive value of preclinical research. Nature. 2012;490(7419):187–91.
10. Kilkenny C, Parsons N, Kadyszewski E, Festing MF, Cuthill IC, Fry D, et al. Survey of the quality of experimental design, statistical analysis and reporting of research using animals. PLoS One. 2009;4(11):e7824.
11. Zhang W, Zhu J, Efferson CL, Ware C, Tammam J, Angagaw M, et al. Inhibition of tumor growth progression by antiandrogens and mTOR inhibitor in a Pten-deficient mouse model of prostate cancer. Cancer Res. 2009;69(18):7466–72.
12. Carver BS, Chapinski C, Wongvipat J, Hieronymus H, Chen Y, Chandarlapaty S, et al. Reciprocal feedback regulation of PI3K and androgen receptor signaling in PTEN-deficient prostate cancer. Cancer Cell. 2011;19(5):575–86.
13. Hollingshead MG. Antitumor efficacy testing in rodents. J Natl Cancer Inst. 2008;100(21):1500–10.
14. El Hilali N, Rubio N, Martinez-Villacampa M, Blanco J. Combined noninvasive imaging and luminometric quantification of luciferase-labeled human prostate tumors and metastases. Lab Investig. 2002;82(11):1563–71.
15. Jiang ZK, Sato M, Wei LH, Kao C, Wu L. Androgen-independent molecular imaging vectors to detect castration-resistant and metastatic prostate cancer. Cancer Res. 2011;71(19):6250–60.
16. Liao CP, Zhong C, Saribekyan G, Bading J, Park R, Conti PS, et al. Mouse models of prostate adenocarcinoma with the capacity to monitor spontaneous carcinogenesis by bioluminescence or fluorescence. Cancer Res. 2007;67(15):7525–33.
17. Seethammagari MR, Xie X, Greenberg NM, Spencer DM. EZC-prostate models offer high sensitivity and specificity for noninvasive imaging of prostate cancer progression and androgen receptor action. Cancer Res. 2006;66(12):6199–209.
18. Baker M. Whole-animal imaging: The whole picture. Nature. 2010;463(7283):977–80.
19. Nastiuk KL, Liu H, Hamamura M, Muftuler LT, Nalcioglu O, Krolewski JJ. In vivo MRI volumetric measurement of prostate regression and growth in mice. BMC Urol. 2007;7:12.
20. Davis JS, Nastiuk KL, Krolewski JJ. TNF is necessary for castration-induced prostate regression, whereas TRAIL and FasL are dispensable. Mol Endocrinol. 2011;25(4):611–20.
21. Greco A, Mancini M, Gargiulo S, Gramanzini M, Claudio PP, Brunetti A, et al. Ultrasound biomicroscopy in small animal research: applications in molecular and preclinical imaging. J Biomed Biotechnol. 2012;2012:519238.
22. Kindblom J, Dillner K, Sahlin L, Robertson F, Ormandy C, Tornell J, et al. Prostate hyperplasia in a transgenic mouse with prostate-specific expression of prolactin. Endocrinology. 2003;144(6):2269–78.
23. Valkenburg KC, Williams BO. Mouse models of prostate cancer. Prostate Cancer. 2011;2011:895238.
24. Lai KP, Huang CK, Fang LY, Izumi K, Lo CW, Wood R, et al. Targeting stromal androgen receptor suppresses prolactin-driven benign prostatic hyperplasia (BPH). Mol Endocrinol. 2013;27(10):1617–31.
25. Sramkoski RM, Pretlow 2nd TG, Giaconia JM, Pretlow TP, Schwartz S, Sy MS, et al. A new human prostate carcinoma cell line, 22Rv1. In Vitro Cell Dev Biol Anim. 1999;35(7):403–9.
26. Alcazar JL, Cabrera C, Galvan R, Guerriero S. Three-dimensional power Doppler vascular network assessment of adnexal masses: intraobserver and interobserver agreement analysis. J Ultrasound Med. 2008;27(7):997–1001.
27. Bland JM, Altman DG. Measurement error and correlation coefficients. BMJ. 1996;313(7048):41–2.
28. Roy-Burman P, Wu H, Powell WC, Hagenkord J, Cohen MB. Genetically defined mouse models that mimic natural aspects of human prostate cancer development. Endocr Relat Cancer. 2004;11(2):225–54.
29. Sharifi N, Gulley JL, Dahut WL. Androgen deprivation therapy for prostate cancer. JAMA. 2005;294(2):238–44.
30. Kasper S, Smith Jr JA. Genetically modified mice and their use in developing therapeutic strategies for prostate cancer. J Urol. 2004;172:12–9.
31. Sugimura Y, Cunha GR, Donjacour AA. Morphological and histological study of castration-induced degeneration and androgen-induced regeneration in the mouse prostate. Biol Reprod. 1986;34(5):973–83.

32. Nastiuk KL, Kim JW, Mann M, Krolewski JJ. Androgen regulation of FLICE-like inhibitory protein gene expression in the rat prostate. J Cell Physiol. 2003;196(2):386–93.
33. Brodoefel H, Burgstahler C, Sabir A, Yam CS, Khosa F, Claussen CD, et al. Coronary plaque quantification by voxel analysis: dual-source MDCT angiography versus intravascular sonography. AJR Am J Roentgenol. 2009;192(3):W84–9.
34. Ayers GD, McKinley ET, Zhao P, Fritz JM, Metry RE, Deal BC, et al. Volume of preclinical xenograft tumors is more accurately assessed by ultrasound imaging than manual caliper measurements. J Ultrasound Med. 2010;29(6):891–901.
35. Wirtzfeld LA, Wu G, Bygrave M, Yamasaki Y, Sakai H, Moussa M, et al. A new three-dimensional ultrasound microimaging technology for preclinical studies using a transgenic prostate cancer mouse model. Cancer Res. 2005;65(14):6337–45.
36. Isaacs JT. Antagonistic effect of androgen on prostatic cell death. Prostate. 1984;5(5):545–57.
37. Kyprianou N, Isaacs J. Activation of programmed cell death in the rat ventral prostate after castration. Endocrinology. 1988;122:552–62.
38. Maini A, Archer C, Wang CY, Haas GP. Comparative pathology of benign prostatic hyperplasia and prostate cancer. In Vivo. 1997;11(4):293–9.
39. Suwa T, Nyska A, Haseman JK, Mahler JF, Maronpot RR. Spontaneous lesions in control B6C3F1 mice and recommended sectioning of male accessory sex organs. Toxicol Pathol. 2002;30(2):228–34.
40. Sugimura Y, Cunha GR, Donjacour AA. Morphogenesis of ductal networks in the mouse prostate. Biol Reprod. 1986;34(5):961–71.
41. Kraaij R, van Weerden WM, de Ridder CM, Gussenhoven EJ, Honkoop J, Nasu Y, et al. Validation of transrectal ultrasonographic volumetry for orthotopic prostate tumours in mice. Lab Anim. 2002;36(2):165–72.
42. Huizen IV, Wu G, Moussa M, Chin JL, Fenster A, Lacefield JC, et al. Establishment of a serum tumor marker for preclinical trials of mouse prostate cancer models. Clin Cancer Res. 2005;11(21):7911–9.
43. Fricke ST, Rodriguez O, Vanmeter J, Dettin LE, Casimiro M, Chien CD, et al. In vivo magnetic resonance volumetric and spectroscopic analysis of mouse prostate Cancer Models. Prostate. 2006;66(7):708–17.
44. Puaux AL, Ong LC, Jin Y, Teh I, Hong M, Chow PK, et al. A comparison of imaging techniques to monitor tumor growth and cancer progression in living animals. Int J Mol Imaging. 2011;2011:321538.
45. Laschke MW, Korbel C, Rudzitis-Auth J, Gashaw I, Reinhardt M, Hauff P, et al. High-resolution ultrasound imaging: a novel technique for the noninvasive in vivo analysis of endometriotic lesion and cyst formation in small animal models. Am J Pathol. 2010;176(2):585–93.
46. Klerk CP, Overmeer RM, Niers TM, Versteeg HH, Richel DJ, Buckle T, et al. Validity of bioluminescence measurements for noninvasive in vivo imaging of tumor load in small animals. Biotechniques. 2007;43(1 Suppl):7–13. 30.
47. Elliot TL, Downey DB, Tong S, McLean CA, Fenster A. Accuracy of prostate volume measurements in vitro using three-dimensional ultrasound. Acad Radiol. 1996;3(5):401–6.
48. Park SY, Hwang SS. Comparison Of Accuracy Of Prostate Model Volume Measurement Between 2 Dimensional And 3 Dimensional Ultrasonography. Int J Radiol. 2010;14(2):n5.
49. Teicher BA. Tumor models for efficacy determination. Mol Cancer Ther. 2006;5(10):2435–43.

9

Benign prostatic enlargement can be influenced by metabolic profile

Mauro Gacci[1*], Arcangelo Sebastianelli[1], Matteo Salvi[1], Cosimo De Nunzio[2], Linda Vignozzi[3], Giovanni Corona[4], Tommaso Jaeger[1], Tommaso Chini[1], Giorgio Ivan Russo[5], Mario Maggi[3], Giuseppe Morgia[5], Andrea Tubaro[2], Marco Carini[1] and Sergio Serni[1]

Abstract

Background: In last years Metabolic Syndrome (MetS) has been closely associated to Benign Prostatic Enlargement (BPE) Aim of our study is to evaluate the effect of MetS and each single MetS parameter on prostate growth in men surgically treated for BPE.

Methods: Overall, 379 men were prospectively enrolled in two tertiary referral centers. *Calculated prostate volume* (PV) was measured with transrectal US defining the antero-posterior (AP), the cranio-caudal (CC) and the latero-lateral (LL) diameters through the ellipsoid formula, while *raw PV* was calculated by suprapubic US. MetS was defined according to the NCEP-ATPIII criteria.

Results: One-hundred and forty men (36.9%) were affected by MetS. The number of MetS parameters (0 to 5) and the presence of MetS were correlated with the *calculated PV*. The number of MetS parameters were also directly related to increasing prostate diameters. At the binary logistic regression, MetS resulted associated to high (>60 cc) raw and calculated PV. Moreover, multivariate analysis suggested that AP diameter was mainly correlated with HDL cholesterol (r:-0.3103, $p = 0.002$) CC diameter with triglycerides (r:-0.191, $p = 0.050$) and LL diameter with systolic blood pressure (r:0.154, $p = 0.044$). However, at the binary logistic regression, only low HDL Cholesterol was the main determinant for the enlargement of all diameters and consequently of the whole PV.

Conclusions: Metabolic factors, specially dyslipidemia, could play a central role in the pathogenesis and progression of BPE/LUTS. Interventional studies are needed to evaluate the impact of early treatment of dyslipidemia on progression of LUTS/BPH.

Keywords: Benign prostatic enlargement, Benign prostatic hyperplasia, Lower urinary tract symptoms, Metabolic syndrome, Dyslipidemia

Background

Benign prostatic hyperplasia (BPH) is one of the most common conditions among middle and advance-aged men [1]. Autopsy studies revealed presence of BPH in 42% of men aged 51–60 year and 85% among men older than 80 year; BPH is characterized by stromal and cell hyperplasia which can lead to the development of prostatic bladder outlet obstruction (BOO) and Lower Urinary Tract Symptoms (LUTS); severe BPH leads to deterioration of QoL and has relevant socio-economic costs [2]. Historically BPH pathogenesis is linked to age and androgens effect but more recently other factors including family history, ethnicity, lifestyle behaviours (reduced physical activity, cigarette smoking and high fat diet) as well as metabolic diseases have been suggested to play an important role [3, 4].

Metabolic syndrome(MetS) is a worldwide complex disorder with high socioeconomic impact. MetS describes the combination of several metabolic abnormalities,

* Correspondence: maurogacci@yahoo.it
[1]Department of Urology, University of Florence, Careggi Hospital, Florence, Italy
Full list of author information is available at the end of the article

including central obesity, hypertension, dyslipidemia, insulin resistance with compensatory hyperinsulinemia, and glucose intolerance [5].

In the last 15 years several MetS components have been closely associated with BPH, suggesting that MetS has very heterogeneous clinical ramifications [6–8].

Although the relationship between BPH/LUTS and MetS is still poorly understood, some findings suggest that men with metabolic alterations faster develop [6] BPH or are more likely to undergo BPH surgery, [7] supporting the hypothesis that pathological alterations typical of MetS also predispose to the development and progression of BPH/LUTS. Indeed, in a recent meta-analysis, we demonstrated that subjects with MetS have significantly higher total and transitional zone prostate volume [9].

Aim of the present study is to evaluate the correlations between the presence of MetS and each single MetS parameter on prostate's anthropometric measures in men surgically treated for BPE.

Methods
Study population and design
Between January 2012 and September 2013, 379 consecutive patients undergone prostatectomy for LUTS due to large BPE, were prospectively enrolled in two tertiary referral centers. In both high volume referral centers, all patients included in this trial were managed by surgeons skilled in diagnosis and treatment of LUTS/BPE. Informed consent for the study was obtained from participants. The study did not require any deviation of the Good Clinical Practice so was conducted in accordance with the principles expressed in the Declaration of Helsinki.

In the study were included patients undergone simple open prostatectomy (OP) or transurethral resection of the prostate (TURP) for moderate to severe LUTS due to BPE refractory to medical treatment. Patients with previous history of prostate surgery, chronic medication for prostatitis and/or urinary infection or bladder stone or known malignant disease including prostate cancer were excluded.

PSA values and prostate volume were evaluated during the pre-hospitalization visits. *Raw prostate volume* was calculated by suprapubic US (by using the "estimated ellipsoid volume" based on prostatic circumference), while *calculated prostate volume* was measured by transrectal US defining the antero-posterior (AP), the cranio-caudal (CC) and the latero-lateral (LL) diameters through the ellipsoid formula (D1xD2xD3xπ/6). OP and TURP were performed as previously reported [10, 11]. LUTS were measured by the International Prostate Symptom Score (IPSS) and categorized as storage and voiding symptoms, immediately before surgery and 6 to 12 months postoperatively.

Definition of MetS
MetS was defined according to criteria defined by the National Cholesterol Education Program-Third Adult Treatment Panel (NCEP-ATPIII) [5, 12]. According these criteria MetS is defined by the presence of at least 3 of the following parameters: (1) waist circumference >102 cm; (2) triglycerides ≥150 mg/dl or treatment for hypetriglyceridemia, (3) HDL-Co < 40 mg/dl or treatment for reduced HDL-C, (4) blood pressure ≥ 130/85 mmHg or current use of antihypertensive medications, and (5) fasting blood glucose >110 mg/dl or previous diagnosis of type 2 diabetes mellitus. All these items of MetS were considered individually (single parameters above vs below cut-off points), as sum of continuous variables (one if the single parameter is positive for MetS, zero if the single parameter is negative), and combined according to MetS (present or absent).

Statistical analyses
Unpaired two-sided Student's t tests has been used for comparisons between men with or without MetS, to compare normally distributed parameters; in all other cases, Mann-Whitney U test has been used. Correlations have been assessed using Pearson's or Spearman's method for normally or non-normally distributed data.

Moreover, we included significant data in a binary logistic model regression to calculate the main determinant of both *raw* and *calculated* prostate volume.

All the analyses were obtained with SPSS statistics 20.0 version for windows XP and a p <0.05 was considered statistically significant.

Results
Three-hundred seventy-nine non selected consecutive men undergone surgical treatment of BPH were recruited in two tertiary referral centers. One-hundred and forty men (36.9%) were affected by MetS: preoperative patient's characteristics, stratified according to MetS diagnosis, are reported in Table 1.

At univariate analysis *raw prostate volume* resulted statistically related with systolic blood pressure and serum trygliceride levels (r = 0.114, *p* = 0.035 and r = 0.126, *p* = 0.013 respectively), while *calculated prostate volume* resulted related with systolic blood pressure, serum trygliceride levels and serum HDL levels (r = 0.179, *p* = 0.015 and r = 0.279, *p* < 0.001 and r = -0.303, *p = p* < 0.001 respectively). The number of metabolic syndrome parameters (0 to 5) and the presence of MetS (≥3/5 parameters) were significantly correlated with the *calculated prostate volume* (r = 0.244, *p* = 0.001 and r = 0.284, *p* < 0.001, respectively). At age-adjusted multivariate analyses, systolic blood pressure, serum HDL levels and the number of MetS parameters were still statistically significantly correlated to

Table 1 Descriptive statistics of population of men included in the study, stratified according to their MetS profile

Patients (n = 379)		With MetS (n = 140)	Without MetS (n = 239)	
		Mean ± SD	Mean ± SD	p value
Demographic	Age (years)	70.0 ± 7.4	68.5 ± 8.8	0.059
	BMI (Kg/m²)	27.5 ± 3.5	25.8 ± 2.4	0.000
	Smokers, Number, (%)	108 (77.1%)	171 (71.5%)	0.417
Prostate Features	Prostate Volume (cc)	88.9 ± 59.1	77.8 ± 41.2	0.053
	PSA (ng/mL)	3.9 ± 3.7	3.0 ± 3.2	0.062
Prostate treatment	α-blockers, Number, (%)	103 (73.5%)	164 (68.6%)	0.200
	5-ARI, Number, (%)	23 (16.4%)	33 (13.8%)	0.467
MetS parameters	WC	104.6 ± 12.9	97.2 ± 7.3	0.000
	Systolic BP	134.9 ± 14.7	131.3 ± 14.6	0.016
	Diastolic BP	78.7 ± 8.5	76.7 ± 8.0	0.020
	Glycemia	108.8 ± 37.1	94.1 ± 16.3	0.000
	Triglyceride	149.8 ± 54.3	111.2 ± 42.7	0.000
	HDL Cholesterol	41.5 ± 11.0	49.1 ± 7.4	0.000

calculated prostate volume (r = 0.175, p = 0.014, r = -0.256, p = 0.004 and r = 0.202, p = 0.007 respectively).

At the binary logistic regression (Table 2) considering all the main determinants of prostate volume, including age, BMI and use of 5-alpha-reductase inhibitors, MetS resulted a statistically significant risk factor for large (>60 cc) raw and calculated prostate volume (OR: 2.43 [95% CI: 1.444.09), p = 0.001 and OR: 4.28 [95% CI: 2.15–8.52), p < 0.001, respectively). A similar data was obtained by using the median (>70 cc) raw volume (OR: 1.82 [95% CI: 1.08–3.09], p = 0.026).

The number of MetS parameters, resulted directly related with the calculated prostate volume (r = 0.244, p = 0.001), with the antero-posterior (r = 0.231, p = 0.002), the cranio-caudal (r = 0.192, p = 0.009) and the latero-lateral diameter (r = 0.171, p = 0.020, see Fig. 1). At the age-adjusted multivariate analysis, including all the diameters, only the AP diameter was significantly related with the number of MetS parameters (r = 2.266, p = 0.025).

Furthermore, at the multivariate analysis based on significant parameters that can influence prostatic growth, the AP diameter was mainly correlated with HDL cholesterol (adjusted r for age, BMI and 5-ARIs: -0.3103, p = 0.002, see Fig. 2a), the CC diameter with triglycerides (adjusted r for age, BMI and 5-ARIs: -0.191, p = 0.050, see Fig. 2b) and the LL diameter with systolic blood pressure (adjusted r for age, BMI and 5-ARIs: 0.154, p = 0.044, see Fig. 2c). However, the binary logistic regression based on a median prostate diameters (AP = 40 mm, CC = 45 mm, LL = 55 mm) adjusted for age, presence of MetS, cigarette smoking and assumption of 5ARI, demonstrated that low HDL Cholesterol was the main determinant for the enlargements of all diameters and consequently of the whole prostate volume (see Fig. 3).

Table 2 Binary logistic regression based on prostate volume ≥ 60 cc vs. prostate volume < 60 cc. Age (< 65 vs. ≥ 65), BMI (< 25 kg/m² vs. ≥ 25 kg/m²), Use of 5 ARI (no vs. yes), Presence of MetS (no vs. yes). OR Odds ratio. LL Lower Limit. UL Upper Limit

	OR	LL 95% CI for OR	UL 95% CI for OR	P value
RAW Prostate volume (N = 379)				
Age	0.995	0.962	1.029	0.769
BMI	0.936	0.859	1.021	0.136
Use of 5ARI	1.054	0.541	2.056	0.877
Presence of MetS	2.430	1.441	4.095	*0.001*
CALCULATED Prostate volume (N = 187)				
Age	0.972	0.930	1.015	0.200
BMI	0.854	0.760	0.959	*0.008*
Use of 5ARI	1.304	0.625	2.719	0.479
Presence of MetS	4.278	2.149	8.519	*0.035*

Italic=statistically significant

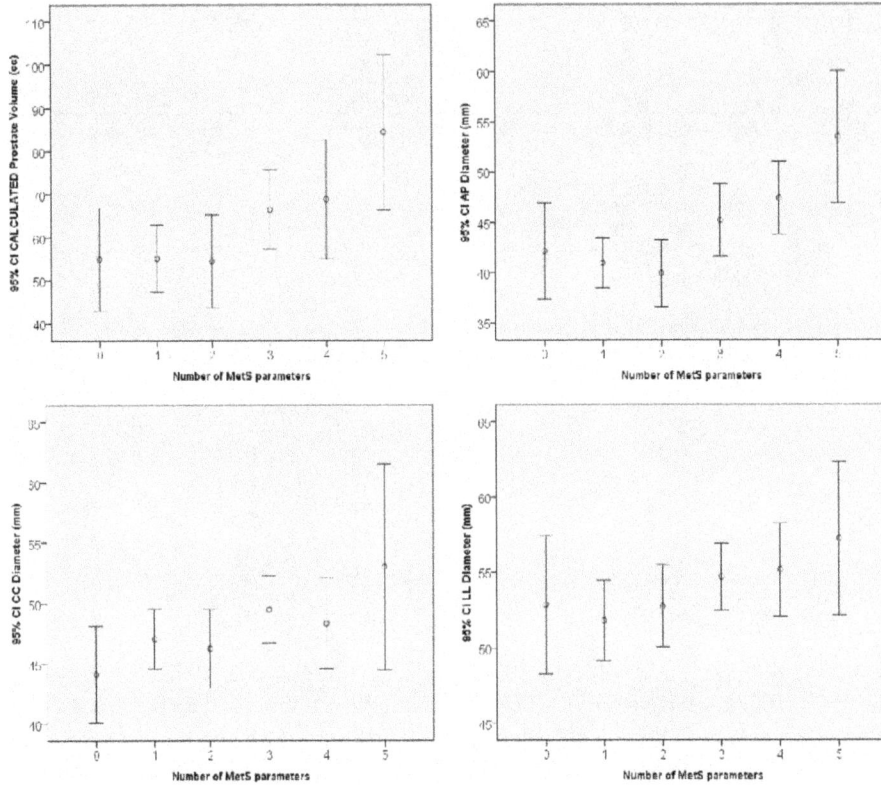

Fig. 1 Mean and 95% confidence interval of the mean of calculated prostate volume, antero-posterior (AP), cranio-caudal (CC) and latero-lateral (LL) diameters, stratified according to the number of MetS parameters

Discussion

Metabolic syndrome (MetS) is a cluster of cardiovascular and metabolic risk factors, associated with insulin resistance [5]. For first in 1998 Hammarsten et al. [13] described the possible relationship between some components of MetS and BPH. In their study, annual transitional prostate volume (TPV) growth rate was significantly higher in BPH patients with MetS as compared with those without MetS (1.019 ml/yr vs 0.699 ml/yr, respectively). After this preliminary work, several authors

have documented a possible association between MetS and BPH [14–16] but other authors didn't confirm this association [17]. Interestingly in a meta-analysis of the available evidence we found that subjects with MetS had significantly higher total prostate volume when compared to those without MetS (+1.8 [95% CI: 0.74;2.87] ml; $p < 0.001$) and these datas are in agreement to the present one. The number of metabolic syndrome parameters (1 to 5) and the presence of MetS itself were related with the prostate diameters as well as *calculated prostate volume,*

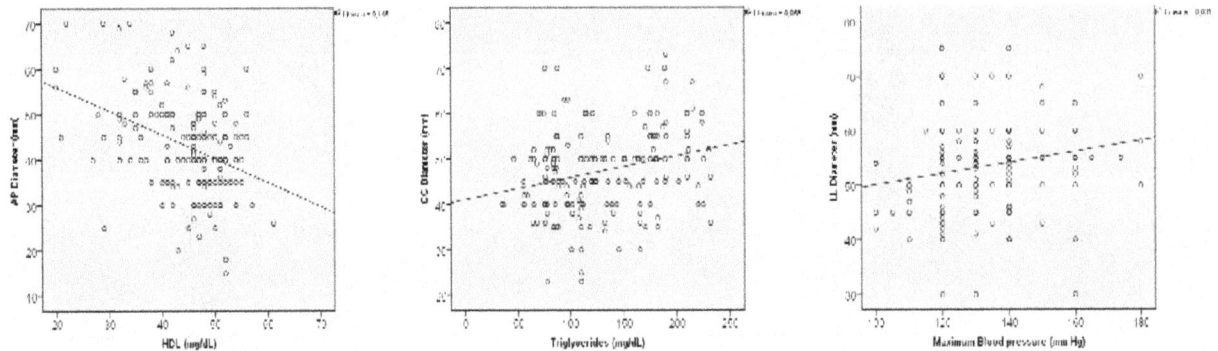

Fig. 2 Scatterplot diagram of correlation between AP diameter and HDL Cholesterol, CC diameter and triglyceride, LL diameter and Systolic blood pressure

AP diameter	p	OR	LL	UL
Elevated WC	1.277	0.492	0.137	1.768
Elevated Systolic BP	0.779	1.119	0.509	2.463
Elevated GLYCEMIA	0.118	0.479	0.190	1.205
Elevated TRIGLYCERIDE	0.017	3.306	1.233	8.864
Reduced HDL-CHOL	0.019	3.887	1.295	12.088

CC diameter	p	OR	LL	UL
Elevated WC	0.181	0.568	0.248	1.301
Elevated Systolic BP	0.333	1.454	0.681	3.106
Elevated GLYCEMIA	0.557	0.765	0.313	1.869
Elevated TRIGLYCERIDE	0.069	2.940	0.936	5.548
Reduced HDL-CHOL	0.028	3.185	1.134	8.941

LL diameter	p	OR	LL	UL
Elevated WC	0.770	0.891	0.410	1.934
Elevated Systolic BP	0.348	0.700	0.332	1.474
Elevated GLYCEMIA	0.737	0.868	0.379	1.987
Elevated TRIGLYCERIDE	0.083	2.126	0.906	4.992
Reduced HDL-CHOL	0.023	2.996	1.167	7.692

Fig. 3 Odds Ratio (OR) based on based on the median prostate diameters (AP = 40 mm, CC = 45 mm, LL = 55 mm) as derived from a logistic regression model adjusted for: Age, PSA, smoking, consumption of finasteride, presence of MetS. p = Pvalue. OR = Odds ratio. LL = Lower Limit. UL = Upper Limit

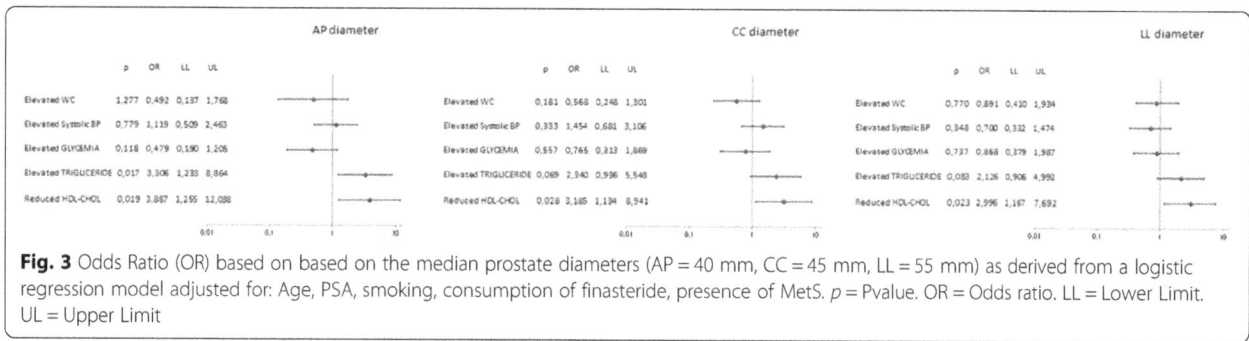

supporting a positive role for metabolic derangements in the progression of BPE.

The pathogenetic mechanisms underlying the association between MetS and BPH/LUTS are not completely understood. Either clinical or experimental evidence supports the role of chronic inflammation as possible link [18]. Although it has been known for at least 30 years that inflammation directly or indirectly contributes to prostate overgrowth, the role of impaired immunoresponse in BPH pathogenesis has been recently accepted [18].

The effect of MetS to BPH pathogenesis probably starts in early adulthood. Indeed, in a previous study on a population of 222 relatively young men seeking medical care for couple infertility, we found a significant association among increasing BMI, higher prostate volume and several sonographic features of prostate inflammation [19]. In addition, higher BMI was significantly related to higher value of IL-8 in seminal vesicle tissues, a reliable surrogate marker of prostate inflammatory diseases [20]. In the same population we also found that MetS severity was associated with increased prostate volume [21]. This association indicates that the effect of MetS on prostate growth begins very early and is detectable even in young adulthood.

We recently developed a non-genomic animal model of MetS, by exposing rabbits to a high-fat diet (HFD) for twelve weeks [22]. Accordingly to the aforementioned epidemiological clinical datas, severe prostatitis-like syndrome, tissue remodeling [22, 23] and bladder dysfunction [22] were demonstrated in animal models of MetS rabbits. Infiltration of inflammatory cells and fibrosis were observed in prostate of MetS rabbits [24]. In addition, we recently demonstrated the capacity of human myofibroblast prostatic cells to secrete several inflammatory cytokines and chemokines, including IL-8, in response to oxidized LDL (oxLDL) and insulin [25, 26]. These datas indicate that different MetS features, mainly dyslipidemia (oxLDL) and insulin resistance, could boost inflammation and tissue-remodelling in BPH. Indeed in a multicentre study on 271 consecutive men treated with simple prostatectomy, the presence of MetS (in particular MetS-associated dyslipidaemia) was associated with more

severe intraprostatic inflammation [27, 28]. Among MetS components, reduced HDL cholesterol and elevated triglycerides were significantly associated with elevated prostate inflammatory score (IS) and CD45 positivity. According to these datas, the present article shows that reduced HDL cholesterol levels were inversely related to all prostatic diameters. Dyslipidemia could have a detrimental effect on prostate cells, boosting prostate inflammation, a key factor in the development and progression of BPH/LUTS. Interestingly, a retrospective population-based cohort study on 2447 men aged 40–79 years, showed that statins assumption was associated with a 6.5 to 7-years delay in the new onset of moderate/severe LUTS/BPE [29]. Similarly, longitudinal datas from Health Professionals Follow up Study (HPFS), a prospective database on more than 18,000 US men, demostrated that men with higher total and abdominal adiposity or who gained weight were more likely to develop LUTS or experience progressive LUTS [30].

Our prospective study has several limitations. Firstly, we included men treated exclusively in two tertiary referral centers for BPH surgery: this population of men with large prostate (≥80 cc), and marked reduction of urinary flow parameters (Qmax < 9 mL/sec) may be very different to that of the general community. Then, we didn't adjust our datas for additional parameters such as physical activity. Finally, we had data on calculated prostate volume only for 187 patients.

Conclusions

In conclusion, present data along with recent evidences, suggest that metabolic factors could play a crucial role in the pathogenesis of LUTS/BPH. Further interventional studies are needed to prove the potential effect of dyslipidemia treatment on LUTS/BPH, and in particular on prostate enlargement.

Abbreviations
BPH: Benign prostatic hyperplasia; BOO: Bladder outlet obstruction; LUTS: Lower urinary tract symptoms; MetS: Metabolic syndrome; OP: Open prostatectomy; TURP: Transurethral resection of the prostate

Acknowledgements
None.

Funding
None.

Authors' contributions
MG, AS and LV have made substantial contributions to conception and design of the study. MG, CDN, AS, MS, LV, GC, TJ, TC and GIR have made substantial contributions to acquisition, analysis and interpretation of data. MG and CDN have been involved in drafting and revising the manuscript. MG, CDN, MM, GM, AT, MC and SS have given final approval of the version to be published.

Competing interests
The authors declare that they have no competing interests.

Author details
[1]Department of Urology, University of Florence, Careggi Hospital, Florence, Italy. [2]Department of Urology, Sant'Andrea Hospital, University "La Sapienza", Rome, Italy. [3]Department of Clinical Physiopathology, University of Florence, Florence, Italy. [4]Endocrinology Unit, Maggiore-Bellaria Hospital, Bologna, Italy. [5]Department of Urology, Policlinico Hospital, University of Catania, Catania, Italy.

References
1. Berry SJ, Coffey DS, Walsh PC, Ewing LL. The development of human benign prostatic hyperplasia with age. J Urol. 1984;132:474–9.
2. Holtgrewe HL. Economic issues and the management of benign prostatic hyperplasia. Urology. 1995;46:23–5.
3. Hammarsten J, Hogstedt B. Hyperinsulinaemia as a risk factor for developing benign prostatic hyperplasia. Eur Urol. 2001;39:151–8.
4. Vignozzi L, Rastrelli G, Corona G, Gacci M, Forti G, Maggi M. Benign prostatic hyperplasia: a new metabolic disease? J Endocrinol Invest. 2014;37(4):313–22.
5. Corona G, Rastrelli G, Morelli A, Vignozzi L, Mannucci E, Maggi M. Hypogonadism and metabolic syndrome. J Endocrinol Invest. 2011;34(7):557–67.
6. De Nunzio C, Aronson W, Freedland SJ, Giovannucci E, Parsons JK. The correlation between metabolic syndrome and prostatic diseases. Eur Urol. 2012;61(3):560–70.
7. Dahle SE, Chokkalingam AP, Gao YT, Deng J, Stanczyk FZ, Hsing AW. Body size and serum levels of insulin and leptin in relation to the risk of benign prostatic hyperplasia. J Urol. 2002;168:599–604.
8. Ozden C, Ozdal OL, Urgancioglu G, Koyuncu H, Gokkaya S, Memis A. The correlation between metabolic syndrome and prostatic growth in patients with benign prostatic hyperplasia. Eur Urol. 2007;51:199–203.
9. Gacci M, Corona G, Vignozzi L, Salvi M, Serni S, De Nunzio C, Tubaro A, Oelke M, Carini M, Maggi M. Metabolic syndrome and benign prostatic enlargement: a systematic review and meta-analysis. BJU Int. 2015;115(1): 24–31.
10. Gacci M, Bartoletti R, Figlioli S, et al. Urinary symptoms, quality of life and sexual function in patients with benign prostatic hypertrophy before and after prostatectomy: a prospective study. BJU Int. 2003;91(3):196–200.
11. Tubaro A, Carter S, Hind A, et al. A prospective study of the safety and efficacy of suprapubictransvesical prostatectomy in patients with benign prostatic hyperplasia. J Urol. 2001;166(1):172–6.
12. Expert Panel on Detection, Evaluation, and Treatment of High Blood Cholesterol in Adults. Executive summary of the third report of the national cholesterol education program (NCEP) expert panel on detection, evaluation, and treatment of high blood cholesterol in adults (adult treatment panel III). JAMA. 2001;285:2486–97.
13. Hammarsten J, Hogstedt B, Holthuis N, Mellstrom D. Components of the metabolic syndrome-risk factors for the development of benign prostatichyperplasia. Prostate Cancer Prostatic Dis. 1998;1:157–62.
14. Parsons JK, Carter HB, Partin AW, et al. Metabolic factors associated with benignprostatic hyperplasia. J Clin Endocrinol Metab. 2006;91:2562–8.
15. Rohrmann S, Smitt E, Giuvanucci E, Platz EA. Associations of obesity withlower urinary tract symptoms andnoncancer prostate surgery in the ThirdNational Health and NutritionExamination Survey. Am J Epidemiol. 2004;159:390–7.
16. Corona G, Gacci M, Maseroli E, Rastrelli G, Vignozzi L, Sforza A, Forti G, Mannucci E, Maggi M. Clinical correlates of enlarged prostate size in subjects with sexual dysfunction. Asian J Androl. 2014;16(5):767–73.
17. Park YW, Min SK, Lee JH. Relationship between lower urinary tract symptoms/benign prostatic hyperplasia and metabolic syndrome in Korean Men. World J Mens Health. 2012;30(3):183–8.
18. Fibbi B, Penna G, Morelli A, Adorini L, Maggi M. Chronic inflammation in the pathogenesis of benign prostatic hyperplasia. Int J Androl. 2010;33(3):475–88.
19. Lotti F, Corona G, Colpi GM, et al. Elevated body mass index correlates with higher seminal plasma interleukin 8 levels and ultrasonographic abnormalities of the prostate in men attending an andrology clinic for infertility. J Endocrinol Invest. 2011;34:e336–4263.
20. Lotti F, Maggi M. Interleukin 8 and the male genital tract. J Reprod Immunol. 2013;100(1):54–65.
21. Lotti F, Corona G, Vignozzi L, et al. Metabolic syndrome and prostate abnormalities in male subjects of infertile couples. Asian J Androl. 2014;16(2):295–304.
22. Filippi S, Vignozzi L, Morelli A, et al. Testosterone partially ameliorates metabolic profile and erectile responsiveness to PDE5 inhibitors in an animal model of male metabolic syndrome. J Sex Med. 2009;6:3274–8872.
23. Vignozzi L, Morelli A, Sarchielli E, et al. Testosterone protects from metabolic syndrome-associated prostate inflammation: an experimental study in rabbit. J Endocrinol. 2012;212:71–84.
24. Morelli A, Comeglio P, Filippi S, et al. Testosterone and farnesoid X receptor agonist INT-747 counteract high fat diet-induced bladder alterations in a rabbit model of metabolic syndrome. J Steroid Biochem Mol Biol. 2012;132:80–9249.
25. Vignozzi L, Gacci M, Cellai I, et al. PDE5 inhibitors blunt inflammation in human BPH: A potential mechanism of action for PDE5 inhibitors in LUTS. Prostate. 2013;73:1391–402.
26. Morelli A, Sarchielli E, Comeglio P, et al. Metabolic syndrome induces inflammation and impairs gonadotropin-releasing hormone neurons in the preoptic area of the hypothalamus in rabbits. Mol Cell Endocrinol. 2014;382(1):107–19.
27. Gacci M, Vignozzi L, Sebastianelli A, et al. Metabolic syndrome and lower urinary tract symptoms: the role of inflammation. Prostate Cancer Prostatic Dis. 2013;16:101–657.
28. Vignozzi L, Gacci M, Cellai I, et al. Fat boosts, while androgen receptor activation counteracts, BPH-associated prostate inflammation. Prostate. 2013;73:789–800.
29. St Sauver JL, Jacobsen SJ, Jacobson DJ, McGree ME, Girman CJ, Nehra A, Roger VL, Lieber MM. Statin use and decreased risk of benign prostatic enlargement and lower urinary tract symptoms. BJU Int. 2011;107(3):443–50.
30. Mondul AM, Giovannucci E, Platz EA. A prospective study of obesity, and the incidence and progression of lower urinary tract symptoms. J Urol. 2014;191(3):715–21.

10

Cost-effectiveness of a fixed-dose combination of solifenacin and oral controlled adsorption system formulation of tamsulosin in men with lower urinary tract symptoms associated with benign prostatic hyperplasia

Jameel Nazir[1*], Lars Heemstra[2], Anke van Engen[2], Zalmai Hakimi[3] and Cristina Ivanescu[2]

Abstract

Background: Storage symptoms, associated with benign prostatic hyperplasia (BPH), often co-exist with voiding symptoms in men with lower urinary tract symptoms (LUTS). Storage symptoms are likely to be most bothersome, and may not be adequately resolved by treatment with α-blocker or antimuscarinic monotherapy. A recent randomised controlled phase 3 trial (NEPTUNE) demonstrated that a fixed-dose combination (FDC) of solifenacin 6 mg plus an oral controlled absorption system (OCAS™) formulation of tamsulosin (TOCAS, 0.4 mg) improved storage symptoms, as well as quality of life, compared with TOCAS alone in men with moderate-to-severe storage symptoms and voiding symptoms. This analysis aimed to assess the cost-effectiveness of a FDC tablet of solifenacin 6 mg plus TOCAS relative to tolterodine plus tamsulosin given concomitantly, from the perspective of the UK National Health Service (NHS).

Methods: A Markov model was developed for men aged ≥45 years with LUTS/BPH who have moderate-to-severe storage symptoms and voiding symptoms. The model calculated cost-effectiveness over an analytical time horizon of 1 year and estimated total treatment costs, quality adjusted life years (QALYs) and incremental cost-effectiveness ratio.

Results: The FDC tablet of solifenacin 6 mg plus TOCAS was associated with lower total annual costs (£860 versus £959) and increased QALYs (0.839 versus 0.836), and was therefore dominant compared with tolterodine plus tamsulosin. Time horizon, discontinuation or withdrawal rates, drug cost and utility values were the main drivers of cost-effectiveness. The probability that the FDC tablet of solifenacin 6 mg plus TOCAS is cost-effective was 100% versus tolterodine plus tamsulosin, at a willingness-to-pay threshold of £20,000/QALY gained.

Conclusions: The FDC tablet of solifenacin 6 mg plus TOCAS provides important clinical benefits and is a cost-effective treatment strategy in the UK NHS compared with tolterodine plus tamsulosin for men with both storage and voiding LUTS/BPH.

Keywords: Benign prostatic hyperplasia, Cost-effectiveness, Fixed-dose combination, Incremental cost-effectiveness ratio, Lower urinary tract symptoms, Quality adjusted life years, Solifenacin, Tamsulosin, Tolterodine

* Correspondence: jameel.nazir@astellas.com
[1]Astellas Pharma Europe Ltd, Chertsey, UK
Full list of author information is available at the end of the article

Background

The term 'lower urinary tract symptoms' (LUTS) is used to describe a condition that encompasses storage, voiding and post-micturition symptoms [1,2]. The aetiology of LUTS can be multifactorial [2,3], but BPH is a common cause in men. Storage symptoms (e.g. urgency, frequency, urgency incontinence and nocturia) and voiding symptoms (e.g. weak or intermittent urinary stream, straining, hesitancy, terminal dribbling and incomplete emptying) are common and frequently co-exist in men with LUTS [4,5]. Storage symptoms represent the most troublesome LUTS, reported in up to 42% of men aged ≥75 years [4]. Storage symptoms are also reported to be the most bothersome LUTS [6].

Overall, the recommended treatment options for men with moderate-to-severe LUTS include α-blockers, 5α-reductase inhibitors (in those with a large prostate, 30 g or 40 mL) and antimuscarinic (in those with predominant storage symptoms) [2,4,7]. In addition, α-blocker plus antimuscarinic combination treatment should be considered for patients not adequately responding to monotherapy of either drug [2,4]. However, the majority of men with moderate-to-severe LUTS associated with BPH receive α-blocker monotherapy only [8], whilst less than 25% are reported to receive an antimuscarinic [8,9]. Additionally, α-blocker monotherapy is reported to improve voiding and storage symptoms in men with LUTS/BPH [10,11]. However, storage symptoms may persist in some men after receiving α-blocker monotherapy, epitomised by data from Lee et al. that reported only 35% of men with storage symptoms were sufficiently controlled by this treatment strategy [12].

Several trials have demonstrated that α-blocker plus antimuscarinic combination treatment is more effective than α-blocker monotherapy for men with moderate-to-severe LUTS and documented storage symptoms [13-19]. The most recent phase 3 trial (NEPTUNE), which included 1,334 men with LUTS/BPH who had moderate-to-severe storage symptoms and voiding symptoms, showed that solifenacin 6 mg plus an oral controlled absorption system (OCAS™) formulation of tamsulosin (TOCAS) improved storage symptoms and quality of life compared with TOCAS alone [18]. The combination treatment was also well tolerated and exhibited an adverse event profile similar to that reported for the individual monotherapies. A once-daily, FDC tablet of solifenacin 6 mg plus TOCAS 0.4 mg aimed at treating both storage and voiding symptoms in men with LUTS/BPH is licensed and available in several countries, including the UK [20].

The aim of this study was to perform a cost-effectiveness analysis for a once-daily FDC tablet of solifenacin 6 mg plus TOCAS (0.4 mg) versus daily tolterodine extended release (ER, 4 mg) plus tamsulosin (0.4 mg) given concomitantly, in men with LUTS/BPH who have moderate-to-severe storage symptoms and voiding symptoms within the UK healthcare setting.

Methods

Model overview

A Markov model was developed to compare the cost-effectiveness of a FDC tablet of solifenacin 6 mg plus TOCAS versus tolterodine plus tamsulosin given concomitantly over an analytical time horizon of 1 year from the perspective of the UK NHS (Table 1). A 4-week cycle period was employed, the minimum time interval used to detect treatment differences in LUTS clinical trials. Inputs for effectiveness data, costs and utilities were extracted from published sources and interviews with clinical experts, as described in detail below. The model provided outcome estimates for total treatment costs, QALYs and incremental cost-effectiveness ratio (ICER). The model was programmed in Microsoft Excel. No ethics or consent were required for this study.

Patients

The model considered men with LUTS/BPH who had moderate-to-severe storage symptoms and voiding symptoms, defined by ≥8 micturitions/day and ≥2 urgency episodes/day (Patient Perception of Intensity of Urgency Scale [PPIUS] grade 3 or 4 [21]).

Treatment pathway

Men entering the model were treated with daily regimens of FDC tablet of solifenacin 6 mg plus TOCAS (0.4 mg) or tolterodine ER (4 mg) plus tamsulosin (0.4 mg) given concomitantly. After a first treatment period of 4 weeks, men could have experienced a treatment response or no response, based on changes in total urgency and frequency score (TUFS) of ≥6 or <6 points, respectively, estimated as the minimally important difference [22]. TUFS is a validated instrument that captures storage symptoms (urgency and frequency) in a single parameter; TUFS is calculated as the sum of the PPIUS scores (grading of 0 to 4 for each void) recorded in a patient's micturition diary divided by the number of days recorded in the diary [18].

Patients, either with or without a response may remain on drug or discontinue the treatment (cope with symptoms or wait for surgery to alleviate symptoms) at any model cycle (Figure 1). After 12 weeks (three cycles), patients were permitted to switch to a different combination regimen. After the first 12 weeks, the treatment effect was assumed to be stable (no improvement or deterioration in TUFS).

Table 1 Cost effectiveness model overview

Aspect	Details
Analytical method	Markov state transition model incorporating a decision tree
Software used	Microsoft Excel 2010
Model perspective	UK NHS
Time horizon	1 year
Cycle length	4 weeks
Patient population	Men with LUTS/BPH who have moderate-to-severe storage symptoms (≥8 micturitions/day and ≥2 urgency episodes/day*) and voiding symptoms
Treatments	Once-daily FDC tablet of solifenacin 6 mg plus TOCAS 0.4 mg
	Tolterodine ER 4 mg plus tamsulosin 0.4 mg daily, given concomitantly
Outcomes	Total treatment costs
	Quality adjusted life years
	Incremental cost-effectiveness ratio

*Patient Perception of Intensity of Urgency Scale, grade 3 or 4.
BPH, benign prostatic hyperplasia; ER, extended release; FDC, fixed-dose combination; LUTS, lower urinary tract symptoms; TOCAS, oral controlled absorption system (OCAS™) formulation of tamsulosin.

Outcomes

The model estimated the following outcomes: total treatment costs; QALYs gained; and ICER. All results are expressed on a per patient basis.

Model input parameters

Assumptions

Several assumptions were made in the model to reflect clinical practice (Additional file 1: Table S1). Input was sought from a group of five clinical experts (two general practitioners [GPs] and three urologists) from the UK, to validate the model input parameters for where data were limited and to fill any data gaps (i.e. surgery, persistence and treatment switching).

Transition probabilities

Transition probabilities for FDC tablet of solifenacin 6 mg plus TOCAS during the first three cycles were derived from the NEPTUNE study (Table 2) [18]. Tolterodine plus tamsulosin was assumed to have the same treatment effect as FDC tablet of solifenacin 6 mg plus TOCAS (Additional file 1: Table S1).

Persistence, switching and surgery

Patients may have discontinued treatment at the end of each cycle due to adverse events or perceptions of efficacy (e.g. satisfaction or dissatisfaction with efficacy; an assumption was made that patients may discontinue treatment despite a positive clinical benefit and/or no

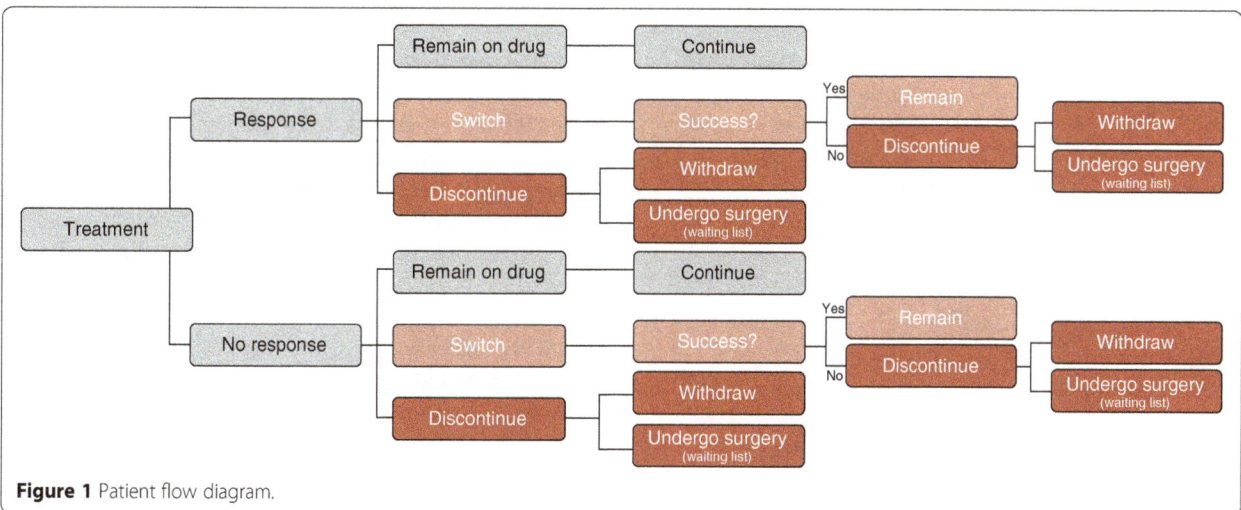

Figure 1 Patient flow diagram.

Table 2 Transition probabilities for the first three cycles [18]

Model cycle	From response to		From no response to	
	Response	No response	Response	No response
1	0.000	0.000	0.539	0.461
2	0.843	0.157	0.278	0.722
3	0.878	0.122	0.248	0.752

tolerability issues). Discontinuation and switching rates were derived from a large observational study of UK primary care between January 2004 and September 2011 (The Health Improvement Network [THIN] database). The analysis included men aged ≥45 years who had an initial diagnosis, symptoms or therapies indicative of LUTS/BPH, and found that over a median follow-up of 2 years, 43.0% and 59.8% of men discontinued solifenacin and tolterodine, respectively [8] (Table 3). In addition, switching rates of 15.3% and 23.3% for solifenacin and tolterodine were reported from the THIN database.

To accommodate the possibility of surgical treatment in the model, it was assumed that 50% of the patients who discontinued the treatment would be eligible for a surgical procedure within 6 months and, consequently, would discontinue drug treatment [4]. Transurethral resection of the prostate (TURP) was chosen as the surgical procedure because it is the current surgical standard procedure for men with LUTS secondary to BPH [2]. The 6-month probability of surgery for TURP was converted into a 1-month probability, assuming that 11% of patients received surgery every month.

Table 3 Discontinuation and switching rates for responders and non-responders [8 and Interviews with clinical experts]

	Responders		Non-responders	
	2 year	4-weekly rate	2 year	4-weekly rate
Discontinuation rates				
FDC tablet solifenacin 6 mg + TOCAS	43.0%	0.023	53.0%	0.031
Tolterodine + tamsulosin	59.8%	0.037	69.8%	0.049
Switching rates				
FDC tablet solifenacin 6 mg + TOCAS	15.3%	0.007	15.3%	0.007
Tolterodine + tamsulosin	23.3%	0.011	23.3%	0.011

FDC, fixed-dose combination; TOCAS, oral controlled absorption system (OCAS™) formulation of tamsulosin.

Quality of life

Utility values were derived from EQ-5D data collected in the NEPTUNE study (Table 4) using the UK tariffs. Withdrawal and discontinuation were assumed to have the same utility as the baseline. The average of the response and non-response health state was used to calculate the second-line treatment utility weight, as specific efficacy data were not available. The utility for the post-surgery health state was derived by combining disutilities from DiSantostefano et al. [23] and the response utility value from the NEPTUNE study [18] with the probabilities of improvement, no improvement and adverse events after surgery [23]. Mapping algorithms were also used to derive utilities from a disease-specific instrument overactive bladder questionnaire (OAB-5D) as part of the sensitivity analysis [Astellas, data on file].

Mortality

The mean age of the men in the model was determined to be 66 years – consistent with the mean age (65.4 years) of the randomised men in the NEPTUNE study [18]. The annual mortality probability for the population was assumed to be the same as that of men aged 66 years from the UK general population (2008–2010) [24].

Costs and resource utilisation

Costs in the model accounted for the resource utilisation associated with all primary care and hospital-based treatments. Costs were considered over the whole model period and were based on the assignment of fixed costs to health states and transitions between health states (Table 5). Direct costs included drug acquisition costs, healthcare professional visits, surgery, hospitalisation time, and treatment of adverse events. All costs were based on 2013 prices and expressed in British pounds (£). Where 2013 unit costs were not available, costs were adapted to 2013 values using the consumer price index. Costs and outcomes were discounted at 3.5% per annum, as recommended by NICE [25].

Drug acquisition costs were obtained from the British National Formulary [26] taking into account the daily dose (Table 5). Patients were assumed to have regular GP/urologist follow-up visits every 6 months; additional visits were planned for the switching or discontinuation of treatment. All surgical procedures were assumed to be TURP based on advice from interviews with clinical experts.

Sensitivity analyses

Deterministic and probabilistic sensitivity analyses were performed to determine the influence of uncertainty on the final results. A standard deterministic univariate sensitivity analysis was performed on all model parameters, varying each parameter through a plausible range whilst holding

Table 4 Utility weights per health state

Health state	Derivation	Utility weight
Baseline	Based on average utilities of patients at baseline	0.848
Response	Value at Week 12	0.887
No response	Value at Week 12	0.870
Second-line treatment	Average of response and no response health states	0.879
Withdrawal	Assumed to be equal to the baseline utility	0.848
Discontinuation	Assumed to be equal to the baseline utility	0.848
Post-surgery	Derived by combining response utility value from NEPTUNE study with disutilities from [23], weighted by probability of improvement, no improvement and adverse events after surgery [23]	0.839
Death	Lowest utility possible	0.000

other parameters fixed and assessing the effect on the overall outcomes and the ICER. Results of these analyses are presented using a tornado diagram. A tornado diagram visualises and orders the model parameters from those that have the highest impact on incremental model results to parameters that have the lowest impact on incremental outcomes.

In the probabilistic sensitivity analyses (PSA), parameter estimates were varied within their uncertainty distributions that best reflect the nature of each specific parameter. Aligned with standard methods [27], gamma distributions were selected for costs, beta distributions for probabilities and utility values, and a Dirichlet distribution was used for transitions in the first 12 weeks of the model. Monte Carlo simulations (n = 1,000) were performed using randomly selected values from the probability distribution assigned to each parameter. The results of the PSA are presented in the form of a graph displaying the results of the 1,000 simulations on the cost-effectiveness plane.

Several scenarios analyses were performed using alternative discontinuation rates, time horizons and utility values. The discontinuation scenario analysis utilised an alternative discontinuation rate for tolterodine, which was based on a report of prescriptions for antimuscarinic therapies in the UK [28]. This report indicated that discontinuation for tolterodine versus solifenacin had a relative ratio of 1:10. Consequently, an alternative 4-weekly discontinuation rate

of 0.026 for tolterodine (46.8% over 2 years) was applied to the model (compared with 0.037 in the base case model). In the time horizon scenario, the cost-effectiveness for FDC tablet of solifenacin plus TOCAS versus tolterodine plus tamsulosin was calculated over four time horizons of 1, 3, 5 and 10 years. Additionally, the utility values for each health state were replaced with OAB-5D-derived utility values (Additional file 1: Table S2).

Results

Base case results

A higher proportion of men treated with the FDC tablet of solifenacin 6 mg plus TOCAS were still on their original treatment compared with tolterodine plus tamsulosin at Week 12 (92.0% versus 87.6%, respectively) and at 1 year (65.0% versus 50.5%, respectively), and a higher proportion of men had a response (56.9% versus 54.4% at 12 weeks, and 41.5% versus 32.8% at 1 year). Additionally, the proportion of men in the post-surgery health state at 1 year was smaller for the FDC tablet of solifenacin 6 mg plus TOCAS (6.9%) compared with tolterodine plus tamsulosin (10.2%) (Table 6).

After 1 year, the FDC tablet of solifenacin 6 mg plus TOCAS was associated with lower annual per patient total costs (£860 versus £959, respectively) and increased QALYs (0.839 versus 0.836) compared with tolterodine plus tamsulosin (Table 7). The FDC tablet of solifenacin

Table 5 Treatment costs

Treatment	Description	Price (£)	Source
FDC tablet solifenacin 6 mg + TOCAS 0.4 mg	One tablet per day	0.92*‡	BNF [26]
Tolterodine 4 mg + tamsulosin 0.4 mg	One tablet + one capsule per day	1.10 (=0.92 + 0.18)‡	BNF [26]
GP visit	Per clinic consultation lasting 17.2 minutes, excl. direct care costs, incl. qualification costs	230.0	PSSRU [41]
Surgery	Prostate transurethral resection procedure 80% without CC, 20% with major CC	2,643.4§	NHS [42]; Antoñanzas et al. [43]

*Price parity with solifenacin 5 mg (£0.92/day); Prescription charge excluded from UK analysis. ‡Price per day. §Price calculated according to Antoñanzas et al. [43]: 20% of LB25F plus 80% of LB25D.

CC, complications and comorbidities; FDC, fixed-dose combination; GP, general practitioner; TOCAS, oral controlled absorption system (OCAS™) formulation of tamsulosin.

Table 6 Base case results: Distribution of patients across the health states

Base case scenario	FDC tablet solifenacin 6 mg + TOCAS	Tolterodine + tamsulosin
Patient in HS1	41.46%	32.76%
Patient in HS2	23.56%	17.76%
Patient on second-line treatment	4.30%	6.50%
Patient withdrawn	14.60%	20.75%
Patient who discontinued treatment	7.71%	10.57%
Patient in post-surgery	6.89%	10.18%
Dead patient	1.48%	1.48%

FDC, fixed-dose combination; HS1, Response health state; HS2, No response health state; TOCAS, oral controlled absorption system (OCAS™) formulation of tamsulosin.

6 mg plus TOCAS was therefore dominant (i.e. more effective and less costly) compared with tolterodine plus tamsulosin (Table 7).

Sensitivity analyses

The univariate analysis showed that the model was most sensitive to time horizon, discontinuation/withdrawal rates, drug cost and EQ-5D-derived utility values (Figure 2). The FDC tablet of solifenacin 6 mg plus TOCAS remained dominant (i.e. costs less and generates more QALYs) or was cost-effective (i.e. ICER below the £20,000 threshold) compared with tolterodine plus tamsulosin in all parameters except time horizon.

The PSA showed that the annual per patient mean incremental cost was −£99 (standard deviation [SD], £33) and the incremental QALYs was 0.0019 (SD, 0.0002), showing that the FDC tablet of solifenacin 6 mg plus TOCAS remained dominant compared with tolterodine plus tamsulosin (mean ICER, −£51,941; Figure 3). At a willingness-to-pay (WTP) threshold of £20,000 per QALY gained, the probability that the FDC tablet of solifenacin 6 mg plus TOCAS is cost-effective was 100% versus tolterodine plus tamsulosin.

Table 7 Base case results: cost-effectiveness

	FDC tablet solifenacin 6 mg + TOCAS	Tolterodine + tamsulosin
Total costs* (£)	860	959
Difference	–	−99
QALYs*	0.840	0.836
Difference	–	0.002
ICER*‡	–	Dominates (−£40,469)

*Per patient at 1 year.
‡FDC tablet solifenacin 6 mg + TOCAS versus tolterodine + tamsulosin.
FDC, fixed-dose combination; ICER, incremental cost effectiveness ratio; QALY, quality of life adjusted years; TOCAS, oral controlled absorption system (OCAS™) formulation of tamsulosin.

Scenario analyses

An analysis that used an alternative discontinuation rate for tolterodine plus tamsulosin, as determined by Wagg et al. [28], indicated that the FDC tablet of solifenacin 6 mg plus TOCAS remained dominant compared with tolterodine plus tamsulosin (Table 8). Similarly, a scenario analysis performed using OAB-5D-derived utilities showed that the FDC tablet of solifenacin 6 mg plus TOCAS remained dominant compared with tolterodine plus tamsulosin with larger incremental QALYs (0.0005) after 1 year (Table 8).

A time horizon analysis up to 5 years showed that the incremental difference in QALYs and total annual costs for the FDC tablet of solifenacin 6 mg plus TOCAS compared with tolterodine plus tamsulosin were proportionally smaller with increasing time (Table 9).

Discussion

There are a few reports of cost-effectiveness of drug treatment in LUTS, but this study represents the first cost-effectiveness analysis of a FDC tablet of solifenacin 6 mg plus TOCAS. Overall, the results of this analysis indicate that the FDC tablet of solifenacin 6 mg plus TOCAS is a cost-effective treatment option for men with LUTS/BPH who have moderate-to-severe storage symptoms and voiding symptoms. The base-case analysis showed that the FDC tablet of solifenacin 6 mg plus TOCAS is dominant (i.e. was associated with improved patient outcomes and lower costs) versus tolterodine plus tamsulosin over a 1-year time horizon.

The robustness of our cost-effectiveness model is demonstrated through the results of the univariate and probabilistic sensitivity analyses, as well as the scenario analyses. The univariate analysis showed that several of the main drivers for superior cost-effectiveness of FDC solifenacin 6 mg plus TOCAS versus tolterodine plus tamsulosin were inputs related to treatment persistence. Data from several areas of medicine describe that adherence/persistence with medication is a key driver of cost-effectiveness [29-32]. Two reports of real-world clinical practice data in the UK indicate improved persistence for solifenacin versus tolterodine in men with LUTS/BPH or overactive bladder (OAB). The THIN database reported that a lower proportion of men with LUTS/BPH discontinued and switched treatment (43% and 15%, respectively) compared with tolterodine (60% and 23%, respectively) over a median follow-up of 2 years [8]. In addition, 35% of patients with OAB were still receiving solifenacin after 12 months compared with 28% for tolterodine ER [28]. Further analyses should be conducted to confirm these observations, and various factors are likely to impact persistence. For example, solifenacin is reported to provide an improved efficacy (urgency and micturitions) and tolerability (dry mouth)

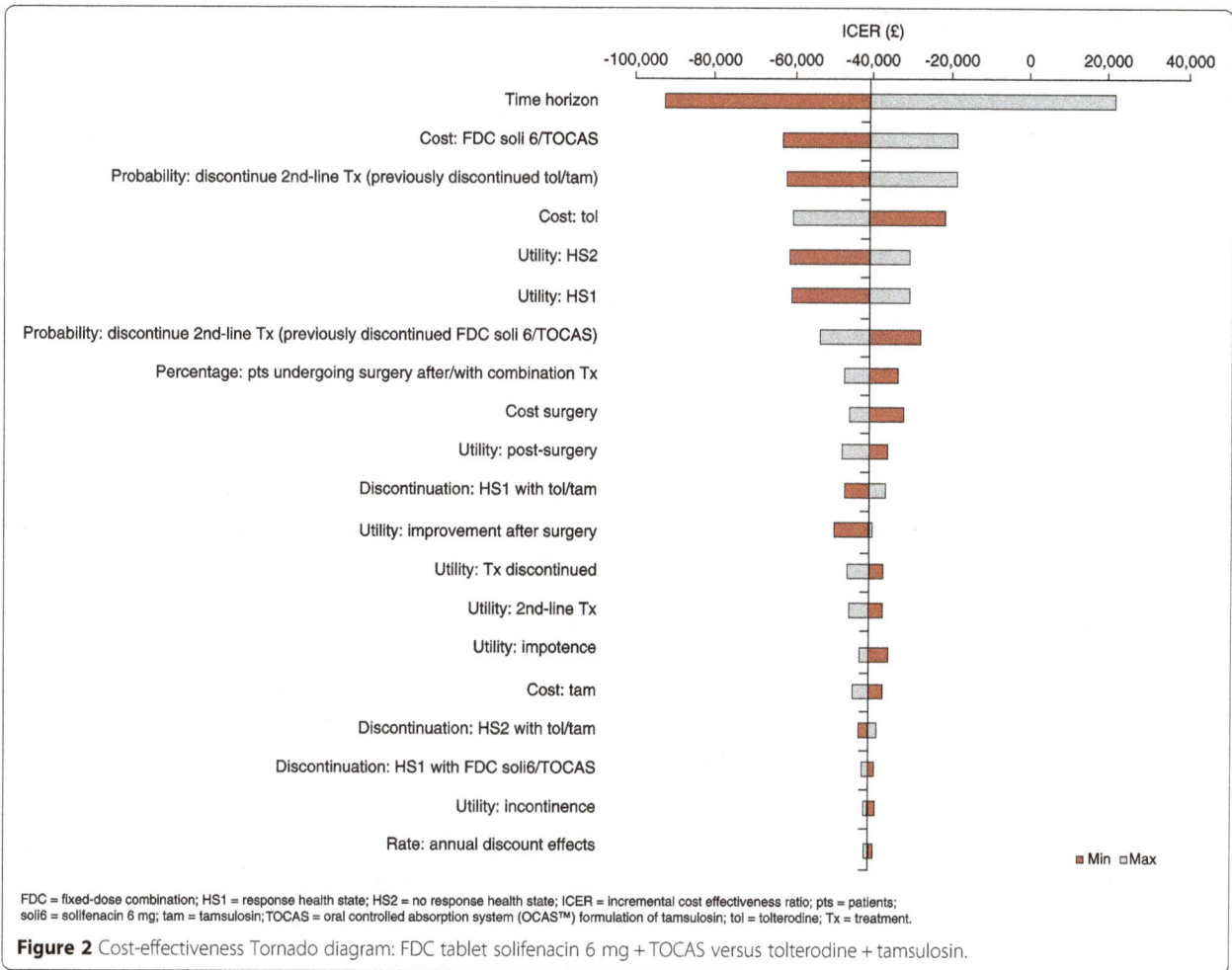

FDC = fixed-dose combination; HS1 = response health state; HS2 = no response health state; ICER = incremental cost effectiveness ratio; pts = patients; soli6 = solifenacin 6 mg; tam = tamsulosin; TOCAS = oral controlled absorption system (OCAS™) formulation of tamsulosin; tol = tolterodine; Tx = treatment.

Figure 2 Cost-effectiveness Tornado diagram: FDC tablet solifenacin 6 mg + TOCAS versus tolterodine + tamsulosin.

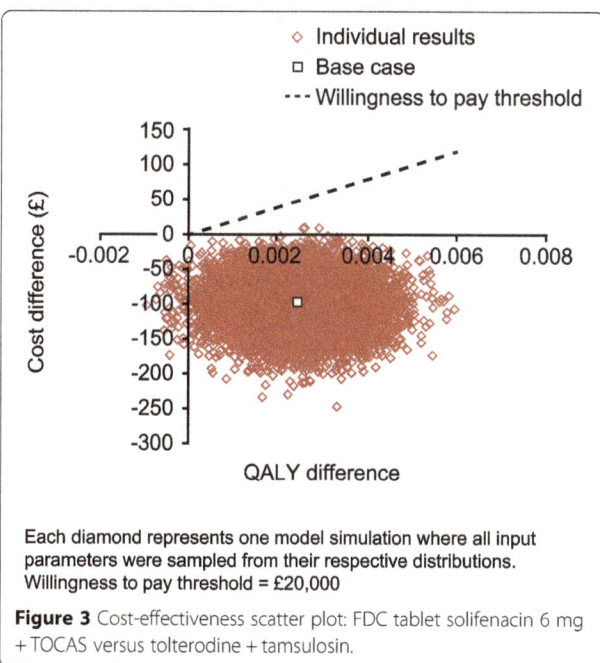

Each diamond represents one model simulation where all input parameters were sampled from their respective distributions. Willingness to pay threshold = £20,000

Figure 3 Cost-effectiveness scatter plot: FDC tablet solifenacin 6 mg + TOCAS versus tolterodine + tamsulosin.

profile compared with tolterodine [33]. Subsequently, this may contribute to the increased persistence with solifenacin, resulting in fewer patients discontinuing medication, reduced switching and/or surgery costs, and improved quality of life. This is supported by the slightly better outcomes, QALY gains and lower overall costs, reported in our analysis.

Time and quality of life utility values were also key drivers of cost-effectiveness in our model. The time horizon analysis showed that the FDC tablet of solifenacin 6 mg plus TOCAS remained dominant at the 3-year time horizon and within a generally acceptable range of cost-effectiveness for up to 10 years. The robustness of our model was also exemplified by data showing that the FDC tablet of solifenacin 6 mg plus TOCAS remained dominant when utilities were derived from both generic (EQ-5D) and disease-specific (OAB-5D) instruments. These data are underscored by the NEPTUNE study quality of life data, which reported significant improvements in International Prostate Symptom Score (IPSS) quality of life and OAB-q health-related quality of life total and coping, sleep, concern, and social subscores

Table 8 Scenario analyses: cost-effectiveness

	Discontinuation analysis		OAB-5D analysis	
	FDC tablet solifenacin 6 mg + TOCAS	Tolterodine + tamsulosin	FDC tablet solifenacin 6 mg + TOCAS	Tolterodine + tamsulosin
Total costs* (£)	860	942	860	959
Difference	–	−82	–	−99
QALYs*	0.839	0.838	0.835	0.831
Difference	–	0.0006	–	0.004
ICER*‡	–	Dominates (−£133,473)	–	Dominates (−£26,143)

*Per patient at 1 year.
‡FDC tablet solifenacin 6 mg + TOCAS versus tolterodine + tamsulosin.
FDC, fixed-dose combination; ICER, incremental cost effectiveness ratio; QALY, quality of life adjusted years; TOCAS, oral controlled absorption system (OCAS™) formulation of tamsulosin.

with FDC tablet of solifenacin 6 mg plus TOCAS compared with TOCAS monotherapy [18].

Data suggest that first-line α-blocker monotherapy may not adequately control symptoms in men with LUTS associated with BPH [12]. As such, current guidelines recommend α-blocker plus antimuscarinic combination as a treatment option for men with moderate-to-severe storage symptoms if symptom relief has been insufficient with the monotherapy of either drug [2,4]. This recommendation is supported by the results of several large randomised trials that have reported improved symptoms and quality of life with combination/add-on therapy compared with α-blocker monotherapy in patients with LUTS [14,15,17,18,34,35]. However, data from a large population-based study, THIN, indicate that α-blocker plus antimuscarinic combination treatment is used in only a small proportion (~15%) of patients with LUTS/BPH who have both storage and voiding symptoms [8]. Overall, these data suggest that there may be an unmet need in this patient population, based on the low use of combination therapy in clinical practice despite its proven effectiveness in men with LUTS/BPH who have both storage and voiding symptoms.

This *de novo* model may have some limitations. First, due to lack of published data, some assumptions were made using expert opinion only, including resource use and the proportion of patients going on to have surgery. Other key assumptions were required, for example due

to the absence of persistence data on FDCs or free combinations in LUTS, and due to there being no head-to-head studies for the combinations assessed in the present study. Additionally, the primary trials for the combination therapies evaluated in our analysis had some notable differences in the patient populations and outcome measures that prohibit an indirect treatment comparison. Patients in these trials had IPSS ≥12 or 13, ≥2 or 3 urgency episodes/24 hours and ≥8 micturitions/24 hours. In contrast to NEPTUNE, TIMES had an inclusion criterion for overactive bladder symptoms but not one for voiding symptoms. In addition, the primary efficacy endpoint in TIMES was the Perception of Treatment benefit question [36] and the secondary endpoints included bladder diary variables, and change in episodes/24 hours of urgency urinary incontinence, urgency, total micturitions and night-time micturitions. In NEPTUNE, the co-primary endpoints were total IPSS and TUFS.

Second, although the model included tamsulosin, solifenacin and tolterodine, which are commonly prescribed for men with LUTS [8], other common α-blockers (e.g. alfuzosin) and antimuscarinics (e.g. oxybutynin) were not considered in our model. Additionally, although men with LUTS may receive α-blocker or antimuscarinic monotherapy, our model was restricted to evaluation of combination treatment only. Therefore, future models will be required to compare the cost-effectiveness of

Table 9 Scenario analysis: time horizon

	FDC tablet solifenacin 6 mg + TOCAS vs tolterodine + tamsulosin			
	1 year	3 years	5 years	10 years
Cost difference* (£)	−99	26	223	404
QALY difference*	0.002	0.011	0.017	0.018
ICER*‡	Dominant (−£40,469)	£2,351	£13,531	£22,224

*Per patient.
‡FDC tablet solifenacin 6 mg + TOCAS versus tolterodine + tamsulosin.
FDC, fixed-dose combination; ICER, incremental cost effectiveness ratio; QALY, quality of life adjusted years; TOCAS, oral controlled absorption system (OCAS™) formulation of tamsulosin.

monotherapy versus combination therapy and to compare other feasible combination therapies.

Third, the model allowed treatment to be discontinued at any cycle (i.e. every 4 weeks), but switching of treatment was not allowed until 12 weeks; this cut-off is consistent with the assessment point of several recent large randomised clinical trials in LUTS [14,18]. However, it is feasible that switching could occur before Week 12 in clinical practice for tolerability, efficacy or other reasons.

Fourth, the switching and discontinuation rates applied to the model were based on data for antimuscarinics only. This was because, to our knowledge, there are no published data reporting the long-term (e.g. ≥1 year) persistence of α-blocker plus antimuscarinic combination therapy in men with LUTS/BPH.

There are a limited number of published cost-effectiveness analyses for combination treatment with α-blockers plus 5α-reductase inhibitors for men with BPH [23,37-39], but only one published report of α-blockers plus antimuscarinic combination therapy in men with LUTS [40]. The cost-effectiveness analyses in BPH found that combination treatment appears to be largely more cost effective than monotherapy [37-39]. Similarly, a secondary analysis of the TIMES study showed that tolterodine plus tamsulosin appears to be more cost-effective compared with tolterodine monotherapy (dominant) or tamsulosin monotherapy (ICER, 10,381/QALY) in patients with LUTS over a 1-year time horizon [40]. Consistent with our analysis, the higher drug acquisition costs of tolterodine plus tamsulosin were offset by the improved efficacy (postponement of surgery) and quality of life benefits with combination treatment. However, there were some differences between these two cost-effectiveness analyses of combination treatment in LUTS, including that the TIMES model did not incorporate resources associated with GP visits.

Conclusion

The FDC tablet of solifenacin 6 mg plus TOCAS has been demonstrated to significantly improve storage symptoms and quality of life compared with TOCAS alone in men with moderate-to-severe storage symptoms and voiding symptoms [18]. This analysis shows that the FDC tablet of solifenacin 6 mg plus TOCAS is also a cost-effective treatment strategy compared with tolterodine plus tamsulosin for this population of men, from the perspective of the UK NHS. Overall, these data suggest that the introduction of a FDC tablet of solifenacin 6 mg plus TOCAS offers clinical and financial benefits for management of men with LUTS/BPH who have both storage and voiding symptoms.

Abbreviations

BNF: British National Formulary; BPH: Benign prostatic hyperplasia; EQ-5D: EuroQol 5-Dimensions; ER: Extended release; FDC: Fixed-dose combination; GP: General practitioner; ICER: Incremental cost-effectiveness ratio; IPSS: International Prostate Symptom Score; LUTS: Lower urinary tract symptoms; NHS: National Health Service; NICE: National Institute for Health and Clinical Excellence; OAB: Overactive bladder; OAB-q: Overactive bladder questionnaire; OCAS™: Oral controlled absorption system; PPIUS: Patient Perception of Intensity of Urgency Scale; PSA: Probabilistic sensitivity analysis; QALYs: Quality-adjusted life years; SD: Standard deviation; THIN: The Health Improvement Network; TOCAS: Oral controlled absorption system (OCAS™) formulation of tamsulosin; TUFS: Total urgency and frequency score; TURP: Transurethral resection of the prostate; UK: United Kingdom; WTP: Willingness to pay.

Competing interests

Zalmai Hakimi is employed by Astellas Pharma Global Development and Jameel Nazir is employed by Astellas Pharma Europe Ltd. Lars Heemstra, Anke van Engen, and Cristina Ivanescu are employed by Quintiles Consulting.

Authors' contributions

All authors contributed to the design of the study, interpretation of the data, critically revised the publication for important intellectual content; and approved the final version for publication. L, A and C collected the data and performed the analyses. All authors have read and approved this manuscript.

Acknowledgements

The model was developed by Anja Prufert and Lars Heemstra from Quintiles, and was funded by Astellas Pharma Europe Ltd. Medical writing support was provided by Tyrone Daniel of Bioscript Medical, and was funded by Astellas Pharma Europe Ltd.

Author details

[1]Astellas Pharma Europe Ltd, Chertsey, UK. [2]Quintiles Consulting, Hoofddorp, Netherlands. [3]Astellas Pharma Global Development, Leiden, Netherlands.

References

1. Abrams P, Cardozo L, Fall M, Griffiths D, Rosier P, Ulmsten U, et al. The standardisation of terminology in lower urinary tract function: report from the Standardisation Sub-committee of the International Continence Society. Urology. 2003;61:37–49.
2. Gravas S, Bachmann A, Descazeaud A, Drake M, Gratzke C, Madersbacher S, et al. Guidelines on the Management of Non-Neurogenic Male Lower Urinary Tract Symptoms (LUTS), incl. Benign Prostatic Obstruction (BPO). Available at: http://uroweb.org/wp-content/uploads/Non-Neurogenic-Male-LUTS_2705.pdf. Last accessed, 20 October 2014.
3. Abrams P, Chapple C, Khoury S, Roehrborn C, de la Rosette J, International Scientific Committee. Evaluation and treatment of lower urinary tract symptoms in older men. J Urol. 2009;181:1779–87.
4. National Institute for Health and Clinical Excellence (NICE). The management of lower urinary tract symptoms in men (June 2010). Available at: https://www.nice.org.uk/guidance/cg97/resources/cg97-lower-urinary-tract-symptoms-full-guideline3. Last accessed, 20 October 2014.
5. Sexton CC, Coyne KS, Kopp ZS, Irwin DE, Milsom I, Aiyer LP, et al. The overlap of storage, voiding and postmicturition symptoms and implications for treatment seeking in the USA, UK and Sweden: EpiLUTS. BJU Int. 2009;103 Suppl 3:12–23.
6. Peters TJ, Donovan JL, Kay HE, Abrams P, de la Rosette JJ, Porru D, et al. The International Continence Society 'Benign Prostatic Hyperplasia' study: the bothersomeness of urinary symptoms. J Urol. 1997;157:885–9.

7. American Urological Association Guideline: Management of Benign Prostatic Hyperplasia (BPH) 2010. Available at: www.auanet.org/education/guidelines/benign-prostatic-hyperplasia.cfm. Last accessed, 20 October 2014.

8. Hakimi Z, Johnson M, Nazir J, Blak BT, Odeyemi IAO. Drug treatment patterns for the management of men with lower urinary tract symptoms associated with benign prostatic hyperplasia who have both storage and voiding symptoms: a study using The Health Improvement Network UK primary care data. Curr Med Res Opin. 2015;31:43–50.

9. Morant SV, Reilly K, Bloomfield GA, Chapple C. Diagnosis and treatment of lower urinary tract symptoms suggestive of overactive bladder and bladder outlet obstruction among men in general practice in the UK. Int J Clin Pract. 2008;62:688–94.

10. Chapple CR, Carter P, Christmas TJ, Kirby RS, Bryan J, Milroy EJ, et al. A three month double-blind study of doxazosin as treatment for benign prostatic bladder outlet obstruction. Br J Urol. 1994;74:50–6.

11. Abrams P, Schulman CC, Vaage S, the European Tamsulosin Study Group. Tamsulosin, a selective alpha 1c-adrenoceptor antagonist: a randomized, controlled trial in patients with benign prostatic 'obstruction' (symptomatic BPH). Br J Urol. 1995;76:325–36.

12. Lee JY, Kim HW, Lee SJ, Koh JS, Suh HJ, Chancellor MB. Comparison of doxazosin with or without tolterodine in men with symptomatic bladder outlet obstruction and an overactive bladder. BJU Int. 2004;94:817–20.

13. Yokoyama T, Uematsu K, Watanabe T, Sasaki K, Kumon H, Nagai A, et al. Naftopidil and propiverine hydrochloride for treatment of male lower urinary tract symptoms suggestive of benign prostatic hyperplasia and concomitant overactive bladder: a prospective randomized controlled study. Scand J Urol Nephrol. 2009;43:307–14.

14. Kaplan SA, Roehrborn CG, Rovner ES, Carlsson M, Bavendam T, Guan Z. Tolterodine and tamsulosin for treatment of men with lower urinary tract symptoms and overactive bladder: a randomized controlled trial. JAMA. 2006;296:2319–28.

15. Kaplan SA, McCammon K, Fincher R, Fakhoury A, He W. Safety and tolerability of solifenacin add-on therapy to alpha-blocker treated men with residual urgency and frequency. J Urol. 2009;182:2825–30.

16. Lee KS, Choo MS, Kim DY, Kim JC, Kim HJ, Min KS, et al. Combination treatment with propiverine hydrochloride plus doxazosin controlled release gastrointestinal therapeutic system formulation for overactive bladder and coexisting benign prostatic obstruction: a prospective, randomized, controlled multicenter study. J Urol. 2005;174:1334–8.

17. Chapple C, Herschorn S, Abrams P, Sun F, Brodsky M, Guan Z. Tolterodine treatment improves storage symptoms suggestive of overactive bladder in men treated with alpha-blockers. Eur Urol. 2009;56:534–41.

18. van Kerrebroeck P, Chapple C, Drogendijk T, Klaver M, Sokol R, Speakman M, et al. Combination therapy with solifenacin and tamsulosin oral controlled absorption system in a single tablet for lower urinary tract symptoms in men: efficacy and safety results from the randomised controlled NEPTUNE trial. Eur Urol. 2013;64:1003–12.

19. van Kerrebroeck P, Haab F, Angulo JC, Vik V, Katona F, Garcia-Hernandez A, et al. Efficacy and safety of solifenacin plus tamsulosin OCAS in men with voiding and storage lower urinary tract symptoms: results from a phase 2, dose-finding study (SATURN). Eur Urol. 2013;64:398–407.

20. Vesomni SPC. Available from https://www.medicines.org.uk/emc/medicine/28535. Last accessed, 20 October 2014.

21. Cartwright R, Srikrishna S, Cardozo L, Robinson D. Validity and reliability of the patient's perception of intensity of urgency scale in overactive bladder. BJU Int. 2011;107:1612–7.

22. Hakimi Z, Mathias SD, Crosby R, Odeyemi IA, Nazir J. Defining clinically meaningful changes for the patient perception of intensity of urgency scale (PPIUS) in men with lower urinary tract symptoms (LUTS) associated with benign prostatic hyperplasia (BPH). Value Health. 2013;16:PRM150.

23. DiSantostefano RL, Biddle AK, Lavelle JP. The long-term cost effectiveness of treatments for benign prostatic hyperplasia. Pharmacoeconomics. 2006;24:171–91.

24. Office for National Statistics: UK Interim Life Tables, 1980–82 to 2008–10. Available at: http://www.ons.gov.uk/ons/taxonomy/index.html?nscl=Interim+Life+Tables. Last accessed, 20 October 2014.

25. National Institute for Health and Care Excellence (NICE): Guide to the methods of technology appraisal (June 2008). Available at: http://www.nice.org.uk/article/pmg9/chapter/Foreword. Last accessed, 20 October 2014.

26. Joint Formulary Committee BNF. British National Formulary (BNF) 66. London: Pharmaceutical Press; 2013.

27. Briggs A, Sculpher M, Claxton K. Decision modelling for health economic evaluation. London: Oxford University Press; 2006.

28. Wagg A, Compion G, Fahey A, Siddiqui E. Persistence with prescribed antimuscarinic therapy for overactive bladder: a UK experience. BJU Int. 2012;110:1767–74.

29. Kanis JA, Cooper C, Hiligsmann M, Rabenda V, Reginster JY, Rizzoli R. Partial adherence: a new perspective on health economic assessment in osteoporosis. Osteoporos Int. 2011;22:2565–73.

30. Hughes DA, Dubois D. Cost-effectiveness analysis of extended-release formulations of oxybutynin and tolterodine for the management of urge incontinence. Pharmacoeconomics. 2004;22:1047–59.

31. Hughes D, Cowell W, Koncz T, Cramer J, International Society for Pharmacoeconomics & Outcomes Research Economics of Medication Compliance Working Group. Methods for integrating medication compliance and persistence in pharmacoeconomic evaluations. Value Health. 2007;10:498–509.

32. Hiligsmann M, Boonen A, Rabenda V, Reginster JY. The importance of integrating medication adherence into pharmacoeconomic analyses: the example of osteoporosis. Expert Rev Pharmacoecon Outcomes Res. 2012;12:159–66.

33. Madhuvrata P, Cody JD, Ellis G, Herbison GP, Hay-Smith EJ. Which anticholinergic drug for overactive bladder symptoms in adults. Cochrane Database Syst Rev. 2012;1:CD005429. doi: 10.1002/14651858.CD005429.pub2.

34. Kaplan SA, Roehrborn CG, Gong J, Sun F, Guan Z. Add-on fesoterodine for residual storage symptoms suggestive of overactive bladder in men receiving α-blocker treatment for lower urinary tract symptoms. BJU Int. 2012;109:1831–40.

35. Yamaguchi O, Kakizaki H, Homma Y, Takeda M, Nishizawa O, Gotoh M, et al. Solifenacin as add-on therapy for overactive bladder symptoms in men treated for lower urinary tract symptoms – ASSIST, randomized controlled study. Urology. 2011;78:126–33.

36. Pleil AM, Coyne KS, Reese PR, Jumadilova Z, Rovner ES, Kelleher CJ. The validation of patient-rated global assessments of treatment benefit, satisfaction, and willingness to continue¯the BSW. Value Health. 2005;8 Suppl 1:S25–34.

37. Ismaila A, Walker A, Sayani A, Laroche B, Nickel JC, Posnett J, et al. Cost-effectiveness of dutasteride-tamsulosin combination therapy for the treatment of symptomatic benign prostatic hyperplasia: a Canadian model based on the CombAT trial. Can Urol Assoc J. 2013;7:E393–401.

38. Walker A, Doyle S, Posnett J, Hunjan M. Cost-effectiveness of single-dose tamsulosin and dutasteride combination therapy compared with tamsulosin monotherapy in patients with benign prostatic hyperplasia in the UK. BJU Int. 2013;112:638–46.

39. Bjerklund Johansen TE, Baker TM, Black LK. Cost-effectiveness of combination therapy for treatment of benign prostatic hyperplasia: a model based on the findings of the combination of avodart and tamsulosin trial. BJU Int. 2012;109:731–8.

40. Verheggen BG, Lee R, Lieuw On MM, Treur MJ, Botteman MF, Kaplan SA, et al. Estimating the quality-of-life impact and cost-effectiveness of alpha-blocker and anti-muscarinic combination treatment in men with lower urinary tract symptoms related to benign prostatic hyperplasia and overactive bladder. J Med Econ. 2012;15:586–600.

41. Personal Social Services Research Unit (PSSRU). Unit Costs of Health and Social Care (2013) University of Kent. Compiled by Lesley Curtis. Available at: http://www.pssru.ac.uk/project-pages/unit-costs/2013/#sections. Last accessed, 20 October 2014.

42. National Health Service (NHS) Reference costs (2012). Available at: http://www.dh.gov.uk/prod_consum_dh/groups/dh_digitalassets/@dh/@en/documents/digitalasset/dh_133578.xls. Last accessed, 20 October 2014.

43. Antoñanzas F, Brenes F, Molero JM, Fernández-Pro A, Huerta A, Palencia R, et al. [Cost-effectiveness of the combination therapy of dutasteride and tamsulosin in the treatment of benign prostatic hyperlasia in Spain]. Actas Urol Esp. 2011;35:65–71.

44. National Institute for Health and Care Excellence (NICE). Pathways for lower urinary tract symptoms in men. Available at: http://pathways.nice.org.uk/pathways/lower-urinary-tract-symptoms-in-men#content=view-node%3Anodes-drug-treatment. Last accessed, 20 October 2014.

45. Kopp RP, Freedland SJ, Parsons JK. Associations of benign prostatic hyperplasia with prostate cancer: the debate continues. Eur Urol. 2011;60:699–700.

46. Ørsted DD, Bojesen SE, Nielsen SF, Nordestgaard BG. Association of clinical benign prostate hyperplasia with prostate cancer incidence and mortality revisited: a nationwide cohort study of 3,009,258 men. Eur Urol. 2011;60:691–8.

11

Prostatic artery embolization versus conventional TUR-P in the treatment of benign prostatic hyperplasia: protocol for a prospective randomized non-inferiority trial

Dominik Abt[1*†], Livio Mordasini[1†], Lukas Hechelhammer[2], Thomas M Kessler[3], Hans-Peter Schmid[1] and Daniel S Engeler[1]

Abstract

Background: Benign prostatic hyperplasia (BPH) is a prevalent entity in elderly men and transurethral resection of the prostate (TURP) still represents the gold standard of surgical treatment despite its considerable perioperative morbidity. Recently, prostatic artery embolization (PAE) was described as a novel effective and less invasive treatment alternative. Despite promising first results, PAE still has to be considered experimental due to a lack of good quality studies. Prospective randomized controlled trials comparing PAE with TUR-P are highly warranted.

Methods/design: This is a single-centre, prospective, randomized, non-inferiority trial comparing treatment effects and adverse events of PAE and TURP in a tertiary referral centre. One hundred patients who are electable for both treatment options are randomized to either PAE or TURP. Changes of the International Prostate Symptom Score (IPSS) after 3 months are defined as primary endpoint. Changes in bladder diaries, laboratory analyses, urodynamic investigations and standardised questionnaires are assessed as secondary outcome measures. In addition contrast-enhanced magnetic resonance imaging of the pelvis before and after the interventions will provide crucial information regarding morphological changes and vascularisation of the prostate. Adverse events will be assessed on every follow-up visit in both treatment arms according to the National Cancer Institute Common Terminology Criteria for Adverse events and the Clavien classification.

Discussion: The aim of this study is to assess whether PAE represents a valid treatment alternative to TURP in patients suffering from BPH in terms of efficacy and safety.

Keywords: Prostate, Benign prostatic hyperplasia, Transurethral resection of the prostate, Embolization, Prostatic artery embolization, Comparative clinical trial

Background

Benign prostatic hyperplasia (BPH) is a prevalent entity, affecting over 50% of men older than 60 years [1]. The clinical picture of the disease includes lower urinary tract symptoms such as interrupted and weak urinary stream, nocturia, urgency and leaking and even

sexual dysfunction in some individuals [2]. Medical therapy is usually the first-line treatment [3]. However, the efficacy of drugs like alpha-blockers is limited, and as disease progresses more invasive treatment options have to be taken into consideration.

In cases with moderate to severe lower urinary tract symptoms transurethral resection of the prostate (TURP) is still the standard treatment. TURP, however, is limited to prostates smaller than 60-80 ml and the procedure is associated with a substantial complication rate. The cumulative short-term morbidity rate is around 11% and

* Correspondence: dominik01.abt@kssg.ch

†Equal contributors

[1]Department of Urology, Cantonal Hospital St. Gallen, Rorschacherstrasse 95, St. Gallen 9007, Switzerland

Full list of author information is available at the end of the article

the necessity for surgical revision is as high as 6%. Bleeding requiring transfusions and transurethral resection syndrome represent potentially serious threats to elderly and frail patients [4]. Prostatic artery embolization (PAE) has been suggested as a minimal invasive alternative procedure, which can be performed in an outpatient setting with rapid recovery and low morbidity [5,6].

PAE was first described in 1979 by Lang et al. [7] as a treatment option in intractable prostatogenic haemorrhage and emerged as a safe and effective treatment thanks to technical refinements throughout the last decades. Using PAE in this purpose, DeMeritt et al. were the first to report on relief of BPH-related bladder outlet obstruction after transarterial polyvinyl alcohol prostate embolization in 2000 [8].

First intentional treatment of BPH by PAE was published in 2008 [9]. Subsequently, promising short- and medium-term results could be shown for patients with symptomatic BPH, refractory to medical treatment: A significant improvement in the International Prostate Symptom Score (IPSS) and maximum urinary flow rate, as well as a reduction of prostate volume and post-void residual urine were reported in several studies [10-13]. Methods and technique to perform PAE are well established and have been described in several publications [14,15]. PAE was shown to be a safe procedure with low morbidity in carefully selected patients [16,17].

However, data concerning PAE has been criticized for different reasons: There is just a small number of studies published by only three research groups with an unclear overlap of the patients that were described so far. Moreover, quality of the studies available was referred to be poor due to study type (cohort), unclear patient selections and dropouts as well as statistical limitations and missing long-term results [17].

Currently, only a single trial was published comparing TURP and PAE: Gao et al. report on promising results of PAE with a post-interventional course outshining the data published so far [18]. This study, however, was devoted little attention most likely due to ambiguities regarding patient selection and good clinical practice issues. TURP still remains clearly the gold standard in surgical treatment of BPH and a prospective randomized trial according to good clinical practice (GCP) comparing PAE and TURP is mandatory, to assess efficacy and safety of PAE in the treatment of BPH.

Methods and design
Study design and location
This is a prospective, randomized, non-inferiority trial conducted at the urological and radiological departments of Cantonal Hospital St. Gallen, St. Gallen, Switzerland.

Study population and recruitment
Recruitment of the study participants is performed at the urological outpatient clinic of Cantonal Hospital St. Gallen by the principle investigator (PI). The PI will check for inclusion and exclusion criteria (Table 1) by reviewing the patient's medical record and by patient-doctor conversation. Study participants are thoroughly informed about the study by the study physician. Possible questions are answered by the PI. If the patient feels well informed and confident to participate in the trial, informed consent can be given within the consultation. If the patient needs further time for consideration, an additional appointment in the outpatient clinic will be arranged within the next 2–3 weeks. Anyway, the patient has got at least 2–3 weeks till admission to the hospital to get clear on study participation and is able to ask further questions at the day of admission.

Study randomisation
Randomisation will be performed using SecuTrial (InterActive Systems GmbH, Berlin, Germany) stratifying on age (<70, ≥70 years) and prostate volume (<50 ml, ≥50 ml).

Study procedures
After baseline visit participants are randomized to TURP or embolisation (Figure 1). Both interventions are performed in an inpatient setting. All subjects receive perioperative antibiotic prophylaxis started one day before procedure and continued for one day after catheter removal (Ciprofloxacin 500 mg twice daily, except infection with different resistance profile was proved before). Moreover, anti-inflammatory (Diclofenac 75 mg twice

Table 1 Inclusion and exclusion criteria

Inclusion criteria	Exclusion criteria
• Men older than 40	• Severe atherosclerosis
• Patient must be a candidate for TURP	• Severe tortuosity in the aortic bifurcation or internal iliac arteries
• Refractory to medical therapy or patient is not willing to consider (further) medical treatment	• Acontractile detrusor
• Patient has a prostate size of at least 25 ml and not more than 80 ml, measured by ultrasound	• Neurogenic lower urinary tract dysfunction
• IPSS ≥8	• Urethral stenosis
• QoL ≥3	• Bladder diverticulum
• Qmax < 12 and/or urinary retention	• Bladder stone with surgical indication
• Written informed consent	• Allergy to intravenous contrast media
	• Contraindication for MRI imaging
	• Preinterventionally proven adenocarcinoma of the prostate
	• Renal failure (GFR < 60 ml/min)

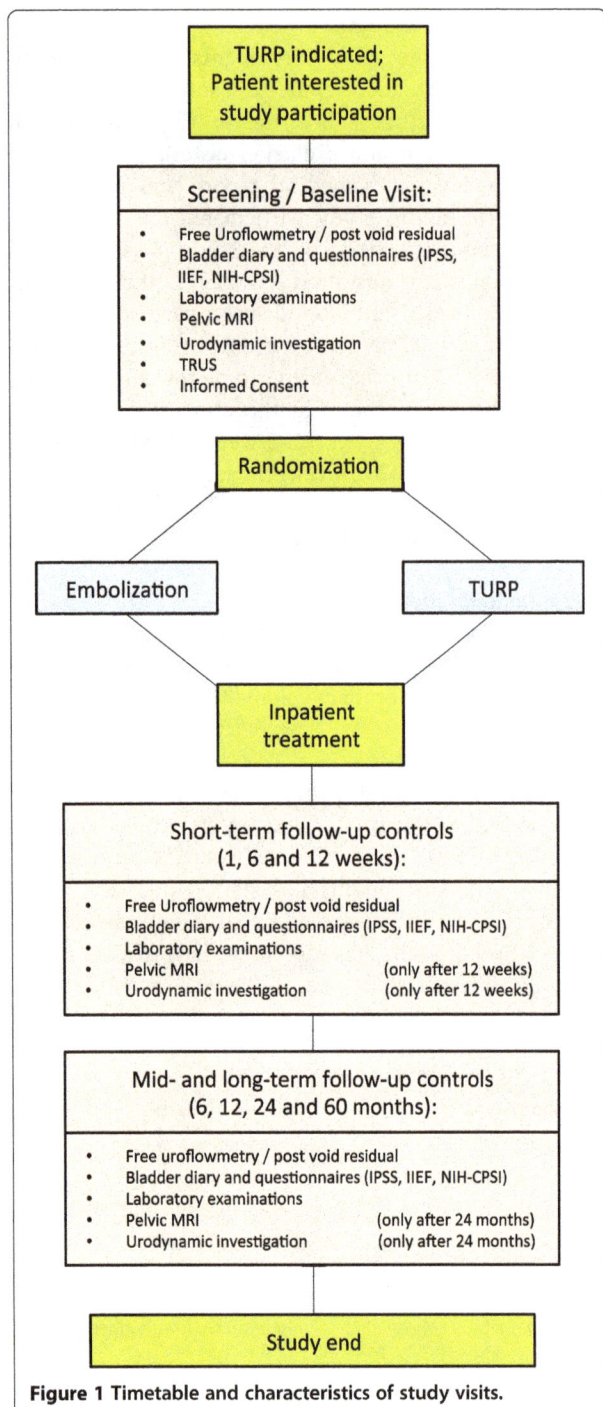

Figure 1 Timetable and characteristics of study visits.

power of 60 W is used. A standard tungsten wire loop (Karl Storz Endoskope; Anklin AG, Binnigen, Switzerland) and electrolyte-free mannitol-sorbitol solution (Purisole, Fresenius Kabi AG, Bad Homburg, Germany) will be used for TURP. Surgery will be performed under spinal or general anaesthesia according to patient's and anaesthetist's preferences by one of the physicians involved into the study (LM, DA, HPS, DSE). A 20 F three-way catheter is inserted for irrigation after resection and left for at least two days depending on bleeding tendency.

PAE

A 16 F transurethral catheter is inserted prior to intervention for better radiological orientation. After local anaesthesia, a unilateral femoral sheath is placed (normally the right common femoral artery) and the patient will have a selective internal iliac arteriogram of the anterior division of both internal iliac arteries by a 5 F catheter to identify the prostatic arterial supply. In special anatomical variants, arteriograms of the external iliac and their branches will be performed. The prostatic vessels, which can derive from every branch of the anterior division, will be selectively catheterized with a 2–3 F micro catheter and subsequent embolization will be performed with 250-400 μm sized Embozene Microspheres (Celonova, San Antonio, TX). The embolization endpoint will be absence of perfusion of the prostate on post embolization angiography and stasis of flow in the prostate arteries. This procedure is performed on both sides whenever possible. Embolization will only be performed by a single interventional radiologist (LH). Transurethral catheter is removed on the first morning after intervention.

Study outcome measures
Characteristics and timing of visits
Regular follow-up controls starting one week after intervention and continued up to 5 years will be performed, assessing the parameters described in Figure 1.

Primary and secondary endpoints
Change of International Prostate Symptom Score (IPSS) 3 months after intervention was defined as primary endpoint. Secondary study endpoints are shown in Table 2.

Statistics, study sample size and power calculation
For the primary endpoint, changes in IPSS at 12 weeks will be compared using a one-sided t-test with significance level 0.025 (equivalent to using the boundaries from a 95% confidence interval (CI)). As long as the t-test is not significant (that is, the 95% CI is entirely above −3), PAE will be considered non-inferior to TURP. A second analysis of the primary endpoint will be adjusted for IPSS at baseline (using linear regression), and

daily) and acid-suppressing medication (Pantoprazole 40 mg once daily) is administered for 1 week starting at the day of intervention. Prostatic medication is abandoned at the day of TURP and 2 weeks after PAE (due to supposed slower efficacy).

TURP
For monopolar transurethral resection, a 24 F Storz resectoscope with a cutting power of 150 W and a coagulation

Table 2 Primary and secondary endpoints

Primary endpoint	• Changes in the IPSS 12 weeks after intervention
Secondary endpoints (see Figure 1 for time points)	
	• Changes in free uroflowmetry and post-void residual
	• Changes in bladder diary
	• Changes in urodynamic investigation
	• Changes in IPSS, CPSI and IIEF
	• Changes of haemoglobin and serum PSA
	• Duration of post procedure catheterisation and hospitalisation
	• Procedure time and radiation parameters
	• Changes of prostate volume, measure of devascularized/resected tissue using MRI
	• Comparison of prostate size, measured preoperatively by TRUS and MRI at baseline

therefore an adjusted confidence interval will also be reported.

Mean differences and corresponding 95% CI will be reported for all secondary endpoints, as well as the p-value from a one-sided t-test. Where an endpoint is clearly not normally distributed, results from a one-sided Mann–Whitney U-test will be substituted. Changes over time will be compared pairwise in the same fashion.

In a study performed at our own institute [19], the standard deviation for IPSS was 4.6. A one-sided t-test with one-sided significance level 0.025 will have 80% power to reject the null hypothesis that the two treatments are not equivalent (that is, the difference in means is −3 or further from zero in the same direction), assuming the expected difference is 0 and the common standard deviation is 4.6, when the sample size is 38 patients in each group. Assuming a dropout rate of 20%, we aim to recruit 100 patients total.

Regulatory issues
Ethical approval
Study was approved by the local ethics committees (EKSG 14/004) and is performed in consideration of the World Medical Association Declaration of Helsinki [20], the guidelines for GCP [21], and the guidelines of the Swiss Academy of Medical Sciences [22]. Handling of all personal data will strictly comply with the federal law of data protection in Switzerland [23].

Quality control, quality assurance and confidentiality
An expert of Clinical Trials Unit (CTU) St. Gallen conducts data monitoring according to GCP. Trial-related

monitoring, audits and regulatory inspections from the ethics committee (EKSG) will be permitted by the principal investigator, providing direct access to source documents. Data collection is performed using electronic case report forms (SecuTrial) programmed by CTU St. Gallen. The respect of the professional secrecy is guaranteed. Insight into the data collected in this trial will only be provided to the involved investigators, the members of the ethics committee experts responsible for the monitoring.

Missing data
Patients will be included in the primary analysis of the primary endpoint, provided that baseline and 12 week IPSS measurements are available. For all other analyses, all collected data will be analyzed.

Safety
All adverse events (AE) and serious adverse events (SAE) which might be related to the study procedures are collected, fully investigated and documented during the entire study period. Assessment of severity of all AEs will be performed according to National Cancer Institute Common Terminology Criteria for Adverse Events v4.0 (CTCAE) and according to the Clavien classification [24]. All SAEs related to study intervention, are reported to the local Ethics Committee. All AEs and SAEs will be followed as long as medically indicated.

Discussion
The aim of this study is to assess whether PAE is a valuable treatment option compared to TURP in patients with BPH, assessing both, short- and long-term treatment effects as well as complications. Using a prospective, randomized, non-inferiority trial design with clearly defined endpoints, as well as inclusion and exclusion criteria and performed according to well-defined quality standards, data will help to estimate treatment efficiency of PAE better. Moreover, potential advantages as well as problems of this emerging intervention can be analysed. The study might also help to define patients that are particularly suitable for PAE and patients that should be treated alternatively. In addition, magnetic resonance imaging performed at different time intervals to intervention might help to get a better understanding of the underlying mechanisms.

Trial status
The trial is in the recruiting phase at the time of manuscript submission.

Abbreviations
BPH: Benign prostate hyperplasia; CI: Confidence interval; GCP: Good clinical practice; IIEF: International index of erectile function; IPSS: International prostate symptom score; MRI: Magnetic resonance imaging; NIH-CPSI: National institute of health – chronic prostatitis symptoms score; PAE: Prostatic artery embolization; PI: Principle investigator; PSA: Prostate

specific antigen; TURP: Transurethral resection of the prostate;
TRUS: Transrectal ultrasound.

Competing interests
The authors declare that they have no competing interests.

Authors' contributions
All authors participated in creating the study design. DA and LM drafted the manuscript. LH, TMK, HPS, and DE provided a critical revision of the manuscript. LM, DA, DE and HPS obtained the funding of this study. All the authors read and approved the final manuscript.

Acknowledgements
We would like to acknowledge Clinical Trials Unit St. Gallen for technical and financial support. Sarah Haile PhD performed the statistical analysis.

Funding
The study is funded by a grant from the CTU commission of Kantonsspital St. Gallen (Nr. 14/08).

Author details
[1]Department of Urology, Cantonal Hospital St. Gallen, Rorschacherstrasse 95, St. Gallen 9007, Switzerland. [2]Department of Radiology and Nuclear Medicine, Cantonal Hospital St. Gallen, Rorschacherstrasse 95, St. Gallen 9007, Switzerland. [3]Neuro-Urology, Spinal Cord Injury Centre & Research, University of Zürich, Balgrist University Hospital, Forchstrasse 340, Zürich 8008, Switzerland.

References
1. Levy A, Samraj GP: Benign prostatic hyperplasia: when to 'watch and wait', when and how to treat. *Cleve Clin J Med* 2007, 74(Suppl 3):S15–S20.
2. Eckhardt MD, Van Venrooij GE, Van Melick HH, Boon TA: Prevalence and bothersomeness of lower urinary tract symptoms in benign prostatic hyperplasia and their impact on well-being. *J Urol* 2001, 166(2):563–568.
3. Michel MC, Mehlburger L, Bressel HU, Schumacher H, Schafers RF, Goepel M: Tamsulosin treatment of 19,365 patients with lower urinary tract symptoms: does co-morbidity alter tolerability? *J Urol* 1998, 160(3 Pt 1):784–791.
4. Reich O, Gratzke C, Bachmann A, Seitz M, Schlenker B, Hermanek P, Lack N, Stief CG: Morbidity, mortality and early outcome of transurethral resection of the prostate: a prospective multicenter evaluation of 10,654 patients. *J Urol* 2008, 180(1):246–249.
5. Sun F, Sanchez FM, Crisostomo V, Lima JR, Luis L, Garcia-Martinez V, Lopez-Sanchez C, Uson J, Maynar M: Benign prostatic hyperplasia: transcatheter arterial embolization as potential treatment–preliminary study in pigs. *Radiology* 2008, 246(3):783–789.
6. Jeon GS, Won JH, Lee BM, Kim JH, Ahn HS, Lee EJ, Park SI, Park SW: The effect of transarterial prostate embolization in hormone-induced benign prostatic hyperplasia in dogs: a pilot study. *J Vasc Interv Radiol* 2009, 20(3):384–390.
7. Lang EK, Deutsch JS, Goodman JR, Barnett TF, Lanasa JA Jr, Duplessis GH: Transcatheter embolization of hypogastric branch arteries in the management of intractable bladder hemorrhage. *J Urol* 1979, 121(1):30–36.
8. DeMeritt JS, Elmasri FF, Esposito MP, Rosenberg GS: Relief of benign prostatic hyperplasia-related bladder outlet obstruction after transarterial polyvinyl alcohol prostate embolization. *J Vasc Interv Radiol* 2000, 11(6):767–770.
9. Carnevale FC, Antunes AA, Da Motta Leal Filho JM, De Oliveira Cerri LM, Baroni RH, Marcelino AS, Freire GC, Moreira AM, Srougi M, Cerri GG: Prostatic artery embolization as a primary treatment for benign prostatic hyperplasia: preliminary results in two patients. *Cardiovasc Intervent Radiol* 2010, 33(2):355–361.
10. Rio Tinto H, Martins Pisco J, Bilhim T, Duarte M, Fernandes L, Pereira J, Campos Pinheiro L: Prostatic artery embolization in the treatment of benign prostatic hyperplasia: short and medium follow-up. *Tech Vasc Interv Radiol* 2012, 15(4):290–293.
11. Carnevale FC, Da Motta-Leal-Filho JM, Antunes AA, Baroni RH, Marcelino AS, Cerri LM, Yoshinaga EM, Cerri GG, Srougi M: Quality of life and clinical symptom improvement support prostatic artery embolization for patients with acute urinary retention caused by benign prostatic hyperplasia. *J Vasc Interv Radiol* 2013, 24(4):535–542.
12. Kurbatov D, Russo GI, Lepetukhin A, Dubsky S, Sitkin I, Morgia G, Rozhivanov R, Cimino S, Sansalone S: Prostatic artery embolization for prostate volume greater than 80 cm(3): results from a single-center prospective study. *Urology* 2014, 84(2):400–404.
13. Bilhim T, Pisco J, Campos Pinheiro L, Rio Tinto H, Fernandes L, Pereira JA, Duarte M, Oliveira AG: Does polyvinyl alcohol particle size change the outcome of prostatic arterial embolization for benign prostatic hyperplasia? Results from a single-center randomized prospective study. *J Vasc Interv Radiol* 2013, 24(11):1595–1602 e1591.
14. Martins Pisco J, Pereira J, Rio Tinto H, Fernandes L, Bilhim T: How to perform prostatic arterial embolization. *Tech Vasc Interv Radiol* 2012, 15(4):286–289.
15. Carnevale FC, Antunes AA: Prostatic artery embolization for enlarged prostates due to benign prostatic hyperplasia. How I do it. *Cardiovasc Intervent Radiol* 2013, 36(6):1452–1463.
16. AP J, Bilhim T, Duarte M, Rio Tinto H, Fernandes L, Martins Pisco J: Patient selection and counseling before prostatic arterial embolization. *Tech Vasc Interv Radiol* 2012, 15(4):270–275.
17. Schreuder SM, Scholtens AE, Reekers JA, Bipat S: The role of prostatic arterial embolization in patients with benign prostatic hyperplasia: a systematic review. *Cardiovasc Intervent Radiol* 2014, 37(5):1198–1219. doi:10.1007/s00270-014-0948-4. Epub 2014 Jul 9. PMID.
18. Gao YA, Huang Y, Zhang R, Yang YD, Zhang Q, Hou M, Wang Y: Benign prostatic hyperplasia: prostatic arterial embolization versus transurethral resection of the prostate–a prospective, randomized, and controlled clinical trial. *Radiology* 2014, 270(3):920–928.
19. Engeler DS, Schwab C, Neyer M, Grun T, Reissigl A, Schmid HP: Bipolar versus monopolar TURP: a prospective controlled study at two urology centers. *Prostate Cancer Prostatic Dis* 2010, 13(3):285–291.
20. World Medical Association: *Declaration of Helsinki - ethical principles for medical research involving human subjects.* 1964. http://www.wma.net/en/30publications/10policies/b3/.
21. *International conference on harmonisation: Good clinical practice guideline.* http://www.ich.org/products/guidelines/efficacy/article/efficacyguidelines.html
22. Swiss Academy of Medical Sciences: *Guideline - concerning scientific research involving human beings.* 2009. http://www.samw.ch/dms/en/Publications/Guidelines/e_Leitfaden_Forschung_def.pdf
23. The Federal Authorities of the Swiss Confederation: *Bundesgesetz über den Datenschutz (DSG) vom 19. Juni 1992, Stand. 01.01.2014.* 1992. http://www.admin.ch/opc/de/classified-compilation/19920153/201401010000/235.1.pdf
24. Dindo D, Demartines N, Clavien PA: Classification of surgical complications: a new proposal with evaluation in a cohort of 6336 patients and results of a survey. *Ann Surg* 2004, 240(2):205–213.

12

A retrospective study of treatment persistence and adherence to α-blocker plus antimuscarinic combination therapies, in men with LUTS/BPH in the Netherlands

Marcus J. Drake[1]* [iD], Sally Bowditch[2], Emilio Arbe[2], Zalmai Hakimi[3], Florent Guelfucci[4], Ikbel Amri[5] and Jameel Nazir[2]

Abstract

Background: To assess treatment persistence and adherence in men ≥45 years of age with lower urinary tract symptoms (LUTS) associated with benign prostatic hyperplasia (BPH), using prescription records from the Netherlands IMS Lifelink™ LRx database.

Methods: In this retrospective, observational cohort study, we identified men who received combination therapy with an α-blocker plus an antimuscarinic (e.g. solifenacin or tolterodine) between 1 November 2013 and 31 October 2014. Treatment could be received as a fixed-dose combination (FDC) tablet or as two drugs administered together (concomitant therapy), if both combination drugs were prescribed within 30 days. The primary objective was to assess treatment persistence, defined as the time from initiation of combination therapy until first discontinuation of the FDC or at least one of the drugs given concomitantly (i.e. ≥30 days without prescription renewal). Subgroup and sensitivity analyses were conducted to assess persistence by antimuscarinic agent, and with different gap lengths used to define discontinuation (45, 60 and 90 days), respectively.

Results: A total of 1891 men received an α-blocker plus an antimuscarinic (FDC, N = 665; concomitant therapy, N = 1226). Median time to discontinuation was significantly longer with FDC versus concomitant therapy (414 vs. 112 days; adjusted hazard ratio [HR] 2.04, 95% confidence interval 1.77, 2.35; p < 0.0001). Persistence at 12 months (51.3% vs. 29.9%) was also significantly greater with FDC compared with concomitant therapy. Assessment of antimuscarinic subgroups showed that median time to discontinuation was longest with solifenacin combinations (214 days) compared with other antimuscarinic combinations (range, 47–164 days; adjusted HR range, 1.27–1.77, p = 0.037). No observable impact on treatment persistence was found by adjusting the gaps used to define discontinuation.

Discussion: This study of real-world evidence of men with LUTS/BPH treated with α-blocker plus antimuscarinic combination therapy in the Netherlands showed that treatment persistence was significantly greater in those who received a FDC tablet compared with combination therapy given concomitantly. The study also shows that treatment persistence was extended in men who received combination therapy containing solifenacin compared with other antimuscarinics.

Conclusions: Overall, these findings may be useful for prescribers, as improved persistence on-treatment may translate into improved outcomes for men with LUTS/BPH. Further study is warranted to establish the key drivers of persistence in men receiving combination therapy for LUTS/BPH.

Keywords: α-blocker, Antimuscarinic, Fixed-dose combination, LUTS/BPH, Treatment persistence

* Correspondence: marcus.drake@bui.ac.uk
[1]Bristol Urological Institute and the School of Clinical Sciences, University of Bristol, Bristol, UK
Full list of author information is available at the end of the article

Background

Lower urinary tract symptoms (LUTS) are most common in the ageing male population, with troublesome LUTS occurring in 30% of men over 65 years of age [1]. LUTS can be divided into voiding, storage and post-micturition symptoms [2]. Although the treatment of LUTS tends to focus on voiding symptoms [1, 2], men typically report storage symptoms (e.g. increased frequency, urgency and nocturia [1, 2]) as the most bothersome [3, 4].

LUTS are commonly associated with benign prostatic hyperplasia (BPH), i.e. LUTS/BPH [1]; together, these conditions have been shown to have a significant impact on men's health-related quality of life and daily activities [5]. Current European recommendations for treatment of LUTS include the use of lifestyle interventions, and pharmacological therapies when these interventions are inappropriate or unsuccessful (i.e. in men with moderate-to-severe LUTS) [2]. Pharmacological treatment options include α-blockers, antimuscarinics and 5α-reductase inhibitors (5-ARIs), which can either be used as monotherapy or in combination, and recent evidence suggests that the use of pharmacological treatments for LUTS/BPH is increasing in some healthcare systems, particularly as combination therapy [6]. The European recommendations suggest different indications for combination therapy, i.e. α-blocker plus an antimuscarinic if relief of storage symptoms has been insufficient with monotherapy of either drug; and α-blocker plus a 5-ARI in men with a substantially enlarged prostate (those more likely to experience disease progression) [2].

Combination therapies can be administered separately (i.e. as concomitant therapy), or as a fixed-dose combination (FDC) in a single tablet. Several randomised, double-blinded trials conducted in men >40 years of age with LUTS/BPH and overactive bladder (OAB) symptoms have demonstrated improved efficacy in those who received α-blocker plus antimuscarinic combination therapy concomitantly compared with monotherapy [7–10]. With regards to FDCs, a randomised, double-blind, multicentre, phase III study of 1690 men ≥45 years of age with moderate-to-severe LUTS/BPH (NEPTUNE; Clinicaltrials.gov identifier: NCT01018511), demonstrated that a FDC of solifenacin 6 mg plus tamsulosin oral controlled absorption system (TOCAS, 0.4 mg) significantly improved voiding and storage symptoms versus placebo, and storage symptoms versus TOCAS alone [11]. The FDC tablet of solifenacin 6 mg plus TOCAS is approved for the treatment of men with moderate-to-severe LUTS/BPH in Europe [12] and was first authorised for marketing in the Netherlands in May 2013 [13]. A FDC of dutasteride and tamsulosin is approved for use in Europe, but only for men with LUTS and an enlarged prostate [14].

Despite the improvements in symptoms of LUTS/BPH, treatment persistence (i.e. the duration from initiation to discontinuation of therapy [15]) and adherence (i.e. the extent to which a patient acts in accordance with the prescribed interval, and dose of a dosing regimen [15]) are reported to be low in men with LUTS/BPH. An observational study of 8694 men ≥45 years of age with LUTS/BPH conducted in the United Kingdom (UK) showed that 38.5% and 53.0% of men discontinued α-blocker and antimuscarinic therapy, respectively, over a median duration of 2.1 years' treatment [16]; and a retrospective study of 670 men with LUTS/BPH in Korea found that approximately two-thirds of men discontinued an α-blocker, a 5-ARI, or both treatments in combination within 1 year of starting treatment) [17]. In the latter study, adverse events (AEs) were among the most common reasons for discontinuation and for switching of treatment.

Overall, there are limited published data regarding treatment patterns in men receiving combination therapy for LUTS/BPH in routine clinical practice. The aims of this study were to assess treatment persistence and adherence with α-blocker plus antimuscarinic combination therapy in men with LUTS/BPH, and compare these endpoints with treatment administered either as a FDC or combination therapy given concomitantly.

Methods
Study design

This was a retrospective, observational cohort study of men with LUTS/BPH who received prescription(s) for combination therapy with an α-blocker plus an antimuscarinic or a 5-ARI. Anonymised patient longitudinal prescription records and demographic data were extracted from the Netherlands IMS LifeLink™ LRx database, which consists of data from pharmacies and dispensing general practitioners (GPs) in the Netherlands (total sample is representative of around 16.5 million people).

The primary objective of the study was to assess treatment persistence in men who received α-blocker plus antimuscarinic combination therapy when prescribed as a FDC, compared with prescriptions of separate combination drugs (concomitant therapy). Adherence was also assessed in these two comparative groups as a secondary objective. Other secondary objectives included: comparing treatment persistence with an α-blocker plus an antimuscarinic combination therapy in subgroups defined by the antimuscarinic drug prescribed; and determining the impact of patient/clinical characteristics associated with persistence to combination therapy. Exploratory objectives were to determine the proportion of men who switched combination therapy (described below); and to compare treatment persistence and adherence in men prescribed with any FDC versus any concomitant therapy (α-blocker plus antimuscarinic or 5-ARI for both types).

Study population

Men ≥45 years of age were treated with combination therapy of an α-blocker plus an antimuscarinic or 5-ARI, prescribed either as a FDC or concomitantly (see Additional file 1: Table S1 for eligible drugs). Combination therapy had to be first prescribed between 1 November 2013 and 31 October 2014 (i.e. the selection period) (Additional file 2: Figure S1), prescriptions had to be received on the same day or within a 30-day window, and all men required continuous enrolment 6 months prior to and 12 months after the start of receiving combination therapy. The end date of database interrogation was 31 October 2015. The start or index date was defined as the date of first prescription of combination therapy – if combination drugs were not received on the same day, the index date was the day on which the second drug in combination was first prescribed. Men were excluded if they received only monotherapy for an eligible drug within the selection period or if they were prescribed the same combination therapy on and prior to the index date.

Endpoints

Treatment persistence (primary endpoint) was defined here as the time from the index date until first discontinuation of at least one of the index combination drugs. The median time to discontinuation, and the proportion of men persistent at 12-months were reported. An index drug was considered discontinued after a period of ≥30 days without prescription renewal; the date of discontinuation was the date of the last prescription of the first discontinued drug in the combination, plus the days of supply of that prescription.

Adherence (secondary endpoint), defined as medical possession ratio (MPR, i.e. the period in which patients have treatment in their possession), was calculated by two methods: the sum of days of supply of the index combination therapy divided by the time to discontinuation (MPR variable) or the sum of days of supply of the index combination therapy divided by 365 days (MPR fixed). The MPR was calculated as mean or median; men were considered as adherent if an MPR of ≥80% was achieved.

Treatment switching (exploratory endpoint), defined as the proportion of men who switched from index combination therapy to another combination therapy (i.e. if at least one drug in the index combination drugs was discontinued and replaced with at least one new drug after the last prescription date, within the 30 days following the discontinuation date).

Statistical analyses

The main analysis was performed in all men who received an α-blocker plus antimuscarinic, either as FDC or as concomitant therapy. Comparisons of persistence and adherence in this population were performed for FDC α-blocker plus an antimuscarinic compared with concomitant α-blocker plus an antimuscarinic; and α-blocker plus antimuscarinic combination therapy defined by the antimuscarinic agent. An exploratory analysis was performed in men who received any FDC therapy versus any concomitant therapy (α-blocker plus antimuscarinic or 5-ARI in both groups).

Baseline demographics and characteristics were reported descriptively. Time to discontinuation was presented using Kaplan-Meier curves. Treatment persistence and adherence were assessed using multivariate Cox regression models that adjusted for potential confounding factors at index date: age, polypharmacy (number of Anatomical Therapeutic Chemical [ATC3] class drugs [defined by the European Pharmaceutical Market Research Association] excluding those approved for the treatment of LUTS/BPH), and type of prescriber. Adjusted hazard ratios (HRs) with associated confidence intervals (CIs) and p-values are reported for comparisons of FDC and concomitant therapy; the FDC was used as the reference. Linear regression models were used for associations of potential confounding factors with MPR.

Several sensitivity analyses of time to discontinuation were performed. One analysis on the definition of time to discontinuation increased the period without prescription renewal from 30 days to 45, 60 and 90 days in the base-case cohort of men (i.e. those who initiated α-blocker and antimuscarinic combination therapy within a 30 day window). Other analyses of time to discontinuation (defined by 30 days without prescription renewal) were performed in men who were treatment-naïve for combination treatment during the pre-index period; men who first received prescriptions for α-blocker and antimuscarinic combination therapy on the same date; and men who first received prescriptions for α-blocker and antimuscarinic combination therapy within an extended 60 day window.

Results

Baseline demographics and characteristics

In total, 377,155 patients were prescribed with a target drug for LUTS/BPH treatment between 1 November 2013 and 31 October 2014. Overall, 371,560 patients were excluded (the most common reason for exclusion was the absence of prescription of an α-blocker and an antimuscarinic or 5-ARI within 30 days of each other during the study period [N = 313,669]), leaving a final study population of 5595 eligible men (Fig. 1). Of these, 1891 men received an α-blocker plus an antimuscarinic

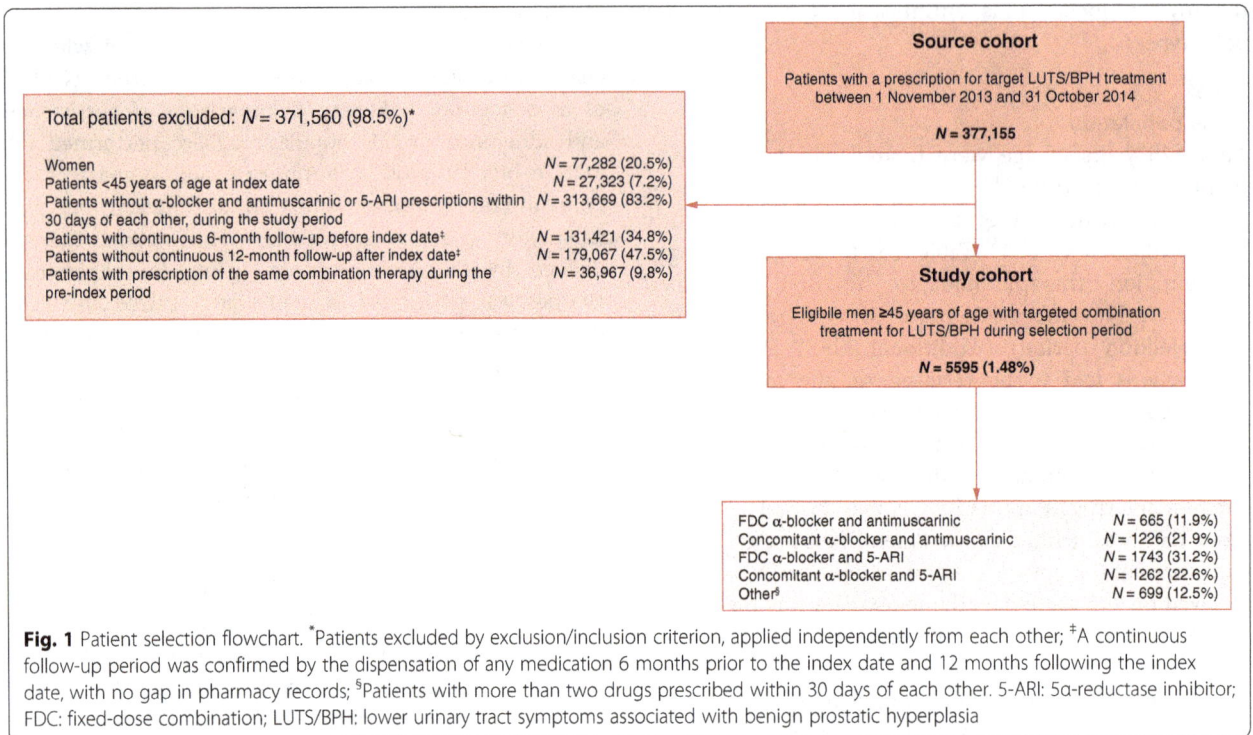

Fig. 1 Patient selection flowchart. *Patients excluded by exclusion/inclusion criterion, applied independently from each other; ‡A continuous follow-up period was confirmed by the dispensation of any medication 6 months prior to the index date and 12 months following the index date, with no gap in pharmacy records; §Patients with more than two drugs prescribed within 30 days of each other. 5-ARI: 5α-reductase inhibitor; FDC: fixed-dose combination; LUTS/BPH: lower urinary tract symptoms associated with benign prostatic hyperplasia

(665 as FDC and 1226 as concomitant therapy). In those receiving an α-blocker plus an antimuscarinic combination, the most common antimuscarinic was solifenacin ($N = 1407$) and flavoxate the least common ($N = 23$).

Baseline characteristics in the cohort that received an α-blocker plus an antimuscarinic are shown in Table 1. The mean age at index date was 71.95 years and a high proportion of men received α-blocker monotherapy (88.2%) and/or antimuscarinic monotherapy (52.3%) prior to the index date. Baseline characteristics were generally similar when comparing men who received either a FDC or concomitant therapy of an α-blocker plus an antimuscarinic. However, a higher proportion of men prescribed with a FDC compared with the concomitant therapy group had received ≤3 different drug classes for conditions other than LUTS/BPH at baseline (74.7% vs. 53.2%); were prescribed combination therapy at index date by a urologist (68.6% vs. 22.0%); and had received any prior combination therapy (34.6% vs. 20.3%) or 5-ARI monotherapy (13.2 vs. 5.6%). Overall, baseline characteristics were similar in subgroups based on the prescribed antimuscarinic at index date (Additional file 3: Table S2).

α-blocker plus antimuscarinic: FDC versus concomitant therapy

Overall time to discontinuation

Median time to discontinuation was significantly longer with α-blocker plus antimuscarinic FDC versus concomitant therapy (414 vs. 112 days; adjusted HR 2.04, 95% CI 1.77, 2.35; $p < 0.0001$) (Fig. 2) and the proportion of men

persistent at 12 months was higher with FDC compared with concomitant therapy (51.3% vs. 29.9%).

Impact of patient/clinical characteristics on time to discontinuation

Median time to discontinuation and persistence at 12 months were greatest in men aged 45–64 years (217 days and 40.3%) compared with those aged 65–74 years (189 days and 38.5%) and ≥75 years (150 days and 35.1%), although the differences were not statistically significant (Fig. 3). When the results were stratified by the number of drugs received at index date, no significant patterns were observed for median time to discontinuation (range, 153–207 days) and persistence at 12 months (range, 34.0%–40.3%) (Fig. 3; Additional file 4: Table S3). Similarly, no significant differences were observed for median time to discontinuation and persistence at 12 months in men prescribed by a urologist (234 days and 41.5%) compared with those prescribed by a GP (148 days and 35.1%; adjusted HR 0.89, 95% CI 0.78, 1.02; $p = 0.095$) or those prescribed by other healthcare providers (181 days and 34.2%; adjusted HR 1.00, 95% CI 0.83, 1.20; $p = 0.976$).

Adherence

Mean MPR and the proportion of men adherent at 12 months were similar for men who received FDC and concomitant therapy (Table 2). Similar adherence data in the FDC and concomitant therapy groups were also evident in the subgroup of men who were persistent at 12 months.

Table 1 Baseline characteristics[a] in those receiving combination therapy with an α-blocker plus an antimuscarinic

	Overall population (N = 1891)[b]	FDC (N = 665)	Concomitant therapy (N = 1226)
Age at index date, mean (SD)	71.95 (9.55)	70.46 (9.11)	72.77 (9.68)
Age at index date, N (%)			
45–64 years	417 (22.1)	172 (25.9)	245 (20.0)
65–74 years	654 (34.6)	260 (39.1)	394 (32.1)
≥75 years	820 (43.4)	233 (35.0)	587 (47.9)
Polypharmacy,[c] mean (SD)	3.38 (3.33)	4.35 (3.18)	5.54 (3.40)
Polypharmacy,[c] N (%)			
0	420 (22.2)	223 (33.5)	197 (16.1)
1–3	729 (38.6)	274 (41.2)	455 (37.1)
4–5	303 (16.0)	79 (11.9)	224 (18.3)
6–8	278 (14.7)	68 (10.2)	210 (17.1)
≥9	161 (8.5)	21 (3.2)	140 (11.4)
Prescriber at index date, N (%)			
Urologist	726 (38.4)	456 (68.6)	270 (22.0)
GP	931 (49.2)	130 (19.6)	801 (65.3)
Other	234 (12.4)	79 (11.9)	155 (12.6)
Prior treatment, N (%)			
Any combination	479 (25.3)	230 (34.6)	249 (20.3)
α-blocker + antimuscarinic	298 (15.8)	121 (18.2)	177 (14.4)
α-blocker	1668 (88.2)	549 (82.6)	1119 (91.3)
Antimuscarinic	989 (52.3)	237 (35.6)	752 (61.3)
5-ARI	157 (8.3)	88 (13.2)	69 (5.6)
Concomitant therapy, N (%)			
Both drugs initiated on the same date	–	–	341 (27.8)
Both drugs initiated within 30 days	–	–	885 (72.2)

5-ARI 5α-reductase inhibitor, FDC fixed-dose combination, GP general practitioner, SD standard deviation
[a]At index date
[b]The overall population comprised men receiving FDC or concomitant therapy of an α-blocker and an antimuscarinic
[c]Number of drugs (classified by Anatomical Therapeutic Chemical code) prescribed, excluding those approved for the treatment of LUTS/BPH.

Sensitivity analyses

Compared with the base-case analysis of 30 days, adjusting the time used to define discontinuation of combination therapy to 45, 60 and 90 days had minimal impact on the results for concomitant therapy but increased median time to discontinuation for the FDC (Additional file 5: Table S4). At each of these timepoints, median time to discontinuation and persistence at 12 months were significantly greater in men who received FDC compared with concomitant therapy ($p < 0.001$ for all assessments). In treatment-naïve men, median time to discontinuation (384 vs. 113 days) and persistence at 12 months (49.6% vs. 30.9%) were significantly greater in those who received FDC versus concomitant therapy (adjusted HR 1.83, 95% CI 1.60, 2.09; $p < 0.0001$) (Additional file 6: Figure S2a). Median time to discontinuation (414 vs. 198 days) and persistence at 12 months (51.3% vs. 38.7%) were also significantly greater in the FDC group compared with men prescribed concomitant combination treatment on the same day (adjusted HR 1.46, 95% CI 1.23, 1.72; $p < 0.0001$) (Additional file 6: Figure S2b). Similarly, in men who received prescriptions for α-blocker and antimuscarinic combination therapy within a 60 day window, median time to discontinuation (424 vs. 90 days) and persistence at 12 months (52.2% vs. 25.7%) were significantly greater in those who received FDC versus concomitant therapy (adjusted HR 2.17; 95% CI 1.90, 2.48; $p < 0.0001$) (Additional file 6: Figure S2c).

Switching

Among the 1183 men who were non-persistent at 12 months, a similar proportion of men who received FDC therapy of an α-blocker plus antimuscarinic switched treatment at 12 months, compared with those receiving concomitant therapy (5.9% vs. 6.5%, respectively) (Table 3), with the majority of men discontinuing

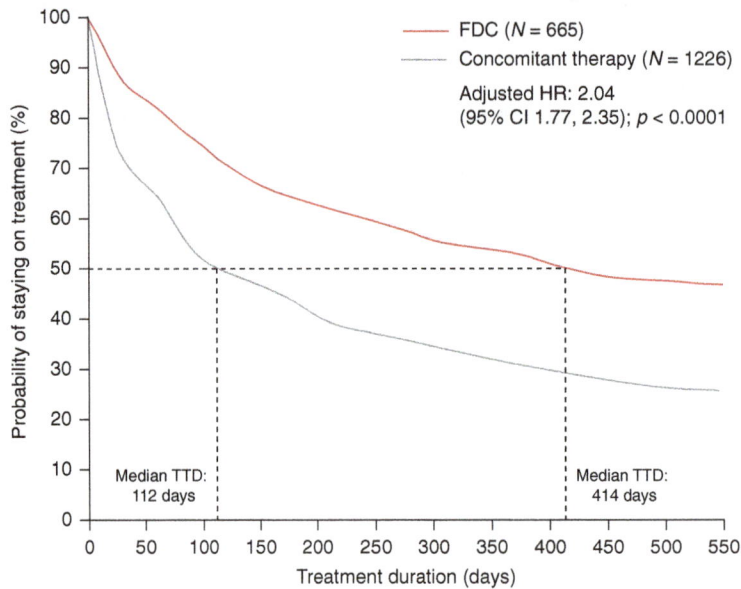

Fig. 2. Median time to discontinuation for FDC versus concomitant therapy α-blocker plus antimuscarinic. CI: confidence intervals; FDC: fixed-dose combination; HR: hazard ratio; TTD: time to discontinuation

treatment and not receiving a prescription for a new combination within 30 days. Due to the low number of men who switched treatment, no clear patterns were observed for the type of treatment men subsequently switched to.

α-blocker plus antimuscarinic: antimuscarinic drug subgroups
Overall time to discontinuation
Median time to discontinuation was significantly longer with FDC or concomitant combination

therapies containing an α-blocker plus solifenacin (214 days), compared with other α-blocker plus antimuscarinic combination therapies (range, 47–164 days; adjusted HR range 1.27–1.77, $p = 0.037$) (Fig. 4a). Similarly, the proportion of men persistent at 12 months was higher with FDC or concomitant combination therapies containing an α-blocker plus solifenacin (40.7%) compared with other α-blocker plus antimuscarinic combinations (range, 24.6%–31.4%). In the subgroup of men who received an α-blocker plus solifenacin, median time to discontinuation

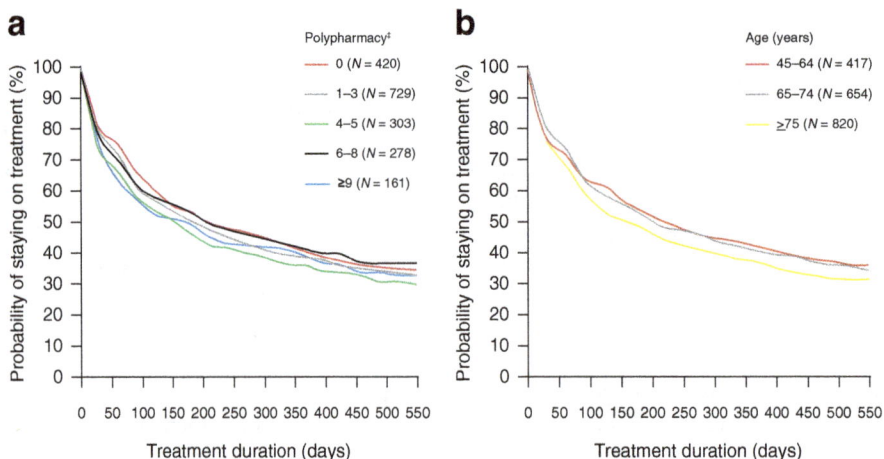

Fig. 3 Median time to discontinuation according to polypharmacy[‡] (**a**) and age (years) at index date (**b**) for all men who received an α-blocker plus antimuscarinic combination therapy (FDC or concomitant therapy). [‡]Number of drugs (classified by Anatomical Therapeutic Chemical code) prescribed, excluding those approved for the treatment of LUTS/BPH. FDC: fixed-dose combination; LUTS/BPH: lower urinary tract symptoms associated with benign prostatic hyperplasia

Table 2 Adherence in men receiving FDC and concomitant therapy with an α-blocker plus an antimuscarinic

	FDC α-blocker and antimuscarinic	Concomitant therapy	
		α-blocker	antimuscarinic
MPR-fixed			
N	566	726	726
Mean (SD)	0.91 (0.52)	0.95 (0.37)	0.89 (0.31)
Adherent,[a] n (%)	453 (80.0)	623 (85.8)	546 (75.2)
MPR-variable			
N	566	726	726
Mean (SD)	0.67 (0.31)	0.69 (0.34)	0.64 (0.32)
Adherent,[a] n (%)	275 (48.6)	358 (49.3)	319 (43.9)
MPR-fixed (persistent men only)			
N	313	380	380
Mean (SD)	0.83 (0.21)	0.93 (0.22)	0.85 (0.22)
Adherent,[a] n (%)	235 (75.1)	324 (85.3)	282 (74.2)

FDC fixed-dose combination, MPR medical possession ratio, SD standard deviation
[a]MPR of ≥80%

(414 vs. 121 days; adjusted HR 1.94, 95% CI 1.67, 2.26; $p < 0.0001$) and persistence at 12 months (51.3% vs. 31.1%) were significantly greater in those treated with FDC compared with concomitant therapy (Fig. 4b).

Table 3 Change of treatment in men initially prescribed an α-blocker plus an antimuscarinic combination treatment and non-persistent at 12 months

	FDC	Concomitant therapy
Change of treatment in men non-persistent at 12 months, N (%)	$N = 324$	$N = 859$
Switch[a]	19 (5.9)	56 (6.5)
No switch/discontinuation[b]	305 (94.1)	803 (93.5)
Switched to, N (%)	$N = 19$	$N = 56$
Combination with new α-blocker	1 (5.3)	5 (8.9)
Combination with new antimuscarinic	6 (31.6)	25 (44.6)
Concomitant therapy with the same drugs	9 (47.4)	3 (5.4)
Concomitant therapy with a new α-blocker and antimuscarinic	3 (15.8)	0
FDC	0	23 (41.1)
No switch/discontinuation, N (%)	$N = 305$	$N = 803$
α-blocker therapy only	58 (19.0)	246 (30.6)
Antimuscarinic therapy only	19 (6.2)	107 (13.3)
No therapy changes	228 (74.8)	450 (56.0)

FDC fixed-dose combination
[a]Alternative combination therapy prescribed within 30 days following discontinuation of index combination therapy
[b]No alternative combination therapy prescribed within 30 days following discontinuation of index combination therapy

Switching

Among the 75 men who switched treatment, a similar proportion of men switched from solifenacin compared with other antimuscarinics (6.9% vs. range, 2.8–6.1%).

α-blocker plus antimuscarinic or 5-ARI: FDC versus concomitant therapy

Overall time to discontinuation

A similar number of men received any FDC ($N = 2408$) or any concomitant therapy ($N = 2488$). The median time to discontinuation was significantly longer in men who received any FDC versus any concomitant combination treatment (not reached vs. 193 days; adjusted HR 2.28, 95% CI 2.10, 2.48; $p < 0.0001$) (Additional file 7: Figure S3); persistence at 12 months was also greater (62.1% vs. 38.1%) in the FDC group.

Discussion

This retrospective study assessed treatment persistence and adherence in over 5000 men with LUTS/BPH and was the first comparison in this population of men receiving treatment with an α-blocker and an antimuscarinic, either as a FDC or as concomitant therapy. Overall, treatment persistence was significantly greater in men who received an α-blocker plus an antimuscarinic as a FDC tablet compared with an α-blocker plus an antimuscarinic given concomitantly. Treatment adherence (assessed by MPR-fixed and -variable) was similar in men who received FDC α-blocker plus antimuscarinic compared with concomitant therapy.

The main study results of improved treatment persistence with FDC α-blocker plus antimuscarinic compared with concomitant therapy were also observed in the sensitivity analyses, which tested adjusting the gaps used to define time to discontinuation. Similar findings were also observed in the subpopulations of treatment-naïve men, those prescribed concomitant combination treatment on the same day, and men who initiated α-blocker and antimuscarinic combination therapy within a 60 day window. Overall, these findings were similar to the base-case analysis and the HRs reported were stable, suggesting that the study results are robust.

The foundation of superior treatment persistence with FDC α-blocker plus antimuscarinic observed in this study is likely to be multifactorial. The results may be partly attributable to the convenience of taking a single tablet (i.e. the FDC) compared with taking two tablets concomitantly. Indeed, patients receiving antihypertensive FDC therapy compared with concomitant therapy have reported significantly increased persistence and adherence in a large, retrospective cohort analysis [18]. In contrast, results from a recent

a

Antimuscarinic (N = 1891)	Median (days)	12-month persistence, N (%)	HR (95% CI); p-value
Solifenacin (N = 1407)	205	572 (40.7)	–
Tolterodine (N = 121)	94	38 (31.4)	1.32 (1.06, 1.65); p = 0.014
Oxybutynin (N = 130)	76	32 (24.6)	1.60 (1.30, 1.98); p < 0.0001
Fesoterodine (N = 95)	163	24 (25.3)	1.38 (1.09, 1.76); p = 0.0082
Flavoxate (N = 23)	47	6 (26.1)	1.77 (1.12, 2.79); p = 0.015
Darifenacin (N = 115)	112	36 (31.3)	1.27 (1.01, 1.60); p = 0.037

b

Fig. 4 Median time to discontinuation according to the antimuscarinic used in combination (α-blocker and antimuscarinic, either as FDC or concomitant therapy) (**a**) and for α-blocker plus solifenacin (FDC vs. concomitant) combination therapy (**b**). CI: confidence intervals; FDC: fixed-dose combination; HR: hazard ratio; TTD: time to discontinuation

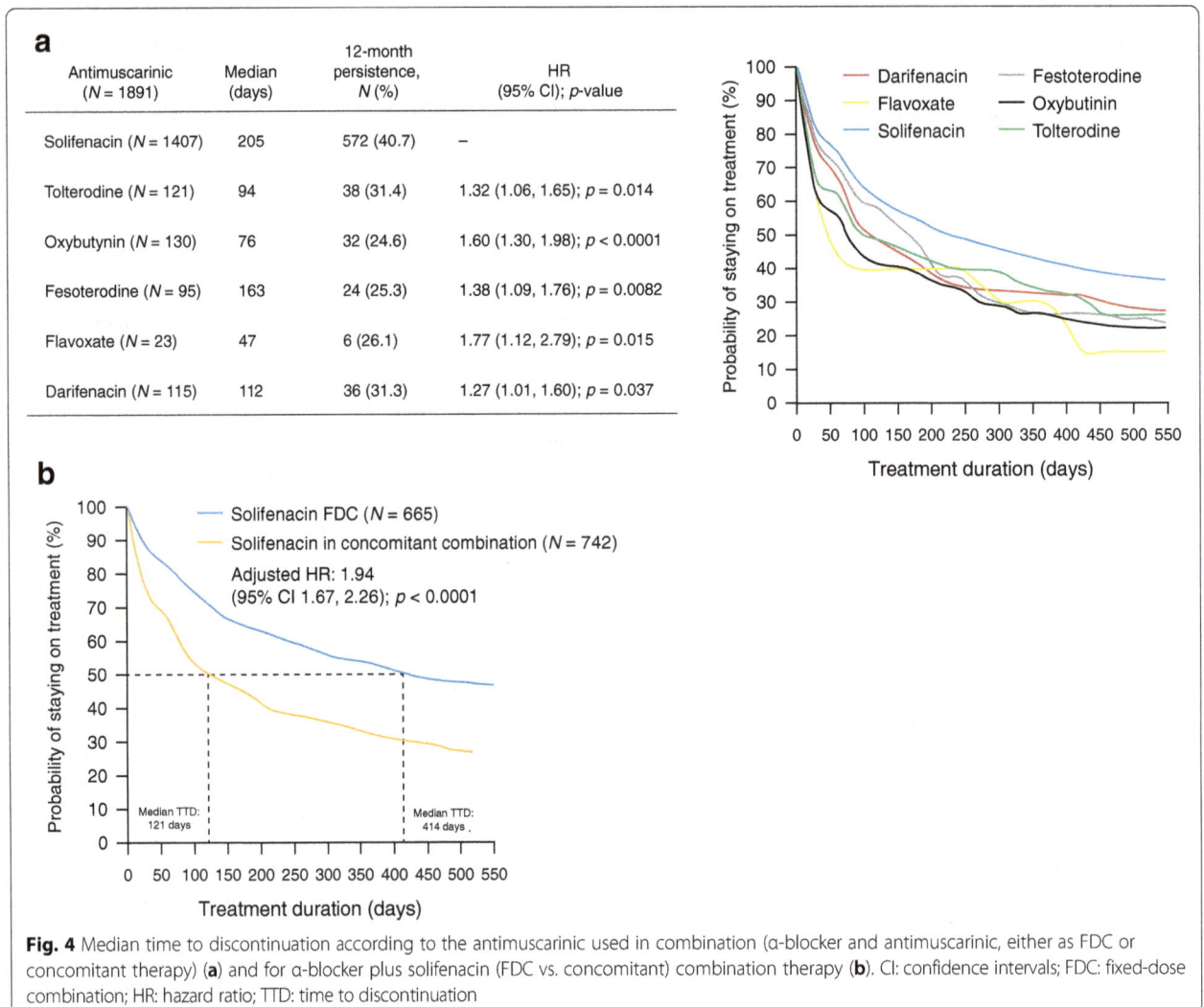

retrospective, population-based cohort study, conducted using prescription records and hospital discharge codes from ~1.5 million men with LUTS/BPH in Italy showed that men were significantly less adherent to, and more likely to discontinue treatment with combination therapy of an α-blocker plus a 5-ARI, compared with monotherapy with either treatment, over 5-years of follow-up [19]. However, there are several notable differences to the current study: Cindolo et al. assessed different drug classes (α-blockers and 5-ARIs), defined discontinuation as no prescriptions for at least two consecutive months, and comparisons were made between combination therapy and the two monotherapies, rather than between FDC and concomitant therapies. In the current study, approximately 40% of the men eligible for inclusion were receiving six or more other drugs types at index date and therefore it is difficult to make conclusions about the impact of convenience from a single tablet on the overall results.

Although the efficacy/tolerability of a FDC has not been directly compared with concomitant combination treatment for LUTS/BPH, studies in other indications have reported improved efficacy and tolerability with FDCs compared with concomitant therapies [20, 21]. The efficacy of FDC therapy in male LUTS has been shown in several studies, for instance, significant improvements in Total Urgency and Frequency Score (TUFS) was observed for FDC solifenacin 6 mg plus TOCAS versus TOCAS alone (p = 0.025) in the NEPTUNE study of 1334 men with storage and voiding LUTS/BPH [11]. In this study, no improvements in efficacy were observed when comparing the FDC solifenacin 6 mg plus TOCAS versus FDC solifenacin 9 mg plus TOCAS. However, our study did not account for different dose strengths or formulations of antimuscarinics used in combination, therefore similar conclusions cannot be drawn with regards to persistence or adherence. An open-label extension of the NEPTUNE trial

(NEPTUNE II) demonstrated that FDC solifenacin 6 mg plus TOCAS was well tolerated (most AEs were mild or moderate) and reductions in International Prostate Symptom Score (IPSS) and TUFS were maintained for up to 52 weeks [22]. In addition, the results from a randomised, open-label, 24-month parallel-group study of 742 men with moderately symptomatic BPH showed significant improvements in IPSS (−5.4 vs. −3.6 [$p < 0.001$]) in men who received FDC dutasteride 0.5 mg plus tamsulosin 0.4 mg versus tamsulosin 0.4 mg (initiated in men whose symptoms did not improve with watchful waiting) [23].

FDC solifenacin 6 mg plus TOCAS 0.4 mg is the only FDC α-blocker plus antimuscarinic approved for the treatment of men with LUTS/BPH [12, 14] and the inclusion of solifenacin within this FDC examined in our study may have contributed to the main findings. Previously reported data from a large, retrospective observational cohort study of 8694 men with LUTS/BPH in the UK showed that fewer patients discontinued (43.0% vs. [mean] 53.0%) or switched treatment (15.3% vs. [mean] 22.0%) from solifenacin compared with most other antimuscarinics, and persisted on-treatment for longer (median duration, 90 days vs. [range] 30–116 days) [16]. These findings are supported by further real-world data in patients with OAB, suggesting that solifenacin provides greater treatment persistence compared with other antimuscarinics (mean persistence 187 vs. 77–157 days; persistence at 12 months, 35% vs. 14%–28%) [24]. The reasons for improved persistence with solifenacin relative to other antimuscarinics are likely attributable to the favourable efficacy and tolerability profile for solifenacin. A long-term open label study of solifenacin for up to 1 year reported that 81% of patients completed 40 weeks of treatment and only 4.7% of patients discontinued treatment due to AEs in patients with OAB [25]. A network meta-analysis of randomised controlled trials conducted in adult patients with OAB showed that solifenacin 5 mg/day provides similar or better efficacy, and a lower or similar risk of dry mouth compared with other common oral antimuscarinics [26]. Patients' perceptions of symptom control/bother may also be a factor in a decision to persist with or discontinue treatment. Patients receiving solifenacin for the treatment of OAB have reported significant improvements in health-related quality of life and perceived bother compared with active comparator treatment or placebo [27, 28]. Indeed, unmet treatment expectations and/or tolerability are the primary reasons for treatment discontinuation in up to 90% of non-persistent patients [29]. In our study, although time to discontinuation and persistence were greater in patients receiving FDC or concomitant combinations containing solifenacin versus other antimuscarinics, the influence of solifenacin on switching could not be assessed

due to low numbers of men ($N = 75$) who met the switching criteria (i.e. replacing a discontinued index drug with at least one new drug within 30 days of the discontinuation date).

Baseline characteristics were well balanced at the index date and few significant differences were observed when the results for persistence were stratified by age, polypharmacy and prescriber. These data suggest that further study is needed to identify the key drivers of persistence in men receiving combination therapy for LUTS/BPH. In particular, it is hard to draw conclusions regarding the true effects of polypharmacy from the results, as men may have been receiving other treatments for a number of different conditions, and the definition of treatment-naïve men was only applied for 6 months prior to the study commencing (as such, the number of previous therapies for LUTS/BPH, including prior receipt of combination therapy, and the time since diagnosis could not be determined). There was a trend (not statistically significant) for greater persistence in men who received prescriptions from urologists compared with GPs. This finding is supported by recent evidence from a retrospective cohort study of 252 men with OAB, which reported that persistence on treatment was higher among men receiving subspecialist supervision, compared with those receiving treatment in internal medicine or general urology departments [30].

Strengths of this study include a large sample of approximately 5000 men with LUTS/BPH and results based on real-world data, using prescription records from a representative sample of pharmacies and dispensing GPs (corresponding to approximately 75% of retail dispensing in the Netherlands). Although real-word data were used, no in-depth clinical information was available regarding diagnosis or reasons for stopping treatment and this was a limitation. Other limitations of the database were that no information was reported on whether men received repeat prescriptions in other pharmacies outside the panel, moved to another address or died (although this was partly addressed by defining the post-index period based on the last available information on other medications). If a patient filed prescriptions at different pharmacies (i.e. one which was not included in the panel), this resulted in missing medication history and misclassification of patients. However, evidence suggests that >90% of patients in the Netherlands are usually loyal to one pharmacy [31]. Also, no information was available about whether drugs were taken correctly, according to the treatment regimen; persistence and adherence were calculated based on the recorded duration of treatment and it was assumed that when a patient was prescribed a medication then it was indeed picked up and used by the patient (however, this limitation is not restricted to retrospective analyses). Therefore, persistence and adherence rates may have been overestimated due to this assumption, although this would have been equivalent in all subcohorts and should not have influenced the comparative results. Although a reasonable number of patients (>100) were prescribed with tolterodine, oxybutynin and darifenacin, solifenacin was the most commonly prescribed antimuscarinic in the primary cohort of our study, and this may have influenced the results of the antimuscarinic subgroup analyses. Observational studies of treatment persistence/adherence with antimuscarinic therapy conducted in the UK and Canada also reported that solifenacin was the most commonly prescribed medication for OAB [24, 32, 33]. However, the pattern of prescriptions across the antimuscarinics was more balanced in these studies, suggesting that the proportion of patients prescribed with solifenacin in the current study (74.4%) may be specific to the Netherlands. Regarding α-blockers, tamsulosin is reported to be the most commonly used for LUTS/BPH [16], but it should also be noted that the impact of individual α-blockers used in combination on persistence, adherence or switching were not assessed in the same way as antimuscarinics in this study; this could perhaps be evaluated in further studies.

Future qualitative studies could also explore the rationale for treatment persistence/switching in LUTS/BPH and the potential benefits which are derived from improved persistence, particularly with regards to efficacy and tolerability, and also healthcare resource use and cost-effectiveness. In such analyses, it should be taken into consideration that patients' medication-taking behaviour (i.e. persistence or adherence) can be attributed to a number of factors, including side effects experienced on-treatment [34, 35], the patient's beliefs, values [35] and perception of the severity of their condition [34], and other behavioural or societal factors [34].

Conclusion

This study suggests that men with LUTS/BPH receiving α-blocker plus antimuscarinic combination therapy as a FDC remain on treatment significantly longer and have superior rates of persistence and adherence compared with men receiving concomitant therapy of an α-blocker plus antimuscarinic. These findings may be useful for prescribers, as improved persistence on-treatment may translate to improved outcomes for men with LUTS/BPH. Further study is warranted to assess the key drivers of persistence in men receiving combination therapy for LUTS/BPH, and also to establish the effects of such therapies on efficacy and tolerability in this patient population.

Additional files

Additional file 1: Table S1. Drugs available for selection using European Pharmaceutical Market Research Association (EphMRA) ATC drug codes [36].

Additional file 2: Figure S1. Study design.

Additional file 3: Table S2. Baseline characteristics* in all men who received combination therapy with an α-blocker plus an antimuscarinic, according to the antimuscarinic drug prescribed (N = 1891)

Additional file 4: Table S3. Persistence in all men who received an α-blocker plus an antimuscarinic (N = 1891): multivariate analysis adjusting baseline characteristics*

Additional file 5: Table S4. Persistence in all men who received an α-blocker blocker plus an antimuscarinic (N = 1891): sensitivity analysis adjusting the gap lengths used to define discontinuation.

Additional file 6: Figure S2. Median time to discontinuation: sensitivity analyses of treatment-naïve men (no prior combination therapy)* (a); index combination first prescribed on the same date* (b); and men who received an α-blocker and an antimuscarinic as combination therapy within 60 days 635 ‡ (c).

Additional file 7: Figure S3. Median time to discontinuation in any FDC* compared with any concomitant therapy*.

Abbreviations

5-ARIs: 5α-reductase inhibitors; AEs: Adverse events; BPH: Benign prostatic hyperplasia; CI: Confidence interval; FDC: Fixed-dose combination; GP: General practitioner; HR: Hazard ratio; IPSS: International Prostate Symptom Score; LUTS: Lower urinary tract symptoms; MPR: Medical possession ratio; OAB: Overactive bladder; TOCAS: Tamsulosin oral controlled absorption system; TUFS: Total Urgency and Frequency Score

Acknowledgements

Medical writing support was provided by David Griffiths, PhD of Bioscript Medical, funded by Astellas Pharma Global Development.

Ethics and consent to participate

In-line with the International Society for Pharmacoeconomics and Outcomes Research guidelines for reporting retrospective database studies (https://www.ispor.org/workpaper/healthscience/FinalReportRetroR.pdf) and the REporting of studies Conducted using Observational Routinely-collected Data (RECORD) checklist (http://record-statement.org/checklist.php), formal ethics approval for this study was not required due to the absence of human data, and the anonymization at source (Netherlands IMS Lifelink™ database) of the prescription data, which were the basis of the study. Consolidated Standards of Reporting Trials (CONSORT) guidelines were also followed for reporting the current study.

Funding

This study (design and collection, analysis and interpretation of data, and writing of the manuscript) was funded by Astellas Pharma Europe Ltd.

Authors' contributions

Conception and design: SB, EA, ZH, FG, IA and JN. Acquisition of data: FG and IA, Analysis and interpretation of the data: All authors (MJD, SB, EA, ZH, FG, IA and JN). Drafting of the manuscript: All authors (MJD, SB, EA, ZH, FG, IA and JN). Critical revision of the manuscript for important intellectual content: All authors (MJD, SB, EA, ZH, FG, IA and JN). Statistical analysis: FG and IA. Obtaining funding: SB, EA and JN. Agreement to be accountable for all aspects of the work in ensuring that questions related to the accuracy or integrity of any part of the work are appropriately investigated and resolved: All authors (MJD, SB, EA, ZH, FG, IA and JN). All authors (MJD, SB, EA, ZH, FG, IA and JN) read and approved the final manuscript.

Competing interests
MD received grants, personal fees and non-financial support from Astellas, Allergan and Ferring, outside of the submitted work. SB, EA, JN are employees of Astellas Pharma Europe Ltd. ZH is an employee of Astellas Pharma Europe B.V. FG and IA received grants from Astellas Pharma Europe Ltd. during the conduct of the study and outside of the submitted work.

Author details
[1]Bristol Urological Institute and the School of Clinical Sciences, University of Bristol, Bristol, UK. [2]Astellas Pharma Europe Ltd, Chertsey, UK. [3]Astellas Pharma Europe B.V, Leiden, the Netherlands. [4]Creativ-Ceutical Ltd, London, UK. [5]Creativ-Ceutical Ltd, Tunis, Tunisia.

References
1. The management of lower urinary tract symptoms in men. Available at: https://www.nice.org.uk/guidance/cg97/chapter/1-recommendations/. Accessed 5 July 2016.
2. Management of non-neurogenic male lower urinary tract symptoms (LUTS), incl. Benign Prostatis Obstruction (BPO). Available at: http://uroweb.org/wp-content/uploads/Non-Neurogenic-Male-LUTS_2705.pdf. Accessed 16 Sept 2016.
3. Chapple CR, Drake MJ, Van Kerrebroeck P, Cardozo L, Drogendijk T, Klaver M, Van Charldorp K, Hakimi Z, Compion G. Total urgency and frequency score as a measure of urgency and frequency in overactive bladder and storage lower urinary tract symptoms. BJU Int. 2014;113(5):696–703.
4. Agarwal A, Eryuzlu LN, Cartwright R, Thorlund K, Tammela TL, Guyatt GH, Auvinen A, Tikkinen KA. What is the most bothersome lower urinary tract symptom? Individual- and population-level perspectives for both men and women. Eur Urol. 2014;65(6):1211_7.
5. Speakman MJ. Lower Urinary Tract Symptoms Suggestive of Benign Prostatic Hyperplasia (LUTS/BPH): More Than Treating Symptoms? Eur Urol Suppl. 2008;7(11):680_9.
6. Cindolo L, Pirozzi L, Fanizza C, Romero M, Sountoulides P, Roehrborn CG, Mirone V, Schips L. Actual medical management of lower urinary tract symptoms related to benign prostatic hyperplasia: temporal trends of prescription and hospitalization rates over 5 years in a large population of Italian men. Int Urol Nephrol. 2014;46(4):695–701.
7. Kaplan SA, McCammon K, Fincher R, Fakhoury A, He W. Safety and tolerability of solifenacin add-on therapy to alpha-blocker treated men with residual urgency and frequency. J Urol. 2009;182(6):2825–30.
8. Lee KS, Choo MS, Kim DY, KIm JC, Kim HJ, Min KS, Lee JB, Jeong HJ, Lee T, Park WH. Combination treatment with propiverine hydrochloride plus doxazosin controlled release gastrointestinal therapeutic system formulation for overactive bladder and coexisting benign prostatic obstruction: a prospective, randomized, controlled multicenter study. J Urol. 2005;174(4 Pt 1):1334–8.
9. Chapple C, Herschorn S, Abrams P, Sun F, Brodsky M, Guan Z. Tolterodine treatment improves storage symptoms suggestive of overactive bladder in men treated with alpha-blockers. Eur Urol. 2009;56(3):534_41.
10. Kaplan SA, Roehrborn CG, Rovner ES, Carlsson M, Bavendam T, Guan Z. Tolterodine and tamsulosin for treatment of men with lower urinary tract symptoms and overactive bladder: a randomized controlled trial. JAMA. 2006;296(19):2319–28.
11. van Kerrebroeck P, Chapple C, Drogendijk T, Klaver M, Sokol R, Speakman M, Traudtner K, Drake MJ. Combination therapy with solifenacin and tamsulosin oral controlled absorption system in a single tablet for lower urinary tract symptoms in men: efficacy and safety results from the randomised controlled NEPTUNE trial. Eur Urol. 2013;64(6):1003–12.

12. European Medicines Committee: Summary of product characteristics for Vesomni 6 mg/0.4 mg modified release tablets. Available at: https://www.medicines.org.uk/emc/medicine/28535/. Accessed 27 Sept 2016.
13. Public Assessment Report for Vesomni 6 mg/0.4 mg modified-release tablets. http://db.cbg-meb.nl/Pars/h111622.pdf/. Accessed 7 May 2017.
14. GlaxoSmithKline UK: European Medicines Committee. Summary of product characteristics for Combodart 0.5 mg/0.4 mg hard capsules. Available at: https://www.medicines.org.uk/emc/medicine/22943. Accessed 8 Nov 2016.
15. Cramer JA, Roy A, Burrell A, Fairchild CJ, Fuldeore MJ, Ollendorf DA, Wong PK. Medication compliance and persistence: terminology and definitions. Value in health : the journal of the International Society for Pharmacoeconomics and Outcomes Research. 2008;11(1):44–7.
16. Hakimi Z, Johnson M, Nazir J, Blak B, Odeyemi IA. Drug treatment patterns for the management of men with lower urinary tract symptoms associated with benign prostatic hyperplasia who have both storage and voiding symptoms: a study using the health improvement network UK primary care data. Curr Med Res Opin. 2015;31(1):43–50.
17. Koh JS, Cho KJ, Kim HS, Kim JC. Twelve-month medication persistence in men with lower urinary tract symptoms suggestive of benign prostatic hyperplasia. Int J Clin Pract. 2014;68(2):197–202.
18. Brixner DI, Jackson KC. 2nd, Sheng X, Nelson RE, Keskinaslan A: Assessment of adherence, persistence, and costs among valsartan and hydrochlorothiazide retrospective cohorts in free-and fixed-dose combinations. Curr Med Res Opin. 2008;24(9):2597–607.
19. Cindolo L, Pirozzi L, Sountoulides P, Fanizza C, Romero M, Castellan P, Antonelli A, Simeone C, Tubaro A, de Nunzio C, et al. Patient's adherence on pharmacological therapy for benign prostatic hyperplasia (BPH)-associated lower urinary tract symptoms (LUTS) is different: is combination therapy better than monotherapy? BMC Urol. 2015;15:96.
20. Gottwald-Hostalek U, Sun N, Barho C, Hildemann S. Management of Hypertension With a Fixed-Dose (Single-Pill) Combination of Bisoprolol and Amlodipine. Clinical pharmacology in drug development. 2017;6(1):9–18.
21. Hatalova K, Pella D, Sidlo R, Hatala R. Switching from a Free Association of Perindopril/Amlodipine to a Fixed-Dose Combination: Increased Antihypertensive Efficacy and Tolerability. Clin Drug Investig. 2016;36(7):591–8.
22. Drake MJ, Chapple C, Sokol R, Oelke M, Traudtner K, Klaver M, Drogendijk T, Van Kerrebroeck P. Long-term safety and efficacy of single-tablet combinations of solifenacin and tamsulosin oral controlled absorption system in men with storage and voiding lower urinary tract symptoms: results from the NEPTUNE Study and NEPTUNE II open-label extension. Eur Urol. 2015;67(2):262–70.
23. Roehrborn CG, Oyarzabal Perez I, Roos EP, Calomfirescu N, Brotherton B, Wang F, Palacios JM, Vasylyev A, Manyak MJ. Efficacy and safety of a fixed-dose combination of dutasteride and tamsulosin treatment (Duodart((R))) compared with watchful waiting with initiation of tamsulosin therapy if symptoms do not improve, both provided with lifestyle advice, in the management of treatment-naive men with moderately symptomatic benign prostatic hyperplasia: 2-year CONDUCT study results. BJU Int. 2015;116(3):450–9.
24. Wagg A, Compion G, Fahey A, Siddiqui E. Persistence with prescribed antimuscarinic therapy for overactive bladder: a UK experience. BJU Int. 2012;110(11):1767–74.
25. Haab F, Cardozo L, Chapple C, Ridder AM. Long-term open-label solifenacin treatment associated with persistence with therapy in patients with overactive bladder syndrome. Eur Urol. 2005;47(3):376–84.
26. Kelleher C, Aballea S, Maman K, Nazir J, Hakimi Z, Chambers C, Odeyemi IA: Comparative Efficacy And Tolerability Of Solifenacin 5mg Versus Oral Antimuscarinic Agents In Overactive Bladder (Oab): A Systematic Literature Review (Slr) And Mixed Treatment Comparison (Mtc). Value in Health. 2014; 17(7):A466.
27. Chancellor MB, Zinner N, Whitmore K, Kobashi K, Snyder JA, Siami P, Karram M, Laramee C, Capo JP Jr, Seifeldin R, et al. Efficacy of solifenacin in patients previously treated with tolterodine extended release 4 mg: results of a 12-week, multicenter, open-label, flexible-dose study. Clin Ther. 2008;30(10):1766–81.
28. Toglia MR, Serels SR, Laramee C, Karram MM, Nandy IM, Andoh M, Seifeldin R, Forero-Schwanhaeuser S. Solifenacin for overactive bladder: patient-reported outcomes from a large placebo-controlled trial. Postgrad Med. 2009;121(5):151–8.

29. Benner JS, Nichol MB, Rovner ES, Jumadilova Z, Alvir J, Hussein M, Fanning K, Trocio JN, Brubaker L. Patient-reported reasons for discontinuing overactive bladder medication. BJU Int. 2010;105(9):1276–82.

30. Tran AM, Sand PK, Seitz MJ, Gafni-Kane A, Zhou Y, Botros SM: Does physician specialty affect persistence to pharmacotherapy among patients with overactive bladder syndrome? Int Urogynecology J. 2016. 2017;28(3): 409–15.

31. Astellas: Analysis of shopping behaviour between 11/2014 and 10/2014, conducted by Netherlands IMS. Data on file. 2017.

32. Chapple CR, Nazir J, Hakimi Z, Bowditch S, Fatoye F, Guelfucci F, Khemiri A, Siddiqui E, Wagg A. Persistence and Adherence with Mirabegron versus Antimuscarinic Agents in Patients with Overactive Bladder: A Retrospective Observational Study in UK Clinical Practice. Eur Urol. 2017;S0302-2838(17): 30062–3 (epub ahead of print).

33. Wagg A, Franks B, Ramos B, Berner T: Persistence and adherence with the new beta-3 receptor agonist, mirabegron, versus antimuscarinics in overactive bladder: Early experience in Canada. Can Urol Assoc J. 2015;9(9–10):343–50.

34. Touchette D, Shapiro N. Medication Compliance, Adherence, and Persistence: Current Status of Behavioral and Educational Interventions to Improve Outcomes. J Manag Care Pharm. 2008;14(6):S2–S10.

35. Shingler SL, Bennett BM, Cramer JA, Towse A, Twelves C, Lloyd AJ. Treatment preference, adherence and outcomes in patients with cancer: literature review and development of a theoretical model. Curr Med Res Opin. 2014;30(11):2329–41.

36. World Health Organization: ATC/DDD Index 2016. Available at: http://www.whocc.no/atc_ddd_index/. Accessed 8 Nov 2016.

13

Impact of preoperative 5α-reductase inhibitors on perioperative blood loss in patients with benign prostatic hyperplasia

Yi-Ping Zhu[1,2], Bo Dai[1,2], Hai-Liang Zhang[1,2], Guo-hai Shi[1,2] and Ding-Wei Ye[1,2]*

Abstract

Background: The ability of 5α-reductase inhibitors (5ARIs) to decrease blood loss during transurethral resection of the prostate (TURP) for benign prostatic hyperplasia (BPH) remains controversial. We aimed to conduct a meta-analysis of all randomized controlled trials (RCTs) to establish the role of 5ARI use prior to TURP.

Methods: We searched studies from the electronic databases PubMed, Embase, Scopus, and Cochrane Library from inception to March 25, 2014. Meta-analysis was performed using the statistical software Review Manager version 5.1.

Results: Seventeen RCTs including 1489 patients were examined. We observed that preoperative treatment with finasteride can decrease total blood loss, blood loss per gram of resected prostate tissue, hemoglobin level alteration, microvessel density (MVD), and vascular endothelial growth factor level. Neither finasteride nor dutasteride reduced operative time, prostate volume, or the weight of gland resected. In contrast, pretreatment with dutasteride before TURP did not decrease the total blood loss or MVD.

Conclusions: Pretreatment with finasteride does seem to reduce perioperative blood loss related to TURP for BPH patients. However, the effect of preoperative dutasteride was inconclusive. Further studies are required to strengthen future recommendations regarding the use of 5ARI as a standard pre-TURP treatment and its optimal regimen.

Keywords: 5α-reductase inhibitor, Benign prostate hyperplasia, Hemorrhage, Meta-analysis

Background

Transurethral resection of the prostate (TURP) remains the gold standard for patients with benign prostatic hyperplasia (BPH) that failed medical therapy. Perioperative hemorrhage is one of the major complications of TURP, and prolonged bleeding will lead to blood transfusion and clot retention [1]. 5α-Reductase inhibitors (5ARIs), including finasteride and dutasteride, can block the conversion of testosterone to dihydrotestosterone (DHT) and has been used to treat BPH and BPH-related hematuria [2].

Since Hagerty et al. [3] first reported that pretreatment with finasteride appears useful in reducing perioperative bleeding in patients undergoing TURP, emerging studies have reported similar results [4–18]. However, the ability of 5ARI to decrease blood loss during TURP for BPH remains controversial, and several studies have reported no significant benefit of preoperative 5ARIs [19–21]. One systematic review also demonstrated that preoperative finasteride can reduce blood loss during TURP while dutasteride cannot [22]. However, the systematic review was criticized for including a nonrandomized trial [23] and a study comparing photoselective vaporization of the prostate (PVP) instead of TURP with controls [24]. Therefore, we aimed to conduct a meta-analysis of all randomized controlled trials (RCTs) to establish the role of 5ARI use prior to TURP.

* Correspondence: dwye.tumor@gmail.com
[1]Department of Urology, Fudan University Shanghai Cancer Center, No. 270 Dong an Road, Shanghai 200032, People's Republic of China
[2]Department of Oncology, Shanghai Medical College, Fudan University, No. 270 Dong an Road, Shanghai 200032, People's Republic of China

Methods

Data sources and search strategy

The present meta-analysis was conducted following the Preferred Reporting Items for Systematic Reviews and Meta-Analyses (PRISMA) statement [25].No protocol exists for this meta-analysis. We searched studies from the electronic databases PubMed, Embase, Scopus, and Cochrane Library from inception to March25, 2014.The search terms used were 5α-reductase inhibitor, TURP, transurethral resection of the prostate, 5ARI, BPH, dutasteride, and finasteride. Meanwhile, references from all retrieved papers were manually searched for further relevant articles. We also searched for abstracts of randomized trials from conference proceedings. If the results of the same population were reported more than one time, only the most recent and complete data were included. No language or other restrictions were used in the search.

Study selection

Studies were considered eligible if they met the following criteria: (1) the study was a RCT, (2) the study participants were BPH patients undergoing monopolar TURP, (3) the main exposure of interest was use of 5ARI in the preoperative period, and (4) the study reported at least one of the following: estimated blood loss(EBL), decrease in hemoglobin (Hb) level, resection weight, blood loss per gram of resected tissue, microvessel density (MVD), and vascular endothelial growth factor (VEGF) level.

We excluded studies if(1) the study was nonrandomized, (2)the full text of the study could not be accessed, (3)outcomes relevant to our interests were not reported, (4) we could not extract data in the appropriate format and failed to obtain the data from the authors, or (5) interventions were bipolar TURP, PVP, or holmium laser enucleation of the prostate (excluded because only one study using PVP and one study using bipolar TURP used 5ARI in the preoperative period, indicating that we could not pool the data into a meta-analysis and perform subgroup analysis because the sample size was too small).

Data extraction and risk of bias assessment

Data were independently extracted from each study applying a standardized form by two reviewers and then cross-checked. Any disagreement was resolved by discussion between the two authors. If these two authors could not reach a consensus, another author was consulted to resolve the dispute and a final decision was made by a majority vote. The quality of the included RCTs was assessed by the Cochrane Risk of Bias Tool.

Data synthesis and analysis

We used the mean difference (MD) and relative risk with a 95% confidence interval (CI) for continuous and dichotomous data, respectively. For studies that presented continuous data as median and range values, the means and standard deviations were calculated using statistical algorithms described by Hozo et al. [26].The DerSimonian and Laird random-effects model was used if there was evidence of heterogeneity between the studies, based on the χ^2 test for heterogeneity and the I^2 test. A P value <0.10 and an I^2 value >50%, respectively, were considered high [27]. Otherwise, the fixed-effect model (Mantel-Haenszel) was selected. Publication bias was assessed using inverted funnel plots. Sensitivity analysis was performed to examine whether the effect estimate was robust to exclusion of different criteria. Analysis was performed using the statistical software Review Manager version 5.1.

Results

Study characteristics

Figure 1 traces the flow of our literature search. Briefly, we retrieved 21 potentially relevant studies for quality evaluation and excluded four RCTs [12, 24, 28, 29] for different reasons. One publication [28] was excluded because it was written in Italian, and we could not contact the author for the English version. Two publications were excluded because the interventions were PVP [24] or transurethral plasmakinetic enucleation of prostate [29]. Two publications by Donohue et al. [8, 12] had overlapping populations, and one study was excluded from meta-analysis because it reported a lower number of cases than the one we included [8]. Finally, 17 RCTs [4–11, 13–21] including 1489 patients met the inclusion criteria (746 with 5ARI and 743 without). The characteristics of included RCTs are summarized in Table 1.

Risk of bias assessment

The results of the risk of bias assessments are reported in Table 2. Overall, most studies had moderate to high risk of bias. The method of randomization was clearly depicted in only three trials. Allocation concealment was adequately stated in six trials. Blinding was evaluated separately for patients and outcome assessors. Blinding of outcome assessment was part of the trial design in only four studies. All but five trials reported incomplete outcome data.

Main outcomes

Estimated blood loss

Nine RCTs including 729 patients evaluated EBL between a 5ARI group and a control group (including seven RCTs for finasteride and two RCTs for dutasteride). Pooling data showed a significant benefit of 5ARI on reducing EBL in the finasteride group, whereas no conspicuous difference was observed in the dutasteride

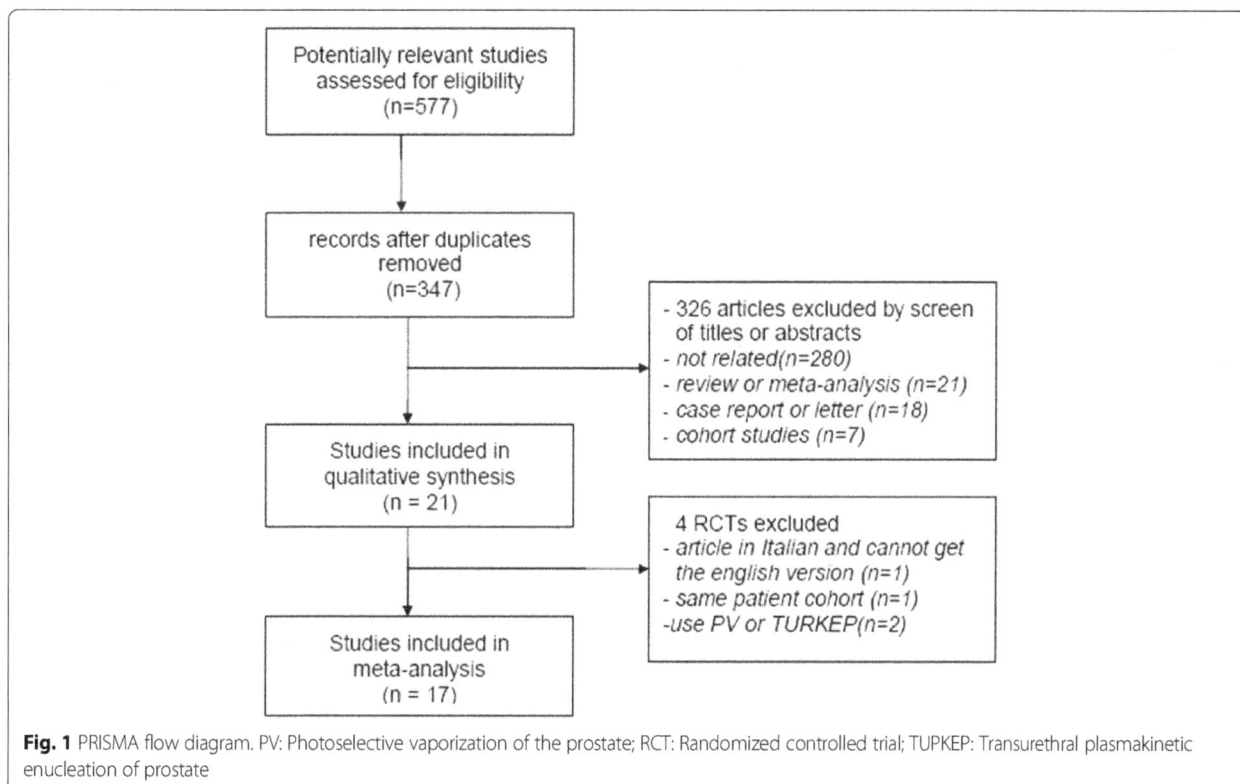

Fig. 1 PRISMA flow diagram. PV: Photoselective vaporization of the prostate; RCT: Randomized controlled trial; TUPKEP: Transurethral plasmakinetic enucleation of prostate

subgroup. The random-effects model was reported because there was evidence of significant heterogeneity (Fig. 2).

Blood loss per gram of resected prostate tissue
Five RCTs that included 323 patients evaluated blood loss per gram of resected prostate tissue between 5ARI and control groups (including four RCTs for finasteride and one RCT for dutasteride). Pooling data showed a significant benefit of 5ARI on reducing blood loss per gram of resected prostate tissue in both the finasteride and dutasteride groups. The random-effects model was reported because there was evidence of significant heterogeneity (Fig. 3).

Hb alteration
Five RCTs including 452patients reported Hb change before and after TURP (including two RCTs for finasteride and three RCTs for dutasteride). When pooled, the results showed that 5ARI reduced the Hb change in the finasteride group but not in the dutasteride group. The random-effects model was selected because there was evidence of significant heterogeneity (Fig. 4).

Blood transfusions needed
Eight RCTs including 565 cases evaluated patients who needed a blood transfusion (including four RCTs for finasteride and four RCTs for dutasteride). When pooled, although there was a trend in favor of the 5ARI

group, the result did not show significant differences between treatment and control groups ($P = 0.05$). According to our analysis, no heterogeneity was found among the trials ($I^2 = 0$); thus, a fixed-effects model was chosen for the analysis (Fig. 5).

MVD and VEGF expression after 5ARI treatment
To elucidate the mechanism of 5ARI action, we identified eight RCTs that evaluated MVD (including six RCTs for finasteride and two RCTs for dutasteride), and six RCTs evaluated VEGF expression after 5ARI treatment (six RCTs including 746 patients for finasteride).The overall result of the meta-analysis showed that the MVD and VEGF of the resected prostate tissue were lower in the finasteride group than in the control group, whereas oral dutasteride did not decrease MVD. The random-effects model was reported because there was evidence of significant heterogeneity (Figs. 6 and 7).

Other parameters
We also evaluated other parameters between the 5ARI and control groups in the present meta-analysis, including operative time, weight of gland resected, and prostate volume. The pooled data showed that both finasteride and dutasteride did not reduce operative time, prostate volume, or weight of gland resected. On the contrary, lesser gland tissue was resected and the prostate volume was smaller in the control group (Table 3).

Table 1 Study characteristics

Study	Country	Age 5ARI	Age Control	Sample size 5ARI	Sample size Control	Intervention 5ARI	Intervention Control	Dose and duration	Outcomes evaluated
Sandfeldt 2001 [10]	Sweden	69	68	26	29	Fin	placebo	5mg daily, 12 weeks	blood loss, operating time, resection weight, MVD
Häggström 2002 [13]	Sweden	NM	NM	15	13	Fin	placebo	5mg daily, 12 weeks	VEGF, MVD
Donohue 2002 [8]	UK	69.9	70.2	32	36	Fin	placebo	5mg daily, 2 weeks	blood loss, resection weight
Liu 2003 [14]	China	68.9	68.4	50	50	Fin	blank	5mg daily, 2 weeks	blood loss, Hb alteration, operating time, resection weight, MVD, VEGF
Li 2004 [6]	China	70.7	72.1	40	40	Fin	blank	5mg daily, 1–2 weeks	blood loss, operating time, resection weigh
Özdal 2005 [4]	Turkey	66.9	66.3	20	20	Fin	blank	5mg daily, 4 weeks	blood loss, Hb alteration, resection weight
Lund 2005 [19]	Denmark	66.5	67	16	17	Fin	placebo	5mg daily, 12 weeks	blood loss, operating time, resection weight
Boccon 2005 [16]	France	NM	NM	32	27	Dut	placebo	0.5mg daily,4 weeks	Hb alteration, resection weight
Lekas 2006 [7]	Greece	68.6	68.8	88	90	Fin	blank	5mg daily, 25.3 weeks	blood loss, MVD ,VEGF
Hahn 2007 [20]	multicenter 3-arm study	67/67	66	72/71	70	Dut	placebo	0.5mg daily, 4 weeks before and 2 weeks after TURP	Hb alteration per gramprostate; MVD
Memis 2008 [11]	Turkey	65	64	13	17	Fin	blank	5mg daily, 4 weeks	MVD
Berardinis 2008 [9]	Italy	68	69	100	100	Fin	placebo	5mg twice, 8 weeks	MVD,VEGF
Tuncel 2009 [21]	Turkey	68.1	67.7	27	21	Dut	blank	0.5mg daily,5 weeks	Blood loss, Hb alteration, MVD
Kravchick 2009 [17]	Israel	67.7	66.15	24	22	Dut	blank	0.5mg daily,6 weeks	blood loss, operating time, resection weight
He 2012 [15]	China	64.5	65.5	30	30	Fin	blank	5mg daily, 2 weeks	blood loss, operating time, resection weight, MVD ,VEGF
Pastore 2013 [18]	Italy	65.66	66.7	71	71	Dut	blank	0.5mg daily,6 weeks	blood loss, operating time, resection weight
Liu 2013 [14]	China	69.2	68.4	90	90	Fin	blank	10mg twice, 2 weeks	blood loss, operating time, resection weight, VEGF

5ARI 5α-reductase inhibitors, Fin finasteride, Dut dutasteride, MVD microvessel density, VEGF vascular endothelial growth factor, RR relative risk, MD mean difference, CI confidence interval

Table 2 Cochrane risk of bias summary of included RCTs

Study	Random Sequence Generation	Allocation Concealment	Blinding of participants and personnel	Blinding of outcome assessment	Incomplete outcome data	Selective outcome reporting	Other sources of bias
Sandfeldt 2001 [10]	Unclear risk	low risk	low risk	low risk	low risk	low risk	low risk
Häggström 2002 [13]	Unclear risk	Unclear risk	high risk	high risk	low risk	low risk	low risk
Donohue 2002 [8]	Unclear risk	Unclear risk	low risk	Unclear risk	low risk	low risk	low risk
Liu 2003 [5]	Unclear risk	Unclear risk	high risk	high risk	high risk	low risk	low risk
Li 2004 [6]	Unclear risk	Unclear risk	high risk	high risk	high risk	low risk	low risk
Özdal 2005 [4]	Unclear risk	Unclear risk	low risk	Unclear risk	low risk	low risk	low risk
Lund 2005 [19]	low risk	low risk	Unclear risk	Unclear risk	low risk	low risk	low risk
Boccon 2005 [16]	Unclear risk	low risk	low risk	low risk	low risk	low risk	low risk
Lekas 2006 [7]	low risk	Unclear risk	high risk	high risk	low risk	low risk	low risk
Hahn 2007 [20]	Unclear risk	low risk	low risk	low risk	low risk	low risk	low risk
Memis 2008 [11]	Unclear risk	Unclear risk	high risk	high risk	low risk	low risk	low risk
Berardinis 2008 [9]	Unclear risk	low risk	low risk	low risk	low risk	low risk	low risk
Tuncel 2009 [21]	Unclear risk	Unclear risk	high risk	high risk	high risk	low risk	low risk
Kravchick 2009 [17]	high risk	low risk	high risk	high risk	high risk	low risk	low risk
He 2012	Unclear risk	Unclear risk	high risk	high risk	high risk	low risk	low risk
Pastore 2013	low risk	Unclear risk	low risk	Unclear risk	low risk	low risk	low risk
Liu 2013 [14]	Unclear risk	Unclear risk	high risk	high risk	low risk	low risk	low risk

5ARI 5α-reductase inhibitors, Fin finasteride, Dut dutasteride, MVD microvessel density, VEGF vascular endothelial growth factor, RR relative risk, MD mean difference, CI confidence interval
afavors control

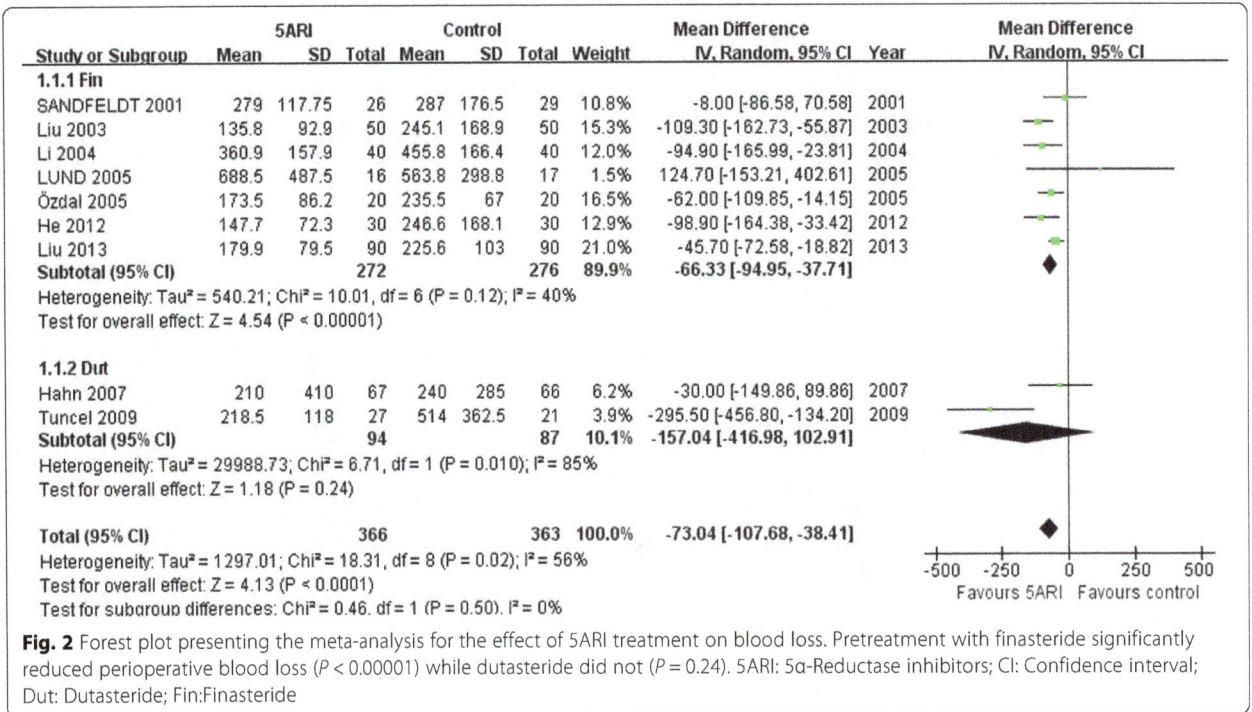

Fig. 2 Forest plot presenting the meta-analysis for the effect of 5ARI treatment on blood loss. Pretreatment with finasteride significantly reduced perioperative blood loss (P < 0.00001) while dutasteride did not (P = 0.24). 5ARI: 5α-Reductase inhibitors; CI: Confidence interval; Dut: Dutasteride; Fin:Finasteride

Sensitivity analysis and publication bias

Sensitivity analysis was performed by sequential removal of individual studies and cumulative statistics for all comparisons of all subjects. The pooled MD was not influenced by the result of any individual study. Funnel plots were used to assess the publication bias. All studies lie inside the 95% CIs, with an even distribution around the vertical, indicating no obvious publication bias (Fig. 8).

Discussion

5ARI is commonly used for treating BPH and hematuria of prostatic origin. However, the concept of preoperatively administering 5ARI to reduce blood loss during TURP has not been accepted by most urologists. In a United Kingdom-based survey, although 98% of urologists used finasteride for hematuria of prostatic origin, only 4% used it before TURP [30]. In the present meta-analysis involving 17 RCTs and 1489 participants, we

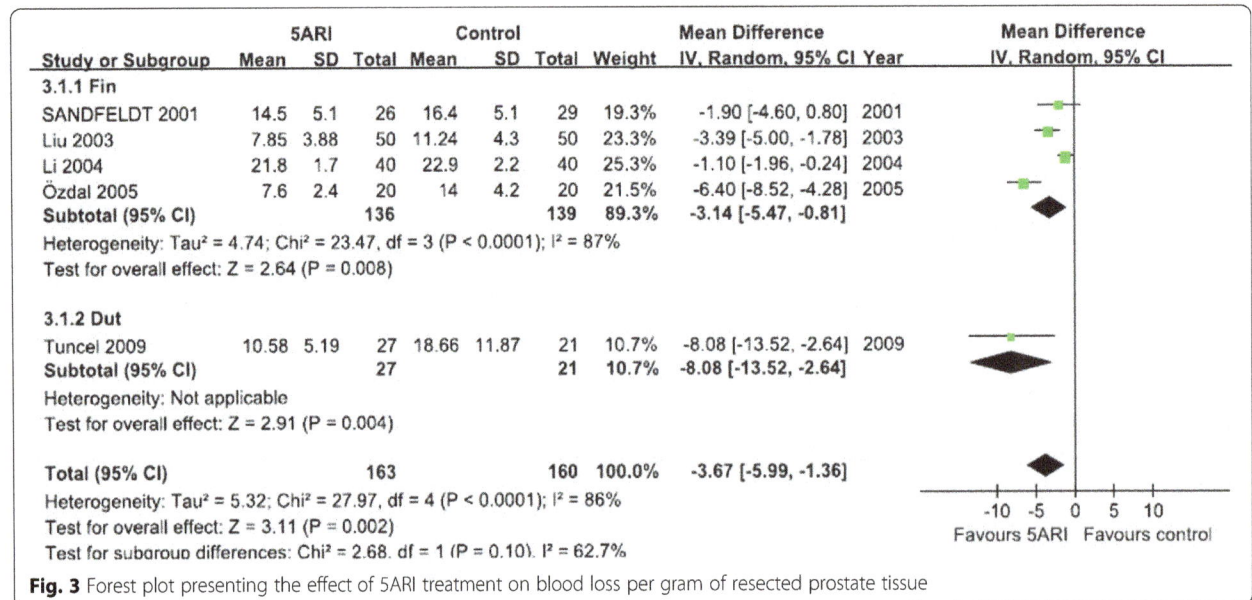

Fig. 3 Forest plot presenting the effect of 5ARI treatment on blood loss per gram of resected prostate tissue

Study or Subgroup	5ARI Mean	SD	Total	Control Mean	SD	Total	Weight	Mean Difference IV, Random, 95% CI	Year	Mean Difference IV, Random, 95% CI
2.1.1 Fin										
DONOHUE 2002/2005	0.99	0.8	32	1.48	0.8	36	21.4%	-0.49 [-0.87, -0.11]	2005	
Özdal 2005	1.88	0.93	20	3.19	1.18	20	16.2%	-1.31 [-1.97, -0.65]	2005	
Subtotal (95% CI)			52			56	37.6%	-0.85 [-1.65, -0.06]		
Heterogeneity: Tau² = 0.26; Chi² = 4.46, df = 1 (P = 0.03); I² = 78%										
Test for overall effect: Z = 2.10 (P = 0.04)										
2.1.2 Dut										
Boccon 2005	1.94	1.81	32	1.4	1	37	15.4%	0.54 [-0.17, 1.25]	2005	
Hahn 2007	2.55	0.39	67	2.55	0.41	66	25.0%	0.00 [-0.14, 0.14]	2007	
Pastore 2013	1.29	0.81	71	1.83	1.25	71	22.0%	-0.54 [-0.89, -0.19]	2013	
Subtotal (95% CI)			170			174	62.4%	-0.07 [-0.54, 0.40]		
Heterogeneity: Tau² = 0.13; Chi² = 10.89, df = 2 (P = 0.004); I² = 82%										
Test for overall effect: Z = 0.30 (P = 0.76)										
Total (95% CI)			222			230	100.0%	-0.35 [-0.79, 0.08]		
Heterogeneity: Tau² = 0.20; Chi² = 28.12, df = 4 (P < 0.0001); I² = 86%										
Test for overall effect: Z = 1.58 (P = 0.11)										
Test for subgroup differences: Chi² = 2.74, df = 1 (P = 0.10), I² = 63.5%										

Favours 5ARI   Favours control   (-2 -1 0 1 2)

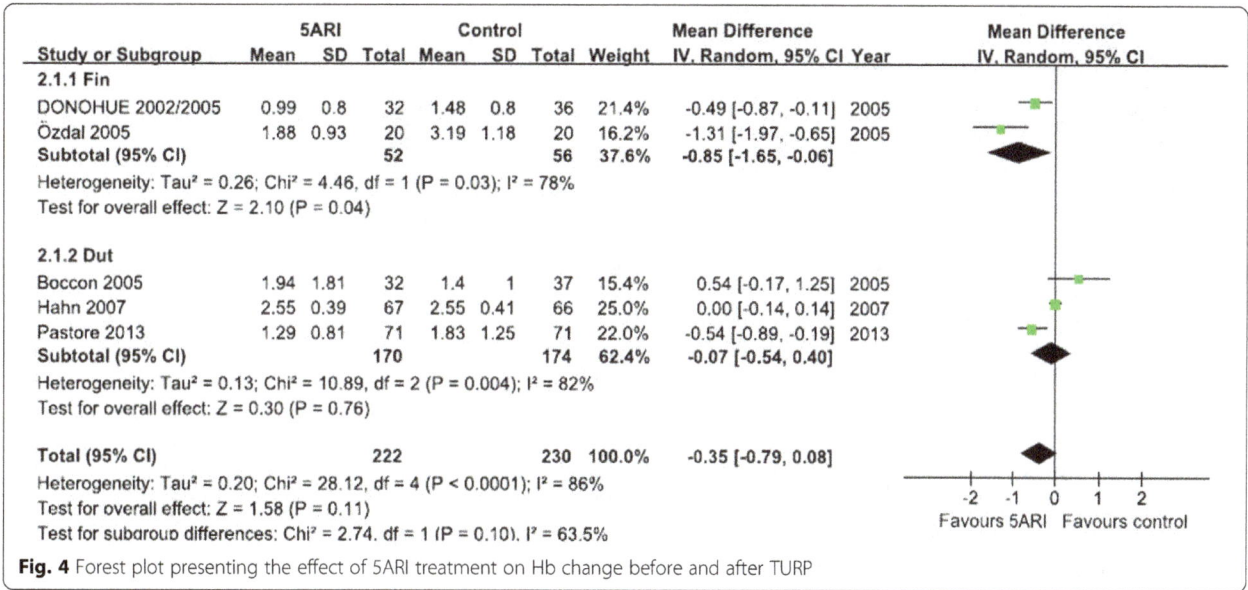

Fig. 4 Forest plot presenting the effect of 5ARI treatment on Hb change before and after TURP

demonstrated that preoperative treatment with finasteride for 2 weeks to 6 months could decrease blood loss during TURP for BPH. In contrast, pretreatment with dutasteride before TURP did not change the total blood loss.

Testosterone is a stimulator of VEGF, and androgen deprivation leads to decreased blood flow in the prostate [31, 32]. Finasteride blocks the conversion of testosterone to DHT, resulting in decreased activity of the androgen-controlled growth factors, such as VEGF. MVD is another histologic indicator of angiogenesis in BPH patients. Emerging data have shown that finasteride treatment prior to TURP significantly decreased MVD in the prostate tissue [9–13]. Our meta-analysis confirmed the results of previous studies, demonstrating that finasteride could significantly decrease MVD and VEGF of the prostate tissue compared with controls.

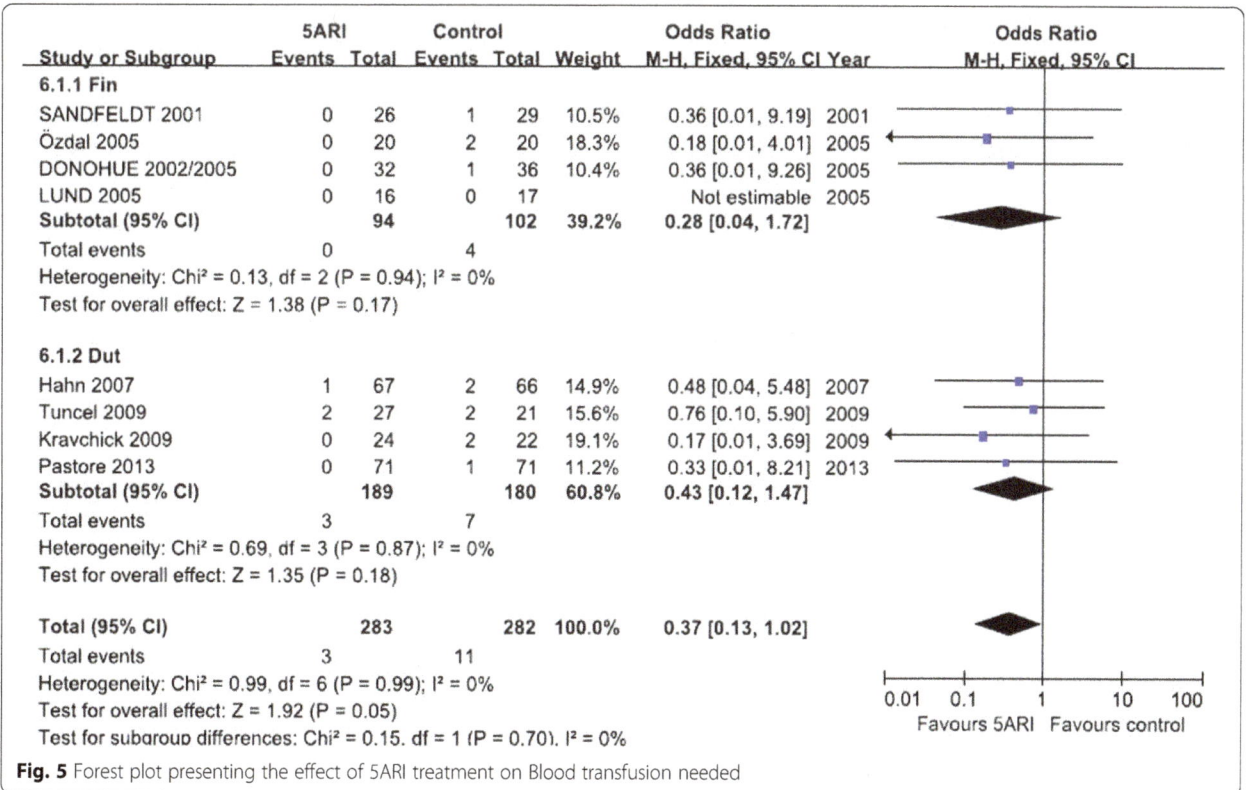

Study or Subgroup	5ARI Events	Total	Control Events	Total	Weight	Odds Ratio M-H, Fixed, 95% CI	Year	Odds Ratio M-H, Fixed, 95% CI
6.1.1 Fin								
SANDFELDT 2001	0	26	1	29	10.5%	0.36 [0.01, 9.19]	2001	
Özdal 2005	0	20	2	20	18.3%	0.18 [0.01, 4.01]	2005	
DONOHUE 2002/2005	0	32	1	36	10.4%	0.36 [0.01, 9.26]	2005	
LUND 2005	0	16	0	17		Not estimable	2005	
Subtotal (95% CI)		94		102	39.2%	0.28 [0.04, 1.72]		
Total events	0		4					
Heterogeneity: Chi² = 0.13, df = 2 (P = 0.94); I² = 0%								
Test for overall effect: Z = 1.38 (P = 0.17)								
6.1.2 Dut								
Hahn 2007	1	67	2	66	14.9%	0.48 [0.04, 5.48]	2007	
Tuncel 2009	2	27	2	21	15.6%	0.76 [0.10, 5.90]	2009	
Kravchick 2009	0	24	2	22	19.1%	0.17 [0.01, 3.69]	2009	
Pastore 2013	0	71	1	71	11.2%	0.33 [0.01, 8.21]	2013	
Subtotal (95% CI)		189		180	60.8%	0.43 [0.12, 1.47]		
Total events	3		7					
Heterogeneity: Chi² = 0.69, df = 3 (P = 0.87); I² = 0%								
Test for overall effect: Z = 1.35 (P = 0.18)								
Total (95% CI)		283		282	100.0%	0.37 [0.13, 1.02]		
Total events	3		11					
Heterogeneity: Chi² = 0.99, df = 6 (P = 0.99); I² = 0%								
Test for overall effect: Z = 1.92 (P = 0.05)								
Test for subgroup differences: Chi² = 0.15, df = 1 (P = 0.70), I² = 0%								

Favours 5ARI   Favours control   (0.01 0.1 1 10 100)

Fig. 5 Forest plot presenting the effect of 5ARI treatment on Blood transfusion needed

Study or Subgroup	5ARI Mean	SD	Total	Control Mean	SD	Total	Weight	Mean Difference IV, Random, 95% CI	Year	Mean Difference IV, Random, 95% CI
4.1.1 Fin										
Haggstrom2002	3.4	0.2	15	3	0.23	13	19.5%	0.40 [0.24, 0.56]	2002	
Liu 2003	21.4	9.7	50	33.4	11.2	50	12.3%	-12.00 [-16.11, -7.89]	2003	
Lekas 2006	37.1	19.8	88	67.4	23.2	90	8.2%	-30.30 [-36.63, -23.97]	2006	
Berardinis2008	16.1	0.4	100	19.2	1.2	100	19.5%	-3.10 [-3.35, -2.85]	2008	
Memis 2008	9.1	5.6	13	13.9	5.9	17	12.2%	-4.80 [-8.94, -0.66]	2008	
He 2012	24.1	9.7	30	37.2	15.3	30	7.9%	-13.10 [-19.58, -6.62]	2012	
Subtotal (95% CI)			296			300	79.7%	-7.66 [-10.31, -5.01]		
Heterogeneity: Tau² = 7.48; Chi² = 670.34, df = 5 (P < 0.00001); I² = 99%										
Test for overall effect: Z = 5.66 (P < 0.00001)										
4.1.2 Dut										
Hahn 2007	48	21	67	44	20	66	7.3%	4.00 [-2.97, 10.97]	2007	
Tuncel 2009	26.9	6.8	27	24.2	6.5	21	13.0%	2.70 [-1.08, 6.48]	2009	
Subtotal (95% CI)			94			87	20.3%	3.00 [-0.33, 6.32]		
Heterogeneity: Tau² = 0.00; Chi² = 0.10, df = 1 (P = 0.75); I² = 0%										
Test for overall effect: Z = 1.77 (P = 0.08)										
Total (95% CI)			390			387	100.0%	-5.46 [-7.83, -3.09]		
Heterogeneity: Tau² = 7.46; Chi² = 675.11, df = 7 (P < 0.00001); I² = 99%										
Test for overall effect: Z = 4.52 (P < 0.00001)										
Test for subgroup differences: Chi² = 24.10. df = 1 (P < 0.00001), I² = 95.9%										

-20 -10 0 10 20
Favours 5ARI   Favours control

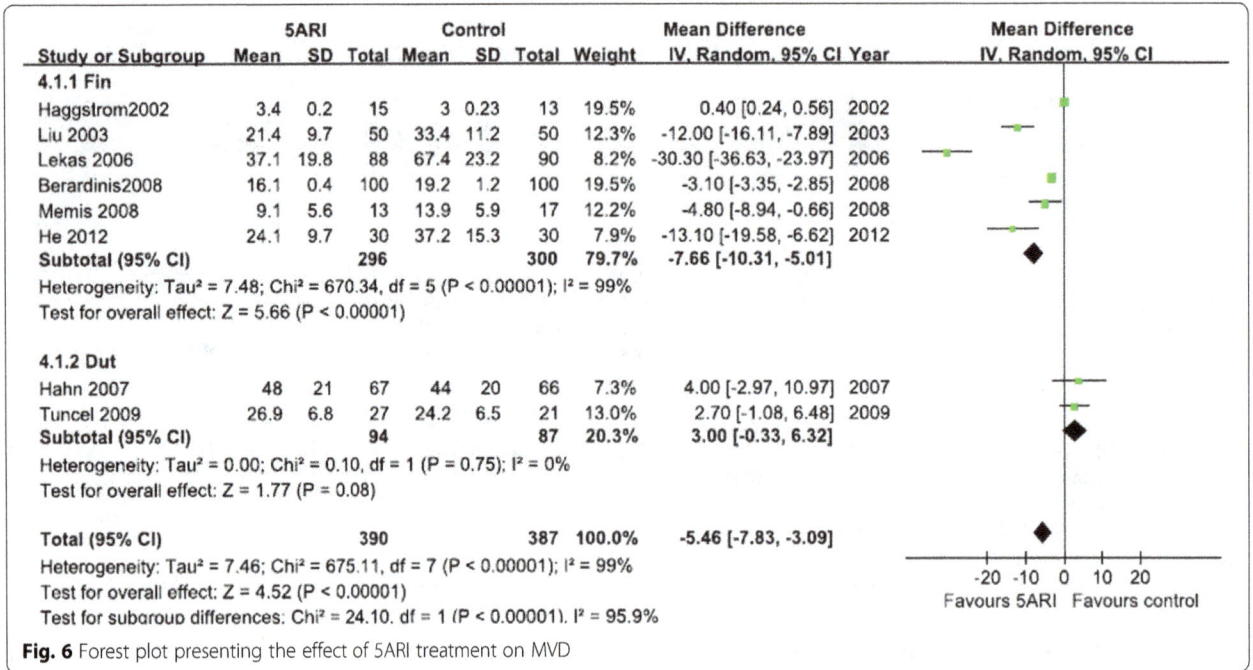

Fig. 6 Forest plot presenting the effect of 5ARI treatment on MVD

Finasteride, a type II 5ARI, has been shown to decrease the size of the prostate, and therefore the operative time might also be decreased secondary to the smaller gland. However, the present meta-analysis showed that neither finasteride nor dutasteride prior to TURP reduced operative time, prostate volume, or weight of the gland resected. One possible explanation is that a decrease in the size of the prostate gland requires up to 6 months of finasteride to occur [33]. However, most RCTs in our meta-analysis used finasteride ranging from 2 to 12 weeks, not enough for shrinkage of the prostate gland. On the contrary, the effect of finasteride on hematuria was more rapid than may reasonably be attributed to decreased prostate size. Liu et al. [5] showed that MVD and VEGF decreased obviously in patients treated with finasteride for 14 days. Taken together, the mechanism by which finasteride decreased blood loss during TURP was probably related to decreased vascularity in the prostate rather than to a smaller prostate and shorter operative time.

Dutasteride, a dual 5ARI, provides greater suppression of 5α-reductase because it antagonizes both type I and II receptors [34]. In theory, it should produce an effect that is better than, or at least similar to, finasteride.

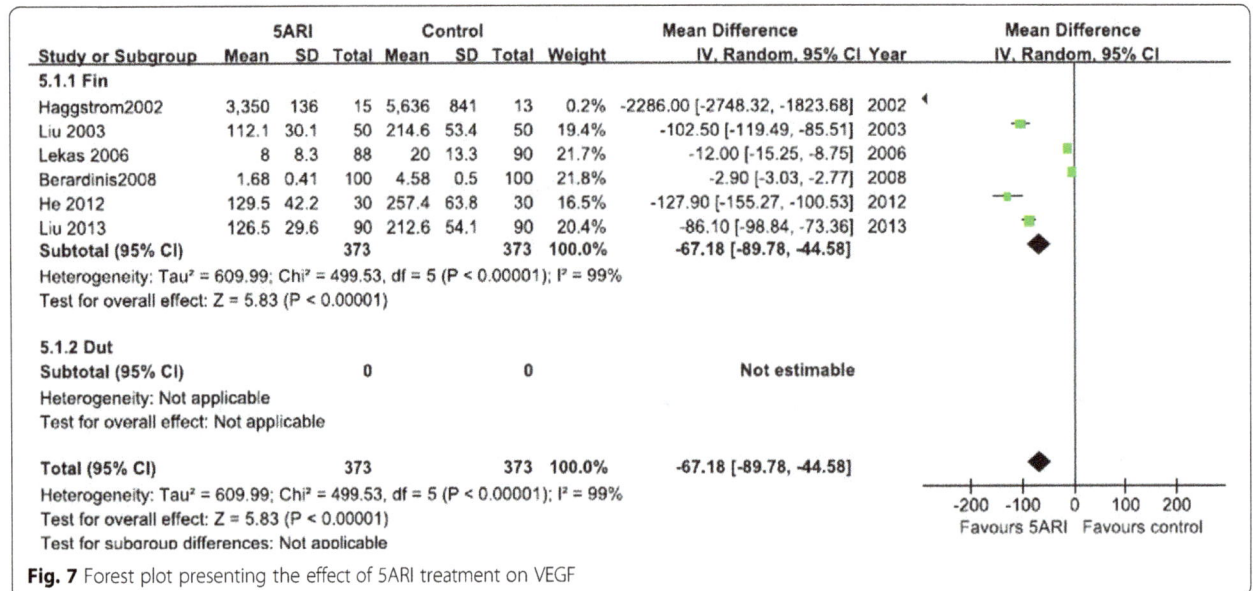

Study or Subgroup	5ARI Mean	SD	Total	Control Mean	SD	Total	Weight	Mean Difference IV, Random, 95% CI	Year	Mean Difference IV, Random, 95% CI
5.1.1 Fin										
Haggstrom2002	3,350	136	15	5,636	841	13	0.2%	-2286.00 [-2748.32, -1823.68]	2002	
Liu 2003	112.1	30.1	50	214.6	53.4	50	19.4%	-102.50 [-119.49, -85.51]	2003	
Lekas 2006	8	8.3	88	20	13.3	90	21.7%	-12.00 [-15.25, -8.75]	2006	
Berardinis2008	1.68	0.41	100	4.58	0.5	100	21.8%	-2.90 [-3.03, -2.77]	2008	
He 2012	129.5	42.2	30	257.4	63.8	30	16.5%	-127.90 [-155.27, -100.53]	2012	
Liu 2013	126.5	29.6	90	212.6	54.1	90	20.4%	-86.10 [-98.84, -73.36]	2013	
Subtotal (95% CI)			373			373	100.0%	-67.18 [-89.78, -44.58]		
Heterogeneity: Tau² = 609.99; Chi² = 499.53, df = 5 (P < 0.00001); I² = 99%										
Test for overall effect: Z = 5.83 (P < 0.0001)										
5.1.2 Dut										
Subtotal (95% CI)			0			0		Not estimable		
Heterogeneity: Not applicable										
Test for overall effect: Not applicable										
Total (95% CI)			373			373	100.0%	-67.18 [-89.78, -44.58]		
Heterogeneity: Tau² = 609.99; Chi² = 499.53, df = 5 (P < 0.00001); I² = 99%										
Test for overall effect: Z = 5.83 (P < 0.0001)										
Test for subgroup differences: Not applicable										

-200 -100 0 100 200
Favours 5ARI   Favours control

Fig. 7 Forest plot presenting the effect of 5ARI treatment on VEGF

Table 3 Study outcomes comparing 5ARI with control

Outcomes	No of studies (Fin/Dut)	No. of patients		RR/MD (Total)	95%CI (Total)	P value (Fin/Dut/Total)	Heterogeneity (Total)			P value
		5ARI(Fin/Dut)	Control(Fin/Dut)				chi^2	df	I^2%	
Blood loss	7/2	272/94	276/87	−73.04	−107.68,−38.41	<0.00001/0.24/<0.0001	18.31	8	56	0.27
Hb alteration	2/3	52/170	56/174	−0.35	−0.79,0.08	0.04/0.76/0.11	28.12	4	86	<0.0001
Blood loss/g tissue	4/1	136/27	139/21	−3.67	−5.99,−1.36	0.008/0.004/0.002	27.97	4	86	<0.0001
MVD	6/2	296/94	300/87	−5.46	−7.83,−3.09	<0.00001/0.08/<0.00001	675.11	7	99	<0.00001
VEGF	6/0	373/0	373/0	−67.18	−89.78,−44.58	<0.00001	499.53	5	99	<0.00001
Operative time	6/4	252/189	256/180	−3.96	−8.17,2.87	0.12/0.35/0.07	32.46	9	72	0.0002
Transfusion needed	4/4	94/189	102/180	0.37	0.13,1.02	0.17/0.18/0.05	0.99	6	0	0.99
Gland resected	7/4	254/189	262/180	1.09	0.3,1.87	0.01[a]/0.4/0.006	8.46	10	0	0.58
Prostate volume	6/2	291/98	297/92	1.85	0.60,3.10	0.003[a]/1.00/0.004	4.33	7	0	0.74

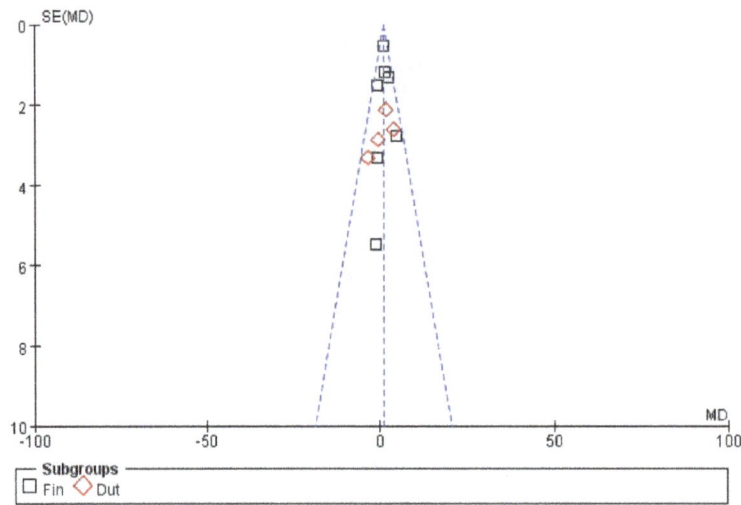

Fig. 8 Funnel plot of the studies represented in our meta-analysis. This funnel plot provided us with a qualitative estimation of publication bias of the studies, and no evidence of bias was found. Dut: Dutasteride; Fin:Finasteride

However, in our meta-analysis, we did not find any differences between the dutasteride and control groups with regard to EBL, decrease in Hb, resection weight, prostate volume, transfusions needed, and operative time. Only one RCT with limited cases showed that pretreatment with dutasteride could decrease blood loss per gram of resected tissue [21].To our surprise, unlike finasteride, pooling data of two RCTs including 181 cases showed that dutasteride treatment did not decrease MVD, which might partially explain why dutasteride was not effective in reducing EBL. In addition, because dutasteride is a newer drug, the patient populations recruited to these RCTs were certainly different from the cohorts that were available for the finasteride RCTs. Thus, selection bias maybe another plausible explanation for the failure to find a difference in the dutasteride group. The exact reason dutasteride was not effective in reducing EBL and MVD remains unclear, and additional well-designed RCTs are needed to establish its actual role.

Because approximately 50% of the variability in blood loss can be accounted for by the amount of resected tissue in TURP, the resection weight and/or prostate size should be taken into account when calculating EBL [35]. In one study by Sandfeldt et al. [10], a positive correlation between EBL and resection weight was reported. According to Hagerty et al. [3], patients with resected weights of >30 g who received finasteride before TURP needed fewer blood transfusions than those who did not receive the drug. Although we found no differences between 5ARI and control groups with regard to transfusions needed, it may be that the trial sample sizes were not large enough to generate enough data for detecting

significant effects. In addition, most RCTs in our meta-analysis did not perform subgroup analysis based on resection weight (e.g.,>30g) or prostate size. Further studies are required to fully assess the hypothesis that the benefit of 5ARI treatment would manifest at resected weights of >30 or >40 g or set a cutoff value for prostate size.

The present meta-analysis had some limitations. First was the quality of the studies assessed; most of the included RCTs did not describe randomization concealment and blinding techniques. Second was the substantial heterogeneity among studies, which was probably caused by the variability among oral 5ARI regimens and outcome measurements. Oral 5ARI regimens were not standardized, and the studies varied in the dose of 5ARI used as well as the drug duration and frequency. Data were therefore analyzed using a random-effects model, which accounts for both within-study and between-study variability. Finally, inherent in any meta-analysis is the possibility of publication bias; that is, small studies with null results tend not to be published. However, several RCTs included in the meta-analysis also contained negative results [11, 19–21], and the funnel plot did not provide any evidence of publication bias.

Conclusion

Pretreatment with finasteride does seem to reduce perioperative blood loss related to TURP for BPH patients. This effect was probably due to decreased vascularity in the prostate rather than a smaller prostate or shorter operative time. However, the effect of preoperative dutasteride was inconclusive. Further studies are required to strengthen future recommendations regarding the use of 5ARI as a standard pre-TURP treatment and its optimal regimen.

Abbreviations

5ARI: 5α-Reductase inhibitor; BPH: Benign prostatic hyperplasia; CI: Confidence interval; DHT: Dihydrotestosterone; EBL: Estimated blood loss; Hb: Hemoglobin; MD: Mean difference; MVD: Microvessel density; PVP: Photoselective vaporization of the prostate; RCT: Randomized controlled trial; TURP: Transurethral resection of the prostate; VEGF: Vascular endothelial growth factor..

Competing interests

The authors declare that they have no competing interests.

Authors' contributions

YPZ and DB performed the systematic review and meta-analysis. HLZ, GHS, and DWY identified the studies and participated in critical evaluation and discussion. All authors read and approved the final manuscript.

Acknowledgements

This project was supported by Shanghai Nature Science Foundation "12ZR1406100."

References

1. Mebust WK, Holtgrewe HL, Cockett ATK, Peters PC. Transurethral prostatectomy: immediate and postoperative complications. Cooperative study of 13 participating institutions evaluating 3,885 patients. J Urol. 1989;141:243–7.
2. Foley SJ, Soloman LZ, Wedderburn AW, Kashif KM, Summerton D, Basketter V, et al. A prospective study of the natural history of hematuria associated with benign prostatic hyperplasia and the effect of finasteride. J Urol. 2000;163:496–8.
3. Hagerty JA, Ginsberg PC, Harmon JD, Harkaway RC. Pretreatment with finasteride decreases perioperative bleeding associated with transurethral resection of prostate. Urology. 2000;55:684–9.
4. Ozdal OL, Ozden C, Benli K, Gokkaya S, Bulut S, Memiş A. Effect of short-term finasteride therapy on preoperative bleeding in patients who were candidates for transurethral resection of the prostate (TUR-P): a randomized controlled study. Prostate Cancer Prostatic Dis. 2005;8:215–8.
5. Liu XD, Yang YR, Lu YP, Zhang XH, Li FY, Wei Q, et al. Preoperative finasteride on decreasing operative bleeding during transurethral resection of prostate. Chin J Urol. 2003;24:694–6.
6. Li GH, He ZF, Yu DM, Li XD, Chen ZD. Effect of finasteride on intraoperative bleeding and irrigating fluid absorption during transurethral resection of prostate: a quantitative study. J Zhejiang Univ (Med Sci). 2004;33:258–60.
7. Lekas AG, Lazaris AC, Chrisofos M, Papatsoris AG, Lappas D, Patsouris E, et al. Finasteride effects on hypoxia and angiogenetic markers in benign prostatic hyperplasia. Urology. 2006;68:436–41.
8. Donohue JF, Sharma H, Abraham R, Natalwala S, Thomas DR, Foster MC. Transurethral prostate resection and bleeding: a randomized, placebo controlled trial of the role of finasteride for decreasing operative blood loss. J Urol. 2002;168:2024–6.
9. Berardinis ED, Antonini G, Busetto GM, Gentile V, Silverio FD, Rossi A. Reduced intraoperative bleeding during transurethral resection of the prostate: evaluation of finasteride, vascular endothelial growth factor, and CD34. Curr Prostate Rep. 2008;6:123–7.
10. Sandfeldt L, Bailey DM, Hahn RG. Blood loss during transurethral resection of the prostate after 3 months of treatment with finasteride. Urology. 2001;58:972–6.
11. Memis A, Ozden C, Ozdal OL, Guzel O, Han O, Seckin S. Effect of finasteride treatment on suburethral prostatic microvessel density in patients with hematuria related to benign prostate hyperplasia. Urol Int. 2008;80:177–80.
12. Donohue JF, Hayne D, Karnik U, Thomas DR, Foster MC. Randomized, placebo controlled trial showing that finasteride reduces prostatic vascularity rapidly within 2 weeks. BJU Int. 2005;96:1319–22.
13. Haggstrom S, Tørring N, Møller K, Jensen E, Lund L, Nielsen JE, et al. Effects of finasteride on vascular endothelial growth factor—a placebo controlled randomized study in BPH patients. Scand J Urol Nephrol. 2002;36:182–7.
14. Liu Y, Hou TH, Jiang HM, Feng YH, Zhang L. Clinical research on preoperative application of finasteride in reducing transurethral resection syndrome. Shan Dong Med drugs. 2013;26:22–4.
15. He EB, Li JF. Effect of different doses of preoperative finasteride on the bleeding during transurethral resection of prostate. J Mod Urol. 2012;17:287–9.
16. Boccon-Gibod L, Valton M, Ibrahim H, Comenducci A. Effect of dutasteride on reduction of intraoperative bleeding related to transurethral resection of the prostate. Prog Urol. 2005;15:1085–9.
17. Kravchick S, Cytron S, Mamonov A, Peled R, Linov L. Effect of short-term dutasteride therapy on prostate vascularity in patients with benign prostatic hyperplasia: a pilot study. Urology. 2009;73:1274–8.
18. Pastore AL, Mariani S, Barrese F, Palleschi G, Valentini AM, Pacini L, et al. Transurethral resection of prostate and the role of pharmacological treatment with dutasteride in decreasing surgical blood loss. J Endourol. 2013;27:68–70.
19. Lund L, Ernst-Jensen KM, Tørring N, Nielsen JE. Impact of finasteride treatment on perioperative bleeding before transurethral resection of the prostate: a prospective randomized study. Scand J Urol Nephrol. 2005;39:160–2.
20. Hahn RG, Fagerstrom T, Tammela TL, Trip OV, Beisland HO, Duggan A, et al. Blood loss and postoperative complications associated with transurethral resection of the prostate after pretreatment with dutasteride. BJU Int. 2007;99:587–94.
21. Tuncel A, Ener K, Han O, Nalcacioglu V, Aydin O, Seckin S, et al. Effects of short-term dutasteride and Serenoa repens on perioperative bleeding and microvessel density in patients undergoing transurethral resection of the prostate. Scand J Urol Nephrol. 2009;43:377–82.
22. Zong HT, Peng XX, Yang CC, Zhang Y. A systematic review of the effects and mechanisms of preoperative 5α-reductase inhibitors on intraoperative haemorrhage during surgery for benign prostatic hyperplasia. Asian J Androl. 2011;13:812–8.
23. Ku JH, Shin JK, Cho MC, Myung JK, Moon KC, Paick JS. Effect of dutasteride on the expression of hypoxia-inducible factor-1a, vascular endothelial growth factor and microvessel density in rat and human prostate tissue. Scand J Urol Nephrol. 2009;43:445–53.
24. Bepple JL, Barone BB, Eure G. The effect of dutasteride on the efficacy of photoselective vaporization of the prostate: results of a randomized, placebo controlled, double-blind study (DOP trial). Urology. 2009;74:1101–4.
25. Moher D, Liberati A, Tetzlaff J, Altman DG. Preferred reporting items for systematic reviews and meta-analyses: the PRISMA statement. Ann Intern Med. 2009;151:264–9.
26. Hozo SP, Djulbegovic B, Hozo I. Estimating the mean and variance from the median, range, and the size of a sample. BMC Med Res Methodol. 2005;5:13.
27. DerSimonian R, Laird N. Meta-analysis in clinical trials. Control Clin Trials. 1986;7:177–88.
28. Arena F. Role of short term treatment with dutasteride in transurethral prostate resection. Trends in Med. 2008;8:103–6.
29. Yu XX, Zhou DQ, Mo ZN, Li WG, Wang J, Liu SW, et al. The clinical application of finasteride in peri-operation of transurethral plasmakinetic enucleation of prostate. Chin J Geriatr. 2011;30:930–3.
30. Donohue JF, Barber NJ. How do we investigate haematuria and what role has finasteride?". BJU Int. 2004;93:3–4.
31. Lekas E, Bergh A, Damber J-E. Effects of finasteride and bicalutamide on prostate blood flow in the rat. BJU Int. 2000;85:962–5.
32. Burchardt M, Burchardt T, Chen MW, Hayek OR, Knight C, Shabsigh A, et al. Vascular endothelial growth factor-a expression in the rat ventral prostate gland and the early effect of castration. Prostate. 2000;43:184–94.
33. Gormley GJ, Stoner E, Bruskewitz RC, Imperato-McGinley J, Walsh PC, McConnell JD, et al. The effect of finasteride in men with benign prostatic hyperplasia. The Finasteride Study Group. N Engl J Med. 1992;327:1185–91.
34. Andriole GL, Kirby R. Safety and tolerability of the 5 alpha reductase inhibitor in dutasteride in the treatment of benign prostatic hyperplasia. Eur Urol. 2003;44:82–8.
35. Ekengren J, Hahn RG. Blood loss during transurethral resection of the prostate as measured by the hemocue photometer. Scand J Urol Nephrol. 1993;27:501–17.

14

Association between self-perception period of lower urinary tract symptoms and International Prostate Symptom Score

Sung Ryul Shim[1†], Jae Heon Kim[2†], Hoon Choi[3], Jae Hyun Bae[3], Hae Joon Kim[5], Soon-Sun Kwon[4], Byung Chul Chun[5] and Won Jin Lee[5*]

Abstract

Background: Most studies focusing on progression of BPH have been limited to the relationship between age and BPH progression, and only few studies have focused on the time duration to start treatment. This study aimed to investigate the association between self-perception period (S-PP) of lower urinary tract symptoms (LUTS) and International Prostate Symptom Score (IPSS).

Methods: This study used data from two large-population surveys: a community-based survey and a university hospital outpatient-based interview survey. Both surveys were conducted in male subjects aged 40 years or older who gave consent to the survey questionnaire and voluntarily expressed their intention to participate. Propensity score matching (PSM) was used to organize the population in both surveys into randomized groups to reduce selection bias. After excluding those who had missing values, 483 subjects were assigned to each group by PSM.

Results: The S-PP of LUTS became significantly longer as the severity of LUTS increased. The S-PP was 4.15 years in the mild group, 4.36 years in the moderate group, and 6.23 years in the severe group. These differences were statistically significant. The correlation between S-PP of LUTS and IPSS was measured by partial correlation while controlling for age (correlation coefficient = 0.20, p <0.001). Multiple regression analysis after controlling for age revealed that one-year increase in the S-PP of LUTS significantly (p <0.001) increased IPSS by 0.322 points.

Conclusions: This study clarified the association between S-PP of LUTS and IPSS in a large-scale population. These findings suggest that, from the perspective of public health, S-PP is an important risk factor for LUTS progression.

Keywords: Lower urinary tract symptoms, Prostatic hyperplasia, Self-concept

Background

Lower urinary tract symptoms (LUTS) of voiding and storage commonly affect middle-aged men. European EPIC study has estimated that LUTS is present in 62.5% of middle-aged men (voiding symptoms, 25.7%; storage symptoms, 51.3%) [1]. Korean EPIC study has estimated that LUTS is present in 53.7% of middle-aged men (void-ing symptoms, 28.5%; storage symptoms, 44.6%) [2].

Benign prostatic hyperplasia (BPH), often causes voiding symptoms, a highly prevalent condition in middle-aged men. In the United States, South Korea, the United Kingdom, and Japan, the prevalence of BPH in age group of 40s to 80s is reported to be 33%, 23%, 41%, and 37%, respectively [3-6]. BPH, representing 80% of causes of geriatric diseases associated with urination, is known to cause decline in sexual function [7] and deterioration in both urination-related [8] and health-related [9] quality of life (QoL). BPH is a progressive disease, with most patients experiencing symptoms worsening over time [10,11]. BPH does not suddenly appear as a disease. It develops slowly in a natural process after subjective

* Correspondence: leewj@korea.ac.kr
†Equal contributors
[5]Department of Preventive Medicine, College of Medicine, Korea University, Seoul, South Korea
Full list of author information is available at the end of the article

perception of LUTS. Therefore, along with age, the self-perception period (S-PP) of LUTS was considered as one of the most important risk factors for BPH [12-14].

Escalating medical expenditures are a major concern in many countries, especially those with populations having high incidence of BPH. In the United States, almost 8 million visits were made with primary or secondary diagnosis of BPH. In 2000, the direct cost of BPH treatment was estimated to be $1.1 billion, exclusive of outpatient pharmaceuticals [15].

From the perspective of public health, identifying risk factors for LUTS is useful to prevent LUTS and to improve QoL. Olmsted County study [16], one of the largest longitudinal studies conducted in America, investigated age as one of many sociodemographic characteristics that may predict the incidence of BPH. Age was also investigated in a study that reanalyzed the same patients of the Olmsted County study [17]. Thus, age is one of the most reliable risk factors for the progression of BPH. Its influence is greater than those of other sociodemographic characteristics. Likewise, most studies focusing on the natural history and progression of BPH have been limited to the relationship between age and BPH progression. In reality, the timing of the first hospital visit after LUTS is different between individuals. In order to explain this more comprehensively, Our previous studies adopted the idea of an S-PP of LUTS from patient's perspective because BPH is characterized by deep involvement of highly subjective symptoms. These studies showed that the S-PP of LUTS, in addition to age, acted as a major risk factor for LUTS [12-14]. However, results from these studies were insufficient to draw general conclusions due to their small sample sizes, even though individuals were sampled equally from large cities, small- and medium-sized cities, and rural areas. The present study attempted to overcome the limitations of previous studies and determine whether S-PP of LUTS is a risk factor for LUTS using data obtained from a community-based interview survey and an interview survey of university hospital outpatients.

Methods
Subjects
The present study used data from two large-population surveys: a community-based interview survey and a university hospital outpatient-based interview survey. Both were conducted with male subjects aged 40 years or older who gave and wrote the informed consents to the survey and voluntarily expressed their intention to participate. This study was approved by the Institutional Review Board of Korea University Ansan Hospital. In order to enhance the validity of International Prostate Symptom Score (IPSS), both surveys excluded the following patients: 1) those who had undergone urological surgery which might affect their IPSS score; 2) those who had

received any treatment for BPH or prostate cancer; 3) those who had evidence of neurological condition, uncontrolled diabetes mellitus, un-controlled hypertension, history of malignancy, urinary tract infection within 3 months, psychiatric illness with medications and alcohol or substance abuse; 4) those who were taking or had taken any drug for the same complaints.

Community-based interview survey
One investigator visited senior welfare centers in South Korea between May 2010 and April 2013 and carried out a survey of 1,030 males using the IPSS questionnaire. During this period, the survey was conducted over a total of 36 times in six metropolitan areas of the country: Seoul, Gyeonggido, Incheon, Daejeon, Daegu, and Busan. In total, the study had a sample size of 518 subjects after excluding those described above.

University hospital outpatients-based survey
Another IPSS questionnaire survey was performed with 2,493 male outpatients who visited university hospitals in South Korea between September 2010 and September 2011. The survey included 20 university hospitals in nine major areas of the country: Seoul, Gyeonggido, Incheon, Daejeon, Daegu, Busan, Gangwondo, Gwangju, and Ulsan. In total, the study had a sample size of 1,278 subjects after excluding those described above.

Study design and measuring tools
This was a cross-sectional study. To evaluate the factors that might affect the severity of LUTS, the study investigated age, S-PP, and IPSS.

IPSS questionnaire
The severity of LUTS was measured by IPSS based on the American Urological Association (AUA) symptom index, with one additional question on quality of life. IPSS questionnaire has been translated into many different world languages and adapted based on the circumstances of each country. IPPS questionnaire is now widely used for objective assessment of LUTS [6,18]. The Korean version of the IPSS verified by Choi et al. in terms of relevance and reliability is now the most typical diagnostic instrument for LUTS in Korea [19].

The IPSS questionnaire consisted of eight items, which included seven 6-point scale questions on symptoms (feeling of incomplete emptying, urinary frequency, interrupted stream, urinary urgency, weak urinary stream, urinary hesitancy, and nocturia) and one 7-point scale question on patient's satisfaction with their urinary condition. Based on the criteria of Barry et al., symptom severity was divided into three groups: mild (a symptom score of 0–7), moderate (8–19), and severe (20–35) [20]. The quality of life or level of satisfaction of LUTS patients was represented by seven grades: "No problem" (0 point = very satisfied), "I'm all right" (1 point), "Somewhat satisfied" (2 points), "Half-satisfied, half-dissatisfied" (3 points), "Somewhat dissatisfied" (4 points), "Distressed" (5 points), and "I can't stand it" (6 points = very dissatisfied).

Age questionnaire
Age as an important factor has impact on generation-specific prevalence, IPSS, and S-PP of LUTS. Therefore, this study queried each participant's date of birth.

S-PP of LUTS
The S-PP of LUTS was defined as the period between the moment the participant perceived any inconvenience resulting from LUTS (feeling of incomplete emptying, interrupted stream, urgency, weak urinary stream, hesitancy, or nocturia) and the time the interview survey was conducted. The longest periods of any LUTS symptoms were regarded as S-PPs.

Reliability
Cronbach's α was 0.652 for the seven 6-point scale questions about symptoms and the one 7-point scale question on satisfaction with urinary conditions, indicating acceptable internal consistency and reliability. Internal consistency with each item excluded did not substantially change the observed value. The reliability of the questionnaire used in this study was estimated to be similar to, or at least not lower than, that in previous studies [14]. This suggested that we used the same method as previous studies. The interview survey of university hospital outpatients was conducted by well-trained professional investigators. The present survey enrolled hospital patients through a formal procedure in compliance with the guidelines of the individual hospitals' institutional ethics committees.

Propensity score matching
Propensity score matching (PSM) was used to organize the population in both surveys into randomized groups to reduce selection bias in sampled population. Since the population of this study included two different groups of people, those "who do not visit hospitals" (in the community-based interview survey) and those "who visit hospitals" (in the interview survey of university hospital outpatients), we allowed Berkson's bias which may result from differences in characteristics between the two groups [21]. PSM typically involves the formation of pairs of treated and untreated subjects with similar propensity score (PS) values. Hence, a logistic regression model was used to calculate and save the predicted probability of the dependent variable and the PS for each observation in the data set. This single score (between 0 and 1) represented the relationship between multiple characteristics and the dependent variable as a single characteristic. Age and S-PP, whose significance was established in previous studies [12-14], were used as independent variables in the analysis.

In this study, in-caliper nearest-neighbor matching proposed by Rosenbaum and Rubin was taken into consideration as a PSM method. Rosenbaum and Rubin suggest use caliper value equal to 0.25 of the standard deviation of the logit of the PS [22]. Accordingly, this study used a caliper of 0.25 times the standard deviation of the PS. Furthermore, one-to-one matching was performed in order to optimize possible effects through several simulations. Excluding those with missing values, 483 subjects were selected from each group using PSM. In this study, the multivariate imbalance measure decreased from 0.50 before PSM to 0.28 after PSM. The implementation of PSM was accordingly evaluated to be appropriate.

Statistical analysis
In order to examine the association between BPH and related risk factors, we analyzed distribution patterns before and after performing PSM. We performed t-test on individual variables to determine whether the confounder was properly controlled between the non-visiting group (for the community-based interview survey) and the visiting group (for the interview survey of university hospital outpatients). For the prevalence of BPH, a frequency analysis was performed on IPSS scores. A one-way ANOVA was carried out to examine the relationships between different BPH severity groups. In an attempt to examine the correlation between the IPSS and the S-PP of LUTS, partial correlation coefficient was measured while controlling for age. A multiple linear regression analysis was conducted to assess how IPSS had changed over a year with respect to risk factors for BPH. In the analysis, independent variables included age and the S-PP of LUTS, both reported to be significant in previous studies [12-14]. The IPSS was used as a dependent variable. The significance of multicollinearity was assessed by comparing the variation inflation factors (VIFs) between independent variables.

All data were presented as mean and standard deviation (SD). Statistical analysis was performed using SPSS version 21.0 software (IBM, New York, NY, USA) with an R module available for PS analysis. All statistics were two-tailed and p-values <0.05 were considered to be significant.

Results
Characteristics of participants before and after PSM
With age and S-PP of LUTS as covariates, propensity scores were estimated as the probability of a hospital visit. The distributions of subjects before and after PSM are shown in Figure 1. The distributions of the non-

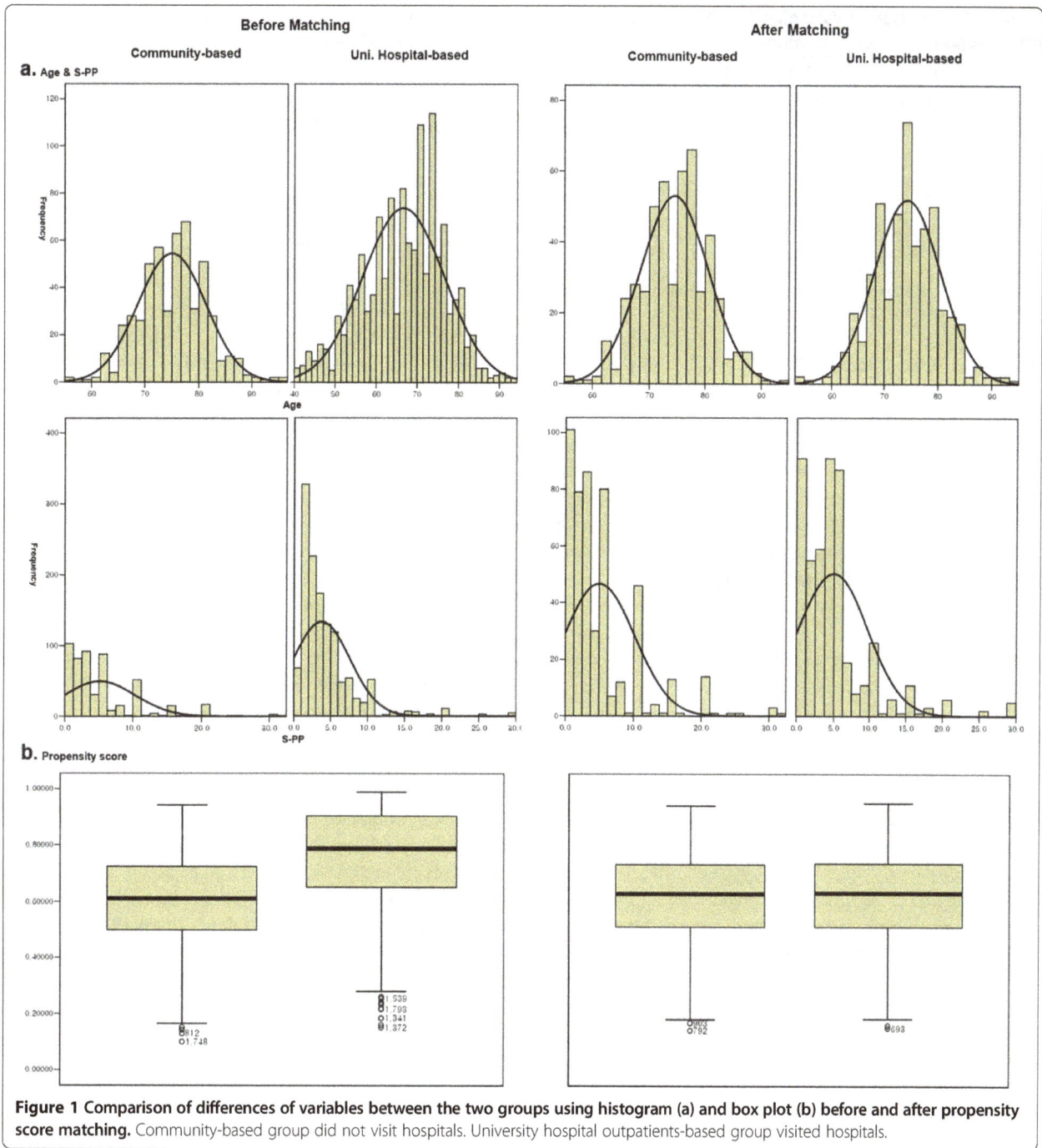

Figure 1 Comparison of differences of variables between the two groups using histogram (a) and box plot (b) before and after propensity score matching. Community-based group did not visit hospitals. University hospital outpatients-based group visited hospitals.

visiting group (subjects in the community-based interview survey) and the visiting group (subjects in the interview survey of university hospital outpatients) before and after PSM were found to be similar to each other in terms of age or S-PP of LUTS (Figure 1a).

Before PSM, the mean propensity scores ranged from 0.46 to 0.72 for the non-visiting group and from 0.64 to 0.92 for the visiting group. The small area of overlap between the two groups indicated that a small number of subjects had similar characteristics. However, when the

non-visiting and visiting group (n = 483 per group) were matched one-to-one after PSM, the two groups had the same mean propensity score of approximately 0.6 with a similar distribution (Figure 1b). After PSM, 483 participants were included in each of the non-visiting and visiting groups. The mean age of community-based survey and hospital outpatients' survey were 74.5 ± 6.06 and 74.3 ± 6.19 years, respectively. There was no statistically significant difference between the two groups in all variables except for IPSS (Table 1).

Table 1 Comparison of variables between the two groups after propensity score matching

	Community* n = 483		Hospital† n = 483		P‡
	Mean	SD	Mean	SD	
Age (years)	74.5	6.06	74.3	6.19	0.560
IPSS	15.3	8.16	18.1	7.61	0.000
S-PP (years)	5.0	5.16	5.0	4.79	0.998
PS§	0.61	0.15	0.62	0.15	0.618

*Community-based group, those who do not visit hospitals. †University hospital outpatient-based group, those who visit hospitals. ‡P-value, student t-test analysis. §Propensity score. IPSS, international prostate symptom score; S-PP, self-perception period of lower urinary tract symptoms.

Prevalence of symptomatic BPH

The distribution of IPSS scores were classified into three groups: mild group (n = 120, 12.4%), moderate group (n = 512, 53.0%), and severe group (n = 334, 34.6%). By age, 87.5% of patients in their 50s, 55.3% of those in their 60s, 53.9% of those in their 70s, and 46.2% of those aged over 80 years belonged to the moderate group. Therefore, as age increased, the proportion of patients in the moderate group was reduced. On the other hand, 12.5% of patients in their 50s, 33.5% of those in their 60s, 34.0% of those in their 70s, and 38.5% of those aged over 80 years belonged to the severe group. Therefore, as age increased, the proportion of patients in the severe group was also increased (Table 2).

S-PP of LUTS

The S-PP was shown to be 4.15 years for the mild group, 4.36 years for the moderate group, and 6.23 years for the severe group. These differences were statistically significant. A post-hoc Tukey's test revealed that the severe group showed a significantly longer perception period than the other groups. However, there was no statistical difference between the mild group and the moderate group. Therefore, as the severity of disease increased, the S-PP of LUTS became longer (Table 3).

Correlation between S-PP of LUTS and IPSS

The correlation between S-PP and IPSS was measured by Pearson's partial correlation while controlling for age,

Table 2 Age-specific IPSS severity and prevalence of LUTS after propensity score matching

IPSS severity	Age groups				
	50-59	60-69	70-79	over 80	Total
Mild	0 (0)	22 (11.2)	70 (12.1)	28 (15.4)	120 (12.4)
Moderate	7 (87.5)	109 (55.3)	312 (53.9)	84 (46.2)	512 (53.0)
Severe	1 (12.5)	66 (33.5)	197 (34.0)	70 (38.5)	334 (34.6)
Total	8 (100)	197 (100)	579 (100)	182 (100)	966 (100)

Values are numbers with percentages in parentheses. IPSS: international prostate symptom score; LUTS: lower urinary tract symptoms.

Table 3 Self-perception period of lower urinary tract symptoms based on severity

	n (966)	S-PP (years)		P*
		Mean	SD	
Mild	120	4.15†	3.95	<0.001
Moderate	512	4.36†	4.27	
Severe	334	6.23	5.97	

*P-value, one-way analysis of variances. †Same letters indicate no statistical significance based on Tukey's multiple comparison. S-PP: self-perception period of lower urinary tract symptoms.

which has a significant impact on both variables, with IPSS and S-PP of LUTS as control variables, S-PP of LUTS as an independent variable, and IPSS as a dependent variable. A weak correlation with a correlation coefficient of 0.20 was found (p <0.001; Table 4).

Association between S-PP of LUTS and IPSS

A multiple linear regression analysis was performed to assess how IPSS had changed over a year with respect to risk factors for LUTS. The IPSS was used as a dependent variable. Result of regression analysis found that a one-year increase in the S-PP of LUTS significantly (p <0.001) increased IPSS by 0.322 points and a standardized coefficient (β) of 0.200 (p <0.001). Age did not show a statistically significant increase in IPSS. The VIF among independent variables was 1.006. Multicollinearity was not significant (Table 5).

Discussion

LUTS is common in elderly men. This was confirmed in the present study. Especially, BPH symptoms become more severe as age increases. This result is similar to those of previous studies [3-6]. BPH can be associated with a number of health-related problems relevant to older men, including increased risk of acute urinary retention, sexual dysfunction, and BPH-related surgery [7,8]. In light of the high prevalence of BPH in older men, increasing life expectancy and retaining a good QoL for older patients requires addressing therapeutic issues and identifying the risk factors of BPH in the general population.

The risk factors for BPH can be seen from two perspectives. The first involves the sociodemographic characteristics of patients, which include age, family history, race, and ambient temperature [10,16,17]. The second

Table 4 Partial correlation between self-perception period of LUTS and IPSS

	n	r*	P
After propensity score matching	966	0.200	<0.001

*Pearson's partial correlation coefficient adjusted for age. IPSS: international prostate symptom score; S-PP: self-perception period of lower urinary tract symptoms.

Table 5 Multiple linear regressions analysis of self-perception period of LUTS and IPSS

	B*	S. E.	β†	P	
Age (years)	0.013	0.041	0.010	0.75	(n = 966)
S-PP (years)	0.322	0.051	0.200	<0.001	

*Unstandardized coefficient. †Standardized coefficient. IPSS: international prostate symptom score; S-PP: self-perception period of lower urinary tract symptoms.

includes biological factors, which include age, peak urine flow, prostate volume, PSA, and sense of residual urine [23]. This study placed its focus on sociodemographic characteristics. The self-perception period of LUTS could be considered as one of the most important risk factors for LUTS along with age. Emberton et al. reported that the natural history of LUTS, such as urinary frequency, urgency, nocturia, interrupted stream, weak urinary stream, and sense of residual urine might vary with age [24].

In the correlation analyses of previous studies, the correlation coefficient between age and IPSS was shown to be 0.17 [25] or 0.377 [26]. Age is one of the reliable risk factors for progression of BPH. Influence of age was the greatest among sociodemographic characteristics. Meanwhile, when controlling for age, partial correlation coefficient in the present study between the S-PP of LUTS and IPSS showed a significant correlation (partial correlation coefficient = 0.20, p <0.001). These findings suggest that S-PP, in addition to age, is an important risk factor for LUTS progression.

Assessing the progression of BPH by natural history and the Olmsted County study, one of the largest longitudinal studies conducted in America, was focused on age. This study was conducted on 2,115 patients over 42 months. In this study, IPSS was increased by 0.18 points on a yearly basis [16]. In a study that reanalyzed the same patients in the 66th and 92nd month, a 0.3 point [17] increase was observed, respectively. Thus, age is one of the most reliable risk factors for the progression of LUTS. Its influence is the greatest of all sociodemographic characteristics. However, in our study, a regression analysis with age and S-PP revealed that yearly increases of age. IPSS was increased by 0.013 points ($p = 0.75$) as age was increased yearly without statistical significance. Age was not a significant predictor of increase in IPSS severity because both large-population surveys did not control for age-generation distributions. Consequently, almost half of the participants were over 70 years old. We also found that as S-PP of LUTS was increased by 1 year, IPSS would increase by 0.322 points (P <0.001), which was a greater change than what was seen for age. The induced regression equation was as follows: IPSS = 14.109 + 0.322 (S-PP) + 0.013 (age). In the event when S-PP and age were increased by 1 year, IPSS could be increased by as much as 0.335 points. This result is smaller than the 0.868 points (p <0.001) found in a previous study using the same methodology [14]. The results of this regression analysis confirmed the results of correlation analysis described above. That is, from the perspective of public health, the S-PP of LUTS might be a more confident sociodemographic characteristic than age.

Emberton et al. raised the issue that, although the notion of disease progression in BPH is generally accepted, there remains uncertainty about the rate and the determinants of progression. In a review on placebo arms of clinical trials of BPH, progression was observed in terms of increasing prostate volume, decrease in urinary flow rate, and an increase in the future risk of acute urinary retention and surgery. By contrast, symptom score was shown to be improved in placebo groups, probably as a result of the "placebo effect" and the "white coat effect" [27,28]. In reality, however, the time of the first visit to a hospital after perceiving LUTS differs between individuals. The S-PP of symptoms could mean the "self-delayed time" before visiting a health provider. It could be affected by various sociodemographic characteristics. Several studies have shown that several sociodemographic risk factors could affect the "self-delayed time" before the first visit to healthcare provider [13,24,29,30]. The S-PP of LUTS before treatment could have a strong relationship with symptom severity at the time of first medical visit. The present study demonstrated that LUTS development depended on the period of patient's subjective perception.

The present study has several limitations. Sample selection bias is unavoidable in observational studies. The general characteristics of patients were uncontrollable in both surveys. There were many missing values in both surveys due to sample selection bias. These results were analyzed using two independent variables (age and the S-PP of LUTS) whose significance was established in previous studies [14]. Therefore, it did not represent the whole population of men aged 40 years or older. Furthermore, PSM only accounted for observed covariates. Unobservable covariates cannot be accounted for in the matching procedure. In addition, there was an obvious correlation between IPSS and the S-PP of LUTS. However, a causal relationship could not be observed. Therefore, in the future, a large-scaled active controlled study is needed using a sociodemographically representative population.

Conclusions

This study clarifies the association between the S-PP of LUTS and IPSS in a large-scale population. These findings suggest that, from the perspective view of public health, S-PP is an important risk factor for LUTS progression. Further longitudinal studies are needed to investigate the real predictive effect of S-PP.

Competing interests

The authors declare that they have no competing interests.

Authors' contributions

SRS and WJL contributed with the conception and design of the study, SRS and JHK drafted the manuscript, SRS, JHK, HC, and JHB collected data, SRS and SSK performed the statistical analyses, and JHB, SSK, HJL, BCC and WJL have contributed on the critical revision of this manuscript. All authors read and approved the final manuscript.

Acknowledgment

This work was supported by Soonchunhyang University Research Fund.

Author details

[1]Department of Epidemiology and Medical Informatics, Korea University, Seoul, South Korea. [2]Department of Urology, Soonchunhyang University College of Medicine, Seoul Hospital, Seoul, South Korea. [3]Department of Urology, Korea University College of Medicine, Ansan Hospital, Ansan, South Korea. [4]Biomedical Research Center, Seoul National University Bundang Hospital, Seongnam, South Korea. [5]Department of Preventive Medicine, College of Medicine, Korea University, Seoul, South Korea.

References

1. Irwin DE, Milsom I, Hunskaar S, Reilly K, Kopp Z, Herschorn S, et al. Population-based survey of urinary incontinence, overactive bladder, and other lower urinary tract symptoms in five countries: results of the EPIC study. Eur Urol. 2006;50(6):1306–14. discussion 1314–1305.
2. Lee YS, Lee KS, Jung JH, Han DH, Oh SJ, Seo JT, et al. Prevalence of overactive bladder, urinary incontinence, and lower urinary tract symptoms: results of Korean EPIC study. World J Urol. 2011;29(2):185–90.
3. Girman CJ, Epstein RS, Jacobsen SJ, Guess HA, Panser LA, Oesterling JE, et al. Natural history of prostatism: impact of urinary symptoms on quality of life in 2115 randomly selected community men. Urology. 1994;44(6):825–31.
4. Lee E, Yoo KY, Kim Y, Shin Y, Lee C. Prevalence of lower urinary tract symptoms in Korean men in a community-based study. Eur Urol. 1998;33(1):17–21.
5. Trueman P, Hood SC, Nayak US, Mrazek MF. Prevalence of lower urinary tract symptoms and self-reported diagnosed 'benign prostatic hyperplasia', and their effect on quality of life in a community-based survey of men in the UK. BJU Int. 1999;83(4):410–5.
6. Tsukamoto T, Kumamoto Y, Masumori N, Miyake H, Rhodes T, Girman CJ, et al. Prevalence of prostatism in Japanese men in a community-based study with comparison to a similar American study. J Urol. 1995;154(2 Pt 1):391–5.
7. Gacci M, Bartoletti R, Figlioli S, Sarti E, Eisner B, Boddi V, et al. Urinary symptoms, quality of life and sexual function in patients with benign prostatic hypertrophy before and after prostatectomy: a prospective study. BJU Int. 2003;91(3):196–200.
8. Yoshimura K, Arai Y, Ichioka K, Terada N, Matsuta Y, Okubo K. Symptom-specific quality of life in patients with benign prostatic hyperplasia. Int J Urol: Off J Japanese Urol Assoc. 2002;9(9):485–90.
9. Hunter DJ, McKee M, Black NA, Sanderson CF. Health status and quality of life of British men with lower urinary tract symptoms: results from the SF-36. Urology. 1995;45(6):962–71.
10. Jacobsen SJ, Jacobson DJ, Girman CJ, Roberts RO, Rhodes T, Guess HA, et al. Treatment for benign prostatic hyperplasia among community dwelling men: the Olmsted county study of urinary symptoms and health status. J Urol. 1999;162(4):1301–6.
11. McConnell JD, Roehrborn CG, Bautista OM, Andriole Jr GL, Dixon CM, Kusek JW, et al. The long-term effect of doxazosin, finasteride, and combination therapy on the clinical progression of benign prostatic hyperplasia. N Engl J Med. 2003;349(25):2387–98.
12. Kim JH, Ham BK, Shim SR, Lee WJ, Kim HJ, Kwon SS, et al. The association between the self-perception period of overactive bladder symptoms and overactive bladder symptom scores in a non-treated population and related sociodemographic and lifestyle factors. Int J Clin Pract. 2013;67(8):795–800.
13. Kim JH, Shim SR, Lee WJ, Kim HJ, Kwon SS, Bae JH. Sociodemographic and lifestyle factors affecting the self-perception period of lower urinary tract symptoms of international prostate symptom score items. Int J Clin Pract. 2012;66(12):1216–23.
14. Shim SR, Kim JH, Kim KH, Yoon SJ, Lee WJ, Kim HJ, et al. Association between the self-perception period of lower urinary tract symptoms and the international prostate symptom score. Urol Int. 2012;88(4):431–7.
15. Wei JT, Calhoun E, Jacobsen SJ. Urologic diseases in america project: benign prostatic hyperplasia. J Urol. 2008;179(5 Suppl):S75–80.
16. Jacobsen SJ, Girman CJ, Guess HA, Rhodes T, Oesterling JE, Lieber MM. Natural history of prostatism: longitudinal changes in voiding symptoms in community dwelling men. J Urol. 1996;155(2):595–600.
17. Sarma AV, Jacobsen SJ, Girman CJ, Jacobson DJ, Roberts RO, Rhodes T, et al. Concomitant longitudinal changes in frequency of and bother from lower urinary tract symptoms in community dwelling men. J Urol. 2002;168(4 Pt 1):1446–52.
18. Sagnier PP, MacFarlane G, Richard F, Botto H, Teillac P, Boyle P. Results of an epidemiological survey using a modified american urological association symptom index for benign prostatic hyperplasia in France. J Urol. 1994;151(5):1266–70.
19. Choi HR CW, Shim BS, Kwon SW, Hong SJ, Chung BH, Sung DH, et al. Translation validity and reliability of IPSS Korean version. Korean J Urol. 1996;37(6):659–65.
20. Barry MJ, Fowler Jr FJ, O'Leary MP, Bruskewitz RC, Holtgrewe HL, Mebust WK, et al. The american urological association symptom index for benign prostatic hyperplasia. The measurement committee of the american urological association. J Urol. 1992;148(5):1549–57. discussion 1564.
21. Berkson J. Limitations of the application of fourfold table analysis to hospital data. Biometrics. 1946;2(3):47–53.
22. D'Agostino Jr RB. Propensity score methods for bias reduction in the comparison of a treatment to a non-randomized control group. Stat Med. 1998;17(19):2265–81.
23. Stuart EA. Matching methods for causal inference: A review and a look forward. Stat Sci. 2010;25(1):1–21.
24. Emberton M, Cornel EB, Bassi PF, Fourcade RO, Gomez JM, Castro R. Benign prostatic hyperplasia as a progressive disease: a guide to the risk factors and options for medical management. Int J Clin Pract. 2008;62(7):1076–86.
25. Lee ELC, Kim YI, Shin YS. Estimation of benign prostatic hyperplasia prevalence in Korea: an epidemiological survey using international prostatic symptom score (IPSS) in Yonchon county. Korean J Urol. 1995;36:1345–52.
26. Cho KSJM, Lim DJ, Son HC, Park SK, Yoo KY, Kim HH, et al. Epidemiologic survey using international prostate symptom score of lower urinary tract symptoms in elderly men above 40 years old in Seoul area. Korean J Urol. 2001;42:840–84.
27. Alwan H, Pruijm M, Ponte B, Ackermann D, Guessous I, Ehret G, et al. Epidemiology of masked and white-coat hypertension: the family-based SKIPOGH study. PLoS One. 2014;9(3):e92522.
28. Emberton M, Fitzpatrick JM, Garcia-Losa M, Qizilbash N, Djavan B. Progression of benign prostatic hyperplasia: systematic review of the placebo arms of clinical trials. BJU Int. 2008;102(8):981–6.
29. Coyne KS, Kaplan SA, Chapple CR, Sexton CC, Kopp ZS, Bush EN. Risk factors and comorbid conditions associated with lower urinary tract symptoms: EpiLUTS. BJU Int. 2009;103 Suppl 3:24–32.
30. Crawford ED, Wilson SS, McConnell JD, Slawin KM, Lieber MC, Smith JA, et al. Baseline factors as predictors of clinical progression of benign prostatic hyperplasia in men treated with placebo. J Urol. 2006;175(4):1422–6. discussion 1426–1427.

15

Clinical evaluation of prostate cancer gene 3 score in diagnosis among Chinese men with prostate cancer and benign prostatic hyperplasia

Jin Huang[1], Kathleen H. Reilly[2], Hui-Zhen Zhang[1]* and Hai-Bo Wang[3]*

Abstract

Background: Prostate cancer is the second most common diagnosed cancer in men. Due to the low specificity of current diagnosis methods for detecting prostate cancer, identification of new biomarkers is highly desirable. The study was conducted to determine the clinical utility of the prostate cancer gene 3 (PCA3) assay to predict biopsy-detected cancers in Chinese men.

Methods: The study included men who had a biopsy at The Affiliated Sixth People's Hospital of Shanghai Jiao Tong University from January 2013 to December 2013. Formalin-fixed, paraffin-embedded tissue blocks were used to test PCA3 and prostate-specific antigen (PSA) mRNA. The diagnostic accuracy of the PCA3 score for predicting a positive biopsy outcome was studied using sensitivity and specificity, and it was compared with PSA.

Results: The probability of a positive biopsy increased with increasing PCA3 scores. The mean PCA3 score was significantly higher in men with prostate cancer (198.03, 95 % confidence interval [CI] 74.79–321.27) vs benign prostatic hyperplasia (BPH) (84.31, 95 % CI 6.47–162.15, $P < 0.01$). The PCA3 score (cutoff 35) had a sensitivity of 85.7 % and specificity of 62.5 %. Receiver operating characteristic analysis showed higher areas under the ROC curve for the PCA3 score vs PSA, but without statistical significance.

Conclusions: Increased PCA3 in biopsy tissue correlated with prostate cancer and the PCA3 assay may improve the diagnosis efficacy as the PCA3 score being independent of PSA level. The diagnostic significance of urinary PCA3 testing should be explored in future study to determine the prediction value in guiding biopsy decision as the clinical relevance of current study was limited for PCA3 testing based on biopsy tissue in a limited number of Chinese men.

Keywords: Prostate cancer, Prostate cancer gene 3, Prostate-specific antigen, China

Background

Prostate cancer is the second most common diagnosed cancer and the sixth leading cause of cancer deaths in men, accounting for 14 % of total new cancer cases [1].

* Correspondence: Liuyuanblz@aliyun.com; hbwang2005@163.com
[1]Department of Pathology, Sixth People's Hospital affiliated to Shanghai Jiaotong University, Yishan Rd 600#, Xuhui District, Shanghai 200233, People's Republic of China
[3]Peking University Clinical Research Institute, Xueyuan Rd 38#, Haidian District, Beijing 100191, People's Republic of China
Full list of author information is available at the end of the article

Prostate cancer diagnosis primarily relies on prostate-specific antigen (PSA) and digital rectal examination (DRE) outcome. The presence of an abnormal DRE or an elevated PSA level is associated with increased risk of prostate cancer, which is followed by a biopsy [2]. The prostate cancer detection rate has greatly increased since the discovery of PSA and widespread PSA testing [3, 4]. Due to the low specificity of PSA, only 25–40 % of patients with a PSA of 2–10 ng/ml are diagnosed with prostate cancer on biopsy, resulting in a substantial number of unnecessary biopsies [5, 6]. Many patients experience pain, discomfort and anxiety following a biopsy, and unnecessary biopsies may lead to complications [7–9]. The identification of biomarkers capable of increasing the probability of a positive biopsy is highly desirable.

Recently the prostate cancer gene 3 (PCA3) has shown promise in identifying men at high probability of a positive biopsy and in guiding repeat biopsy decisions [10–15]. PCA3, which has been measured in urine in men at risk of prostate cancer, is over-expressed in prostate cancer cells compared with benign prostatic tissues [16]. Elevated PCA3 scores have been associated with a positive biopsy outcome [11], and the performance of PCA3 screening is maintained through repeat biopsies [10, 17]. In addition, PCA3 scores may be correlated with the tumor indexes of prostate cancer, such as tumor volume and Gleason score [18, 19].

Unfortunately, limited studies on the application of PCA3 scores in prostate cancer detection in the Chinese population are available in the literature [20]. Chinese men differ significantly from the Western population genetically. The clinical applicability of PCA3 scores in Chinese men should be investigated thoroughly. There was a high variability in cancer detection rates even among Asian populations, and Chinese-specific data is necessary to provide adequate information in counseling Chinese men who would consider prostate biopsy for suspected prostate cancer. Hence, the prostate biopsy database was set up in Department of Pathology, Sixth People's Hospital affiliated to Shanghai Jiaotong University. The objective of the present study was to examine the performance characteristics of the PCA3 score in predicting biopsy-detected prostate cancer in the Chinese population. We also compared the performance of the PCA3 assay to that of PSA.

Methods
Study design
The study included men who had a biopsy at The Affiliated Sixth People's Hospital of Shanghai Jiao Tong University from January 2013 to December 2013, excluding men with medical therapy known to affect PSA or invasive treatment for benign prostatic hyperplasia (BPH). The study was reviewed and approved by the Ethics Committee of The Affiliated Sixth People's Hospital of Shanghai Jiao Tong University. All subjects received a detailed explanation of the study and written informed consent was obtained from all participants.

The histological slides were blinded and evaluated independently of the results of the other assays by two experienced pathologists. If the diagnosis differed between two pathologists, histological slides were reviewed again and a consensus diagnosis was obtained.

Specimen collection and PCA3 assay procedure
Prostate cancer and BPH specimens were obtained from formalin-fixed, paraffin-embedded tissue blocks.

We examined a series of 136 primary specimens collected by needle biopsy at the hospital. After adding 800 μl dimethylbenzene, tissue sections were incubated at 65 °C for 10 min to remove the paraffin. When tissue was to be manually dissected or scraped, the sections were immediately transferred to a microcentrifuge tube. The tube was centrifuged at 13,000 rpm for 3 min and the supernatant was sucked up. Then 800 μl 100 % ethanol was added and centrifuged again at 13,000 rpm for 5 min with the supernatant discarded. Then 800 μl 50 % ethanol was added and centrifuged at 14,000 rpm for 10 min with the supernatant discarded. Then 500 μL lysis mixture and proteinase K 5 μL were added to the centrifuge tube and incubated at 65 °C for 3 h. The sample tube was shaken at 1 h intervals during the incubation.

These samples after incubation were used for the detection of PCA3 and PSA mRNA according to the manufacturer's instructions. The detection was based on branched DNA (bDNA) technology (DiaCarta, CA, USA), which is a sandwich nucleic acid hybridization procedure for the direct quantitation without RNA purification or reverse transcription polymerase chain reaction. The capture plate containing sample and bifunctional oligonucleotide probe sets was read on the Kodia QuantiVirus® Luminometer System by the supplied analysis software. The PCA3 score was calculated as (PCA3 mRNA)/(PSA mRNA) × 1000. Transrectal ultrasound guided biopsy with at least 10 peripheral zone cores was performed, and the specimens were reviewed by local pathologists.

Statistical analyses
The age, values for the PCA3 scores, PSA levels, and % free PSA between prostate cancer patients and subjects with BPH were compared using the Wilcoxon rank sum test. In men with positive biopsy, the same test was used to examine the significance of differences in marker values from patients with Gleason scores ≤7 and with Gleason scores ≥8. Pearson correlation coefficients examined the relationship between PCA3 score and PSA level. Univariate associations of biopsy outcome with base predictors age, PSA and PCA3 score were evaluated using simple logistic regression analysis. In addition, adjusted odds ratios (aORs) were calculated for predictors that were statistically significant in the multivariate model.

The performance of PCA3 score for detecting prostate cancer was evaluated by sensitivity and specificity and their associated 95 % confidence intervals (CI) at various cutoff points using the receiver operating characteristic (ROC) analysis. The diagnostic accuracy of the PCA3 score was compared to that of PSA using the areas under the ROC curve (AUC) using the nonparametric method of Delong et al. [21]. The Youden index, calculated as sensitivity + specificity-1, was used for capturing the maximum vertical distance of the ROC curve and for determining cut-offs points. Statistical tests were performed using SAS 9.1 software (Cary,NC, USA). All tests were 2-tailed and $P < 0.05$ was considered the cut-off level for statistical significance for all analyses.

Results

Study population

Of the 136 included patients, 112 (82.4 %) had prostate cancer and 24 (17.6 %) were BPH on positive biopsy (Table 1). Ages ranged from 51 to 88 years and the median age was 70 years (interquartile range, IQR 66–77). Among the subjects with prostate cancer, the pathological biopsy Gleason score was ≤7 in 67.0 % and ≥8 in 33.0 % of men.

The probability of a positive biopsy increased with increasing PCA3 scores. The median PCA3 score was significantly higher in men with positive biopsy (111.37, IQR 42.64–320.90) vs BPH (17.76, IQR 9.19–81.90, $P < 0.01$). However, there was no significant difference in PCA3 scores between prostate cancer patients with biopsy Gleason score ≤7 (113.68, IQR 49.38–326.44) and patients with biopsy Gleason score ≥8 (102.59, IQR 12.07–278.23, $P = 0.27$). There was also no significant difference in PCA3 scores between prostate cancer patients with biopsy Gleason score ≤6 (94.26, IQR 41.81–326.44) and patients with biopsy Gleason score ≥7 (139.02, IQR 42.66–295.69, $P = 0.56$).

The probability of a positive biopsy also increased with increasing PSA. The median PSA was 13.67 (IQR, 7.98–29.02), and the prostate cancer patients had a significantly higher median PSA level (15.54, IQR 8.49–47.70) than BPH subjects (8.70, IQR 6.39–12.17, $P < 0.01$). The prostate cancer patients with Gleason score ≥8 had a significantly higher PSA level (54.09, IQR 13.46–100.00) than those with Gleason score ≤7 (13.21, IQR 8.43–21.25, $P < 0.01$). The PSA was <4 ng/ml in 9 men (6.6 %), 4–10 ng/ml in 37 men (27.2 %) and ≥10 ng/ml in 90 men (66.2 %). There was no significant difference

in PCA3 scores among 3 groups of subjects with different PSA level. No relationship was found between PCA3 score and PSA based on correlation analysis (r = 0.08, $P = 0.33$).

ROC curve

A ROC curve was used to demonstrate the diagnostic performance of PCA3 score and PSA for detecting prostate cancer (Fig. 1). The figure included the sensitivity and specificity of the two assays. The AUC of PCA3 score and PSA was 0.775 (95 % CI, 0.695–0.842) and 0.736 (95 % CI, 0.653–0.808), respectively. ROC analysis showed that there was no significant difference in AUC between PCA3 score vs PSA ($P = 0.60$).

Correlation of PCA3 score and PSA with diagnosis of prostate cancer

Results in terms of sensitivity and specificity are shown in Table 2. The PCA3 score cutoff of 35 provided the optimal balance (i.e., the maximum sum of sensitivity and specificity) between sensitivity (80.4 %) and specificity (62.5 %). Subjects with a PCA3 score of 35 or greater had a 6.8-fold higher probability of a positive biopsy than those with a PCA3 score less than 35 ($P < 0.01$) (Table 3).

The sensitivity of PCA3 score (≥35) was 80.4 % (90/112) (95 % CI 71.8–87.3) and the specificity was 62.5 % (15/24) (95 % CI, 40.6–81.2). The sensitivity and specificity of PSA (≥4 ng/ml) were 95.5 % (107/112) (95 % CI 89.9–98.5) and 16.7 % (4/24) (95 % CI 4.7–37.4), respectively; while the sensitivity and specificity of PSA (≥10 ng/ml) were 71.4 % (80/112) (95 % CI 62.1–79.6) and 58.3 % (14/24) (95 % CI 36.6–77.9). The sensitivity

Table 1 The characteristics of the study population

	Prostate cancer	BPH[a]	P value
Age (Years)[b]	71.00 ± 11.00	67.00 ± 13.00	0.12
PSA(ng/ml)[b]	15.54 ± 39.21	8.70 ± 5.78	<0.01
PCA3 score	111.37 ± 278.26	17.76 ± 72.71	<0.01
<35	22 (19.6)	15 (62.5)	<0.01
≥35	90 (80.4)	9 (37.5)	
% free PSA[b]	0.12 ± 0.08	0.18 ± 0.17	0.03
Biopsy Gleason score			
≤7	75 (67.0)		
≥8	37 (33.0)		

[a]BPH, benign prostatic hyperplasia
[b]Median ± interquartile range

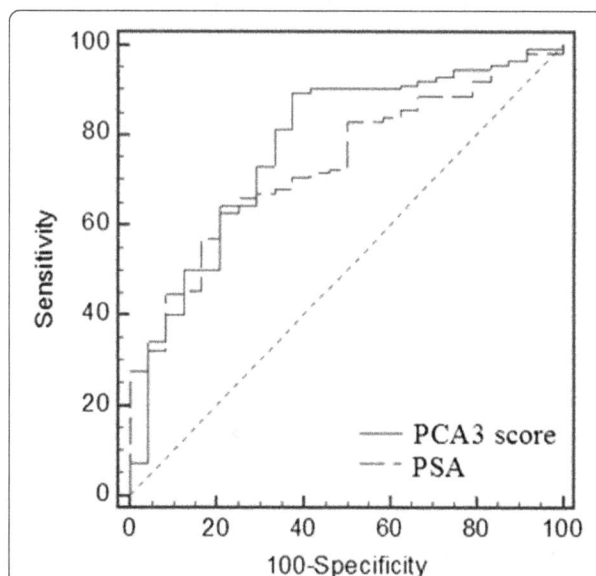

Fig. 1 ROC curve of PCA3 score and PSA for detecting prostate cancer. PCA3: prostate cancer gene 3; PSA: prostate-specific antigen. ROC: receiver operating characteristic

Table 2 Sensitivity and specificity of the PCA3 score and PSA

	% Sensitivity (95 % CI)	% Specificity (95 % CI)
PCA3 score cutoff 20	83.0 (74.8–89.5)	58.3 (36.6–77.9)
PCA3 score cutoff 35	80.4 (71.8–87.3)	62.5 (40.6–81.2)
PSA cutoff 4	95.5 (89.9–98.5)	16.7 (4.7–37.4)
PSA cutoff 10	71.4 (62.1–79.6)	58.3 (36.6–77.9)

for detecting prostate cancer was comparable, but the specificity was significantly lower for PSA (≥4 ng/ml) than PCA3 score (≥35). Although without statistical significance, both sensitivity and specificity of PSA (≥10 ng/ml) were lower than PCA3 score (≥35).

Univariate and multivariate logistic regression analyses

In univariate analysis, PSA >10 ng/ml (vs. <4 ng/ml) and a PCA3 score of ≥35 were significant independent predictors of positive biopsies (Table 3). In multivariate analysis, a PCA3 score of ≥35 remained significant independent predictor of positive biopsies (adjusted OR 6.73; 95 % CI 2.49–18.14). PSA >10 ng/ml (vs. <4 ng/ml) was also significant ($P = 0.02$).

Discussion

Due to the low specificity of PSA for detecting prostate cancer, unnecessary biopsy remains substantial [5]. The discovery and the development of novel biomarkers for prostate cancer diagnosis remains a challenge, despite the widespread use of PSA and DRE. The study evaluated the PCA3 assay as an additional tool in facilitating diagnosis of prostate cancer in Chinese men. An increasing PCA3 score corresponded with an increasing probability of a positive biopsy. The mean PCA3 score was

Table 3 Univariate and multivariate logistic regression analyses in predicting prostate cancer detection upon prostate biopsy

	OR (95 % CI)	P value
Univariate logistic regression model		
Age	1.05 (0.99–1.11)	0.14
% free PSA	1.22 (0.75–1.98)	0.43
PSA level (ng/ml)		
<4	1.0	
4 ~ 10	2.16 (0.48–9.70)	0.31
>10	6.40 (1.47–27.83)	0.01
PCA3 score		
<35	1.0	
≥35	6.82 (2.64–17.61)	<0.01
Multivariate logistic regression model		
PSA level 4 ~ 10 ng/ml	2.66 (0.50–14.08)	0.25
PSA level >10 ng/ml	6.99 (1.38–35.33)	0.02
PCA3 score ≥35	6.73 (2.49–18.14)	<0.01

significantly higher in men with positive biopsy *vs* a negative biopsy. The slight superiority of diagnostic accuracy of PCA3 score over PSA level was shown in this study, although without statistical significance. Data was also consistent with the PCA3 score being independent of PSA level [10, 11].

In a European multicenter study, the diagnostic accuracy of the PCA3 score was evaluated in men undergoing an initial biopsy [22]. The AUC ROC for the PCA3 score for predicting biopsy outcome was 0.761 and comparable to that in this study at 0.775. In European PCA3 studies, the AUC ROC was 0.761 in the initial and 0.658 in the repeat biopsy study [10]. These results suggested that the PCA3 assay can be used to guide both initial and repeat biopsy decisions. Therefore, PCA3 score may be considered clinically meaningful and its application in clinical practice can be justified [22, 23]. The PCA3 score cutoff of 35 provided the optimal balance between sensitivity (80.4 %) and specificity (62.5 %). Subjects with a PCA3 score of 35 or greater had a 6.8-fold higher probability of a positive biopsy than those with a PCA3 score less than 35 ($P < 0.01$). However, the additive value of PCA3 score in predicting biopsy outcome and the most optimal PCA3 score cutoff should be further evaluated by prospective studies to identify men with a high probability of a positive biopsy.

Multiple studies have also compared the diagnostic performance of the PCA3 assay to that of the traditional biomarkers, such as PSA and % free PSA [10, 11, 19]. These studies have shown the superiority of the PCA3 score over PSA level, although with slight improvement [19]. In our study, the AUC of PCA3 score and PSA was 0.775 (95 % CI, 0.695–0.842) and 0.736 (95 % CI, 0.653–0.808), respectively; and there was no significant difference ($P = 0.60$). This discrepancy can be explained by the smaller sample of men and by the restricted proportion of negative biopsy studied in the present report (82.4 % positive biopsy); this resulted in a decrease of statistical power. However, the sensitivity for detecting prostate cancer was comparable, but the specificity was significantly lower for PSA (≥4 ng/ml) than PCA3 score (≥35); both sensitivity and specificity of PSA (≥10 ng/ml) were lower than PCA3 score (≥35), although without statistical significance. Most importantly, data were also consistent with the PCA3 score being independent of PSA level, i.e., the diagnostic accuracy of the PCA3 score was not affected by PSA levels, confirming the findings of prior studies [10, 11, 22]. It was demonstrated that PCA3 fulfilled the most stringent criteria for a novel marker, i.e., in addition to univariate discriminatory ability it improved sensitivity and specificity and confirmed its independent predictor status [23].

In the analysis of the overall cohort of the European study, Haese et al. found that the PCA3 score was significantly higher in men with high Gleason scores [10]. Studies evaluating men undergoing radical prostatectomy showed an association between PCA3 score, tumor volume and Gleason score [24]. Our findings did not confirm this. This discrepancy can be explained by the smaller sample of men. Men at higher risk of aggressive and high Gleason score prostate cancer were studied in the present study (33.0 % patients with Gleason score ≥8). This resulted in a decrease of statistical power. However, other studies also questioned the relationship between the PCA3 score and aggressive prostate cancer [10, 11, 18, 19]. The association between PCA3 score and aggressive prostate cancer needs further evaluation in controlled studies to confirm the utility in selecting men with clinically insignificant prostate cancer.

The current study was subject to several limitations. The study population was referred to a PCA3 test for several reasons (i.e., a high PSA level or suspicious prostate cancer), therefore, those who were selected to have a PCA3 test because of a clinical concern for prostate cancer may differ from screening populations referred to triage testing. These subjects in the study had a median age of 70 years (IQR 66–77) with a relatively high PSA level (median 13.67; IQR 7.98–29.02), which is higher than that of a typical screening population [15]. The subjects recruited with high clinical suspicion for prostate cancer could not represent the population in China, more unlikely to reflect the actual situation in China. Secondly, the study sample was relatively small (especially the number of participants with negative biopsy) to compare the clinical performance of PCA3 score and serum PSA testing. Finally, PCA3 testing was based on formalin-fixed, paraffin-embedded tissue blocks collected before biopsy, therefore the clinical relevance was limited. To help determine the need for biopsy decision in screening populations, the diagnostic significance of urinary PCA3 testing will be explored in a future study.

Conclusions

This study showed that increased PCA3 in biopsy tissue correlated with prostate cancer and that the PCA3 assay could aid in diagnosis of prostate cancer in a limited number of Chinese men. The probability of a positive biopsy increased with increasing PCA3 score. In this population, the PCA3 score had a comparable diagnostic accuracy with PSA as there was no significant difference in ROC AUC between PCA3 score and PSA. Most importantly, the PCA3 assay confirmed its independent diagnosis value and may improve the diagnosis efficacy as the PCA3 score being independent of PSA level. However, the clinical relevance was limited as PCA3 testing was based on biopsy tissue. To help determine the prediction value in guiding biopsy decision, the diagnostic significance of urinary PCA3 testing should be explored in future study.

Abbreviations
PSA: Prostate-specific antigen; DRE: Digital rectal examination; PCA3: Prostate cancer gene 3; BPH: Benign prostatic hyperplasia; aORs: Adjusted odds ratios; CI: Confidence intervals; ROC: Receiver operating characteristic; IQR: Interquartile range.

Competing interests
The authors declare no conflict of interest.

Authors' contributions
Authors JH and H-ZZ conceived and designed the experiments. JH and H-ZZ performed the experiments. JH, KH.R and H-BW analyzed the data. JH, KH.R and H-BW contributed to the writing of the manuscript. All authors contributed to and have approved the final manuscript.

Acknowledgments
We would like to appreciate the reviewers for their helpful suggestions or commons on this paper.

Fundings
No funding.

Author details
[1]Department of Pathology, Sixth People's Hospital affiliated to Shanghai Jiaotong University, Yishan Rd 600#, Xuhui District, Shanghai 200233, People's Republic of China. [2]New York City, NY, USA. [3]Peking University Clinical Research Institute, Xueyuan Rd 38#, Haidian District, Beijing 100191, People's Republic of China.

References
1. Torre LA, Bray F, Siegel RL, Ferlay J, Lortet-Tieulent J, Jemal A. Global cancer statistics, 2012. CA Cancer J Clin. 2015. doi:10.3322/caac.21262.
2. Catalona WJ, Hudson MA, Scardino PT, Richie JP, Ahmann FR, Flanigan RC, et al. Selection of optimal prostate specific antigen cutoffs for early detection of prostate cancer: receiver operating characteristic curves. J Urol. 1994;152(6 Pt 1):2037–42.
3. Nadji M, Tabei SZ, Castro A, Chu TM, Murphy GP, Wang MC, et al. Prostatic-specific antigen: an immunohistologic marker for prostatic neoplasms. Cancer. 1981;48(5):1229–32.
4. Pelzer AE, Horninger W. How should PSA screening efforts be focused to prevent underdiagnosis and overdiagnosis of prostate cancer? Nat Clin Pract Urol. 2008;5(4):172–3. doi:10.1038/ncpuro1051.
5. Nath A, Singh JK, Vendan SE, Priyanka, Sinha S. Elevated level of prostate specific antigen among prostate cancer patients and high prevalence in the Gangetic zone of Bihar, India. Asian Pac J Cancer Prev. 2012;13(1):221–3.
6. Thompson IM, Pauler DK, Goodman PJ, Tangen CM, Lucia MS, Parnes HL, et al. Prevalence of prostate cancer among men with a prostate-specific antigen level < or =4.0 ng per milliliter. N Engl J Med. 2004;350(22):2239–46. doi:10.1056/NEJMoa031918.
7. Raja J, Ramachandran N, Munneke G, Patel U. Current status of transrectal ultrasound-guided prostate biopsy in the diagnosis of prostate cancer. Clin Radiol. 2006;61(2):142–53. doi:10.1016/j.crad.2005.10.002.
8. Ozden E, Bostanci Y, Yakupoglu KY, Akdeniz E, Yilmaz AF, Tulek N, et al. Incidence of acute prostatitis caused by extended-spectrum beta-lactamase-producing Escherichia coli after transrectal prostate biopsy. Urology. 2009;74(1):119–23. doi:10.1016/j.urology.2008.12.067.
9. Raaijmakers R, Kirkels WJ, Roobol MJ, Wildhagen MF, Schröder FH. Complication rates and risk factors of 5802 transrectal ultrasound-guided sextant biopsies of the prostate within a population-based screening program. Urology. 2002;60(5):826–30.
10. Haese A, de la Taille A, van Poppel H, Marberger M, Stenzl A, Mulders PF, et al. Clinical utility of the PCA3 urine assay in European men scheduled for repeat biopsy. Eur Urol. 2008;54(5):1081–8. doi:10.1016/j.eururo.2008.06.071.
11. Deras IL, Aubin SM, Blase A, Day JR, Koo S, Partin AW, et al. PCA3: a molecular urine assay for predicting prostate biopsy outcome. J Urol. 2008; 179(4):1587–92. doi:10.1016/j.juro.2007.11.038.
12. Chun FK, de la Taille A, van Poppel H, Marberger M, Stenzl A, Mulders PF, et al. Prostate cancer gene 3 (PCA3): development and internal validation of

a novel biopsy nomogram. Eur Urol. 2009;56(4):659–67. doi:10.1016/j.eururo.2009.03.029.

13. Hessels D, Schalken JA. The use of PCA3 in the diagnosis of prostate cancer. Nat Rev Urol. 2009;6(5):255–61. doi:10.1038/nrurol.2009.40.

14. Klatte T, Waldert M, de Martino M, Schatzl G, Mannhalter C, Remzi M. Age-specific PCA3 score reference values for diagnosis of prostate cancer. World J Urol. 2012;30(3):405–10. doi:10.1007/s00345-011-0749-1.

15. Salami SS, Schmidt F, Laxman B, Regan MM, Rickman DS, Scherr D, et al. Combining urinary detection of TMPRSS2:ERG and PCA3 with serum PSA to predict diagnosis of prostate cancer. Urol Oncol. 2013;31(5):566–71. doi:10.1016/j.urolonc.2011.04.001.

16. de Kok JB, Verhaegh GW, Roelofs RW, Hessels D, Kiemeney LA, Aalders TW, et al. DD3(PCA3), a very sensitive and specific marker to detect prostate tumors. Cancer Res. 2002;62(9):2695–8.

17. Aubin SM, Reid J, Sarno MJ, Blase A, Aussie J, Rittenhouse H, et al. Prostate cancer gene 3 score predicts prostate biopsy outcome in men receiving dutasteride for prevention of prostate cancer: results from the REDUCE trial. Urology. 2011;78(2):380–5. doi:10.1016/j.urology.2011.03.033.

18. Nakanishi H, Groskopf J, Fritsche HA, Bhadkamkar V, Blase A, Kumar SV, et al. PCA3 molecular urine assay correlates with prostate cancer tumor volume: implication in selecting candidates for active surveillance. J Urol. 2008;179(5):1804–9. doi:10.1016/j.juro.2008.01.013. discussion 9–10.

19. Ploussard G, Haese A, Van Poppel H, Marberger M, Stenzl A, Mulders PF, et al. The prostate cancer gene 3 (PCA3) urine test in men with previous negative biopsies: does free-to-total prostate-specific antigen ratio influence the performance of the PCA3 score in predicting positive biopsies? BJU Int. 2010;106(8):1143–7. doi:10.1111/j.1464-410X.2010.09286.x.

20. Shen M, Chen W, Yu K, Chen Z, Zhou W, Lin X, et al. The diagnostic value of PCA3 gene-based analysis of urine sediments after digital rectal examination for prostate cancer in a Chinese population. Exp Mol Pathol. 2011;90(1):97–100. doi:10.1016/j.yexmp.2010.10.009.

21. DeLong ER, DeLong DM, Clarke-Pearson DL. Comparing the areas under two or more correlated receiver operating characteristic curves: a nonparametric approach. Biometrics. 1988;44(3):837–45.

22. de la Taille A, Irani J, Graefen M, Chun F, de Reijke T, Kil P, et al. Clinical evaluation of the PCA3 assay in guiding initial biopsy decisions. J Urol. 2011;185(6):2119–25. doi:10.1016/j.juro.2011.01.075.

23. Kattan MW. Evaluating a new marker's predictive contribution. Clin Cancer Res. 2004;10(3):822–4.

24. De Luca S, Passera R, Bollito E, Milillo A, Scarpa RM, Papotti M, et al. Biopsy and radical prostatectomy pathological patterns influence Prostate cancer gene 3 (PCA3) score. Anticancer Res. 2013;33(10):4657–62.

16

Prostatic arterial embolization for the treatment of lower urinary tract symptoms due to large (>80 mL) benign prostatic hyperplasia

Mao Qiang Wang[*†], Li Ping Guo[†], Guo Dong Zhang, Kai Yuan, Kai Li, Feng Duan[†], Jie Yu Yan, Yan Wang, Hai Yan Kang and Zhi Jun Wang

Abstract

Background: Currently, large prostate size (>80 mL) of benign prostatic hyperplasia (BPH) still pose technical challenges for surgical treatment. This prospective study was designed to explore the safety and efficacy of prostatic arterial embolization (PAE) as an alternative treatment for patients with lower urinary tract symptoms (LUTS) due to largeBPH.

Methods: A total of 117 patients with prostates >80 mL were included in the study; all were failure of medical treatment and unsuited for surgery. PAE was performed using combination of 50-μm and 100-μm particles in size, under local anaesthesia by a unilateral femoral approach. Clinical follow-up was performed using the international prostate symptoms score (IPSS), quality of life (QoL), peak urinary flow (Qmax), post-void residual volume (PVR), international index of erectile function short form (IIEF-5), prostatic specific antigen (PSA) and prostatic volume (PV) measured by magnetic resonance (MR) imaging, at 1, 3, 6 and every 6 months thereafter.

Results: The prostatic artery origins in this study population were different from previously published results. PAE was technically successful in 109 of 117 patients (93.2%). Follow-up data were available for the 105 patients with a mean follow-up of 24 months. The clinical improvements in IPSS, QoL, Qmax, PVR, and PV at 1, 3, 6, 12, and 24 months was 94.3%, 94.3%, 93.3%, 92.6%, and 91.7%, respectively. The mean IPSS (pre-PAE vs post-PAE 26.0 vs 9.0; $P < .0.01$), the mean QoL (5.0 vs 3.0; $P < 0.01$), the mean Qmax (8.5 vs 14.5; $P < 0.01$), the mean PVR (125.0 vs 40.0; $P < 0.01$), and PV (118.0 vs 69.0, with a mean reduction of 41.5%; $P < 0.01$) at 24-month after PAE were significantly different with respect to baseline. The mean IIEF-5 was not statistically different from baseline. No major complications were noted.

Conclusions: PAE is a safe and effective treatment method for patients with LUTS due to large volume BPH. PAE may play an important role in patients in whom medical therapy has failed, who are not candidates for open surgery or TURP or refuse any surgical treatment.

Keywords: Angiography, Benign prostatic hyperplasia (BPH), Lower urinary tract symptoms (LUTS), Prostatic artery embolization (PAE)

* Correspondence: wangmq@vip.sina.com
[†]Equal contributors
Department of Interventional Radiology, Chinese PLA General Hospital
Beijing, 100853 Beijing, People's Republic of China

Background

Lower urinary tract symptoms (LUTS) are common complaints resulting from benign prostatic hyperplasia (BPH), is one of the most common diseases of aging men [1,2]. LUTS can reduce quality of life by impeding normal activities and causing complications such as acute urinary retention or urinary tract infection. The indication for treatment depends on the severity and bother of urinary symptoms. Treatment options include medical treatment, minimally invasive management, and surgical therapies.

Although both medical and surgical therapies for syptomatic BPH are effective, they are associated with significant morbidity rates and some degree of sexual dysfunction [3,4]. In addition, patients with LUTS due to BPH are often elderly and some patients may have severe comorbidities. Because of the increasing operative risk of undergoing transurethral resection of the prostate (TURP) or open surgery for these patients, especially in patients with large-volume BPH (>80 mL) [5,6], non-surgical treatment alternatives are required to meet their needs. Several minimally invasive treatments were originally conceived as an attempt to offer equivalent efficacy as operative therapy but without the burden and risk of operative morbidity [7,8]. Therefore, the development of new minimally invasive modalities for treatment of BPH has constituted an interesting field of research.

Recently, prostatic artery embolisation (PAE) for BPH has been shown to be a safe and effective procedure that improves lower urinary tract symptoms related to BPH and is associated with a decrease in prostate volume [9-11]. However, the rate of clinical failure after PAE was relatively high. As many as 25% of patients may not show a significant reduction in the international prostate symptoms score (IPSS) or improvement in peak flow rate (Qmax). In addition, the average of reduction rate in the prostatic volume after PAE varies from 20% to 32% [9-12]. One component of PAE where best practice remains to be defined is the choice of embolic agent size. In theory, embolization with larger particles (ie, >200 µm), as previously reported results [10,11], may not a optimal size for PAE because of early proximal occlusion. We assumed that smaller-size particles (<100 µm) may induce greater ischemia with a more distal penetration into the prostate, and hence lead to a better clinical outcome. In the present study, we designed to investigate the safety and efficacy of PAE with combined polyvinyl alcohol particles (PVA) 50-µm and 100-µm in size as a primary treatment for patients with LUTS due to large-volume BPH after failure of medical treatment.

Methods
Study population
Ethics statement
This prospective study was approved by the hospital review boards of Chinese Peoples Liberation Army General Hospital, and has been performed in accordance with the ethical standards laid down in the 1964 Declaration of Helsinki and its later amendments. Written informed consent was obtained from all the patients for the study.

From February 2009 to July 2013, a total of 117 patients (age range, 57–87 years; mean, 71.5 years) diagnosed with severe LUTS due to large-volume BPH (>80 mL) that was refractory to medical treatment underwent PAE. The base line data of these patients were provided in Table 1.

Inclusion criteria included men older than 50 years with a diagnosis of severe LUTS (International Prostate Symptom Score [IPSS] >18 points, quality of life [QoL] score >3, Qmax <12 mL/sec) due to BPH refractory to medical treatment for at least 6 months (alpha-1-adrenergic receptor antagonist or/and 5-alpha-reductase inhibitor) and a prostatic volume (PV) >80 mL (86-164 mL). The patient selection was achieved in a multidisciplinary manner in conjunction with urologists and interventional radiologists. All patients were assessed by an urologist and anesthesiologist as being unsuited for surgery owing to pulmonary disease (chronic obstructive pulmonary disease [COPD] in 33 patients) and cardiovascular diseases on antiplatelet therapy (coronary artery stent placement in 57, coronary bypass in 14 and cardiac valve replacement in 3 patients). Fifteen patients underwent transrectal US-guided prostate biopsy due to a PSA level >4.0 ng/mL with negative results for malignancy. Exclusion criteria included malignancy, large bladder diverticula (>5 cm), large bladder stones (>2 cm), chronic renal failure, active urinary tract infection, neurogenic bladder and detrusor failure, urethral stricture, and unregulated coagulation parameters.

Patient evaluation
Efficacy variables of IPSS, QoL score (scored as delighted = 0, pleased = 1, mostly satisfied = 2, mixed-about equally satisfied and dissatisfied = 3, mostly dissatisfied = 4, unhappy = 5, and terrible =6), the International Index

Table 1 Pre-PAE baseline data (N = 117)

Characteristics	Values Mean ± SD	Range
Age (year)	71.5 ± 13.5	57.0–87.0
IPSS (point)	26.0 ± 5.5	21.0-35.0
QoL score	5.0 ± 1.0	4.0-6.0
PV (mL)	118.0 ± 35.0	86.0-164.0
PSA (ng/mL)	3.9 ± 3.0	1.0-7.2
Qmax (mL/s)	8.5 ± 2.0	5.0-10.0
PVR (mL)	125.0 ± 50.0	85.0-180.0
IIEF-5 (point)	11.0 ± 6.5	5.0-17.0

International Index of Erectile Function short form = IIEF-5, IPSS = International Prostate Symptom Score, PAE = prostaic arterial embolization, PSA = prostatic specific antigen, PV = prostatic volume, PVR = postvoid residual urine, Q_{max}=peak urinary flow rate, QoL = quality of life.

of Erectile Function short form (IIEF-5), Qmax, post-void residual volume (PVR), and PV were assessed before PAE and at 1, 3, 6 and every 6 months after the procedure. Serum prostatic specific antigen (PSA) was assessed before PAE and at 24 hours, 1 week, 1, 3, 6 and every 6 months after the procedure. The PV was measured by magnetic resonance (MR) imaging. The MR imaging protocol for all examinations was the same, including axial and sagittal T2-weighted and non–contrast-enhanced and contrast-enhanced T1-weighted pulse sequences, and a 1.5-T magnet was used with a phased-array 12-channel body coil (GE Healthcare, Milwaukee, Wisconsin). The volume of prostate was determined using the standard ellipsoid formula: length × width × height × 0.52. All MR images were assessed independently by two radiologists who were unaware of the outcomes of PAE, and disparate measurements were resolved by consensus.

Embolization technique

Patients stopped taking all prostatic medications 3 days before embolization. After undergoing successful PAE, all prostatic medications were stopped during the entire follow-up period if there was consistent clinical improvement. Patients started an acid-suppressing drug (omeprazole 20 mg, AstraZeneca Pharmaceutical Co. Ltd., China, once daily), an anti-inflammatory (naproxen 750 mg, Guangzhou Baiyun Mountain Pharmaceutical Co. Ltd., China, twice daily) and an antibiotic (ciprofloxacin, 500 mg, Guangzhou Xin Pharmaceutical Co. Ltd., China, twice daily) 1 day before the procedure and continued for 7 days following PAE. During PAE, we did not us the analgesic drugs routinely because all the patients were well tolerated to the procedures.

Angiography

Patients underwent angiography and PAE in a therapeutic angiography unit equipped with a digital flat-panel detector system (INNOVA 4100 IQ; GE Healthcare, Milwaukee, Wis, USA) with nonionic contrast medium (Visipaque 320 mgI/mL; GE Healthcare). Embolization was performed with a unilateral femoral approach in all patients. After local anesthesia was achieved, the femoral artery was cannulated using a 4-Fr vascular sheath (Radifocus, Terumo, Japan) with Seldinger's technique.

Initial pelvic angiography was performed with a 4-Fr pigtail type catheter (Cordis, USA) to evaluate iliac vessels. Selective digital subtraction angiography (DSA) was performed with a 4-Fr Simmons I catheter (Cordis, USA) to evaluate the hypogastric and prostatic arteries (PAs) by using the ipsilateral anterior oblique projection of 30°. The PAs were identified with DSA and Cone-beam computed tomography (CB-CT), and selectively catheterized with a coaxial 2.7-F microcatheter (Progreat

2.7; Terumo, Tokyo, Japan). Selective PA angiography before embolization was performed (3–5 mL contrast medium at 0.5-1 mL/s) in neutral and ipsilateral anterior oblique projections (35°) to ensure that the tip of the microcatheter was inside or at the ostium of the prostatic arteries. CB-CT was performed with a 3–5-second delay after injection of 4–6 mL contrast medium at 0.5-1 mL/s to evaluate for sites of nontarget embolization.

The origin of the prostatic arteries, revealed by the DSA, rotational angiography (images from a rotational scan acquired with a C-arm equipped with a flat panel detector) and Cone-beam CT, was assessed independently by two interventional radiologists with more than 10 years of experience; and the disparate findings were resolved by consensus.

Embolization

We started PAE with smaller PVA particles (47 ~ 90-μm, mean 50-μm; Polyvinyl alcohol foam embolization particles, PVA, Cook Incorporated, Bloomington, IN, USA)) for the distal or intra-prostate embolization; when reaching near stasis in the intra-prostate arterial branchese, we switched to larger PVA particles (90 ~ 180-μm, mean 100-μm; PVA, Cook Incorporated, Bloomington, IN, USA) for the proximal of the prostatic arterial embolization. This technique was modified from the suggestion by Bilhim T et al. [13]. We believe that using the smaller-sized particles firstly is essential to avoid early proximal occlusion of the prostatic arteries and to achieve the goal of diffuse gland parenchymal ischemia.

Each vial of PVA (1 mL) was diluted in a 40-mL solution of nonionic contrast medium (iodixanol 320 mgI/mL; Visipaque; GE Healthcare). The particles were slowly injected through a 2-mL syringe under fluoroscopic control. Before embolization, vasodilator with nitroglycerin (200-300 μg) was used intra-arterially through the microcatheter to prevent vasospasm and to increase artery size to facilitate super-selective catheterization. The end point of embolization was near stasis; after it was achieved, a waiting time of 4-5 min followed for the particles to be redistributed in the feeding vessels; and then more embolic material was injected until complete stasis of the feeding artery was seen fluoroscopically. After PAE, angiography was performed using the power injector, with the 4-F catheter at the anterior branch of the internal iliac artery to check for any further blood supply to the prostate. Embolization was then performed on the contralateral side by using the same technique.

Post-procedural management

The patients stayed in the hospital for 1-6 days for observation. The patients were monitored for adverse effects. Appropriate hydration was administered 2 to

3 days after PAE. In all individuals, antibiotics were given to prevent infection as described before.

Outcome measures

Technical success was defined as unilateral or bilateral PAE, as successful embolization of all angiographically and/or CBCT-visible arterial supply to the prostate. Primary end points were the reduction of 7 points of the IPSS (or at least reduction of 25 % of the total score) and the increase of Qmax (>3 mL/sec) at 24-month after PAE. Secondary end points were the reduction of PV, PVR, and QoL at 24 months after PAE. Clinical failure after PAE was defined when one of the following criteria was met: IPSS ≥ 20, QoL ≥ 4, Qmax improvement <3 mL/s.

Postembolization symptoms and complications were registered and classified according to the quality improvement guidelines for percutaneous transcatheter embolization [14]. Complications were considered minor if they could be addressed by ambulatory medical treatment and major if they resulted in prolonged hospitalization, hospital readmission, or required surgery.

Statistical analysis

The study's quantitative variables were expressed as mean values, standard deviation, and minimum and maximum values, whereas the qualitative variables were expressed as numbers and percentages. A Student t test for paired samples was used when appropriate. A P value of 0.05 or lower was considered to indicate statistical significance. Statistical analysis was performed using SPSS 16.0 software for Windows (Chicago, Illinois).

Results

PAE was technically successful in 109 of 117 patients (93.2%). Technical failure was seen in 8 patients (6.8%): the embolization was impossible owing to severe tortuosity and atherosclerotic changes of the iliac arteries in 6 patients, none of the prostatic arteries were revealed in 2 patients. Bilateral PAE was performed in 101 (92.7%) patients; the remaining 8 (7.3%) patients underwent unilateral PAE due to severe atherosclerotic stenosis of an unilateral PA. Mean procedural time was 105 min (range 65–180 min) with a mean fluoroscopy time of 30.0 min (range 20–45 min).

Based on the analysis of selective DSA, rotational angiography, and CB-CT of the internal iliac arteries, it was possible to identify the number of independent PAs and their origin in 109 patients with 218 pelvic sides. There was one PA in 95.0% of the pelvic sides (207/218) and two independent PAs in 5.1% (11/218). The most frequent PA origin was the gluteal-pudendal trunk (39.5%; 86/218; Figure 1). Other common origins were the superior vesical artery (31.7%; 69/219; Figure 2), the middle third of internal pudendal artery (27.5%; 60/218;

Figure 3). Three PAs (1.4%) arise from the middle rectal artery (Table 2).

Follow-up data were available for the 105 patients, who were observed for a mean of 24 months (range 17–36 months). Four patients were lost to follow-up. The proportion of patients who demonstrated clinical success at 1, 3, 6, 12, and 24 months was 94.3% (99 of 105 patients), 94.3% (99/105 patients), 93.3% (98 of 105 patients), 92.6% (87 of 94 patients), and 91.7% (77 of 84 patients), respectively. As shown in Table 3, the LUTS of the patients showed significant improvements. Significant infarcts (mean 60%, range 55 %-90 %) were seen in all patients with clinical success as measured by MRI at 1-month after PAE, exclusively in the prostatic central zone; the infarct areas were reduced progressively in size. At 6-12 months after PAE, the infarcts could not be detected clearly in the majority of patients, resulting from the netrotic tissue absorption (Figures 4 and 5).

At 24-month follow-up of these 84 patients, the mean IPSS decreased from 26.0 ± 5.5 points to 9.0 ± 5.5 points ($P < 0.01$), mean QoL decreased from 5.0 ± 1.0 points to 3.0 ± 1.0 points ($P < 0.01$), mean Qmax increased from 8.5 ± 2.0 to 14.5 ± 3.5 mL/s ($P < 0.01$), mean PVR decreased from 125.0 ± 50.0 mL to 40.0 ± 15.0 mL ($P < 0.01$), and mean PV decreased from 118.0 ± 35.0 mL to 69.0 ± 18.0 mL (with a mean reduction of 41.5%, P < 0.01). Sixty-two patients were followed more than 24 months and these changes were sustained throughout the observation period. No significant differences ($P = 0.6$) were observed in IIEF-5 scores during the follow-up period compared with preoperative data.

The serum total PSA values before and after PAE were provided in Table 4. At 24 h after embolization, the mean serum total PSA increased from 4.00 ± 2.50 ng/mL to 87.50 ± 45.00 ng/mL (with s mean of 21.9 times relative to the mean baseline values; $P < 0.01$). By 1 week after embolization, mean PSA dropped to 30.5 ± 20.0 ng/mL (mean, 7.6 times; $P < 0.01$). By 1 month after embolization, mean PSA dropped to the baseline values ($P = 0.6$); by 3-month and 6-month of follow-up, the mean PSA was statistically significantly lower than at baseline ($P < 0.05$), and was almost sustained over time.

Poor outcome after PAE was observed in 7 (8.3%) patients at 24 months after PAE: unilateral PAE in 6 patients and bilateral PAE in one patient. The PAS values in the 7 patients were increased by 4.9-8.5 times (mean, 7.0 times) relative to their mean baseline values at 24 h after embolization. The prostate infarction rate detected by MRI at 1 month after PAE in the 7 patients was 10%-25%; the PV reduction rate at 3-month follow-up was 10%-17% (mean, 15%). The clinical failure had direct relationship with the PAS values at 24 h after PAE, the prostate infarction rate at 1 month after PAE, and the PV reduction rate at 3-month follow-up.

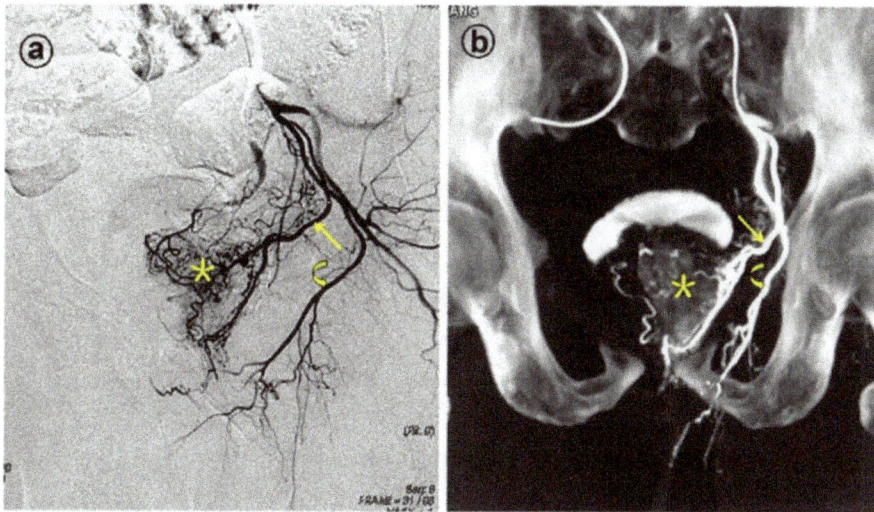

Figure 1 Prostatic artery arise from the gluteal-pudendal trunk. Images from a patient with significant lower urinary tract symptoms due to benign prostatic hyperplasia (92 mL) underwent bilateral PAE. **a**. Digital subtraction angiography (DSA) after selective catheterization of the anterior division of the left internal iliac artery with ipsilateral oblique view demonstrated the left prostatic artery (straight arrow) arising from gluteal-pudendal trunk; the curved arrow indicates the left internal pudendal artery; and the asterisk indicates the contrast staining in the left prostate lobe. **b**. Cone-beam CT image with coronal view after selective catheterization of the anterior division of the left internal iliac artery demonstrates the left prostatic artery (straight arrow) and the left internal pudendal artery (curved arrow). The asterisk indicates the contrast staining in the left prostate lobe.

No major adverse events were noted in this series. As minor complications (Table 5), urethral burning occurred in 19 (17.4%) patients, transient hematuria occurred in 11 (10.9%) patients, transient hemospermia occurred in 9 (8.1%) patients, transient rectal bleeding occurred in 8 (7.34%) patients, and small inguinal hematoma at the punctured site occurred in 3 (2.8%) patients. These patients with small amount of rectal bleeding may be attributed to ischemic rectal complication, resulted as the rectal nontarget embolization. All these

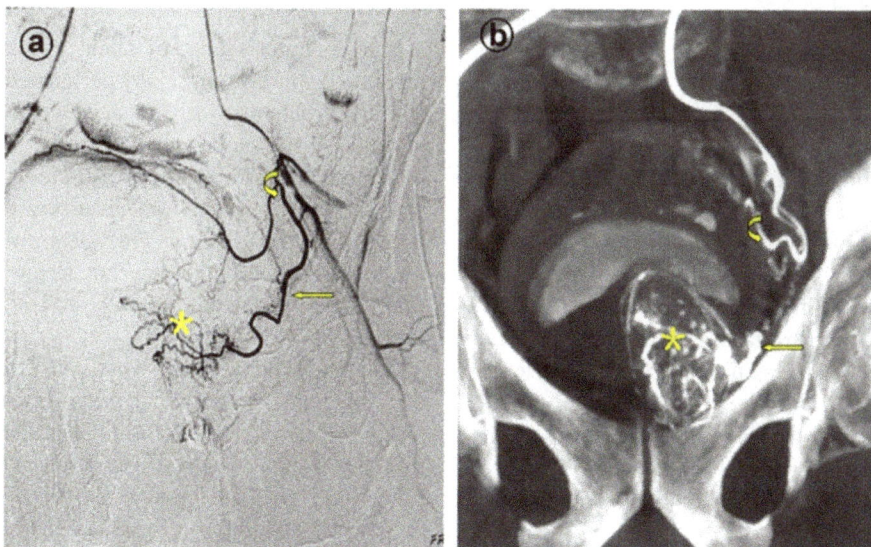

Figure 2 Prostatic artery arise from the superior vesical artery. Image from a patient with lower urinary tract symptoms due to benign prostatic hyperplasia (121 mL) underwent PAE. **a**. Digital subtraction angiography (DSA) of the anterior division of the left internal iliac artery with ipsilateral oblique view demonstrates the left prostatic artery (straight arrow) and the superior vesical artery (curved arrow). The asterisk indicates the corkscrew pattern of intra-prostate arteriola. **b**. Cone-beam CT image with coronal view after selective catheterization of the anterior division of the left internal iliac artery demonstrates the left prostatic artery (straight arrow) and the superior vesical artery (curved arrow). The asterisk indicates the corkscrew pattern of intra-prostate arteriola.

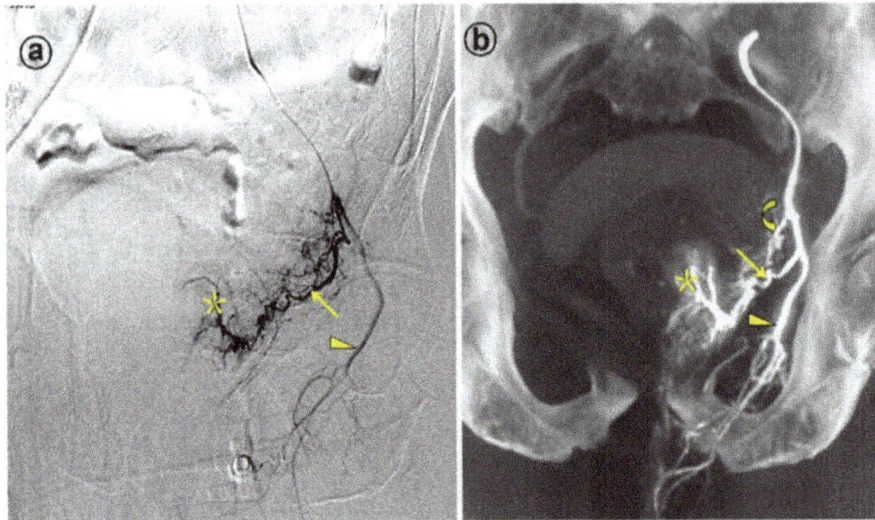

Figures 3 Prostatic artery arise from the internal pudendal artery. Images from a patient with severe lower urinary tract symptoms due to benign prostatic hyperplasia (117 mL) underwent PAE. **a**. Digital subtraction angiography (DSA) of the anterior division of the left internal iliac artery with ipsilateral oblique view demonstrates the left prostatic artery (straight arrow) and the left internal pudendal artery (arrowhead). The asterisk indicates the contrast staining in the left prostate lobe. **b**. Cone-beam CT image with coronal view after selective catheterization of the anterior division of the left internal iliac artery demonstrates the left prostatic artery (straight arrow) and the left internal pudendal artery (arrowhead). The curved arrow indicates the inferior vesical artery, which is difficult to identifying on the DSA. The asterisk indicates the contrast staining in the left prostate lobe.

minor complications disappeared during the first 1 week. Thirty-one patients (28.4%) experienced acute urinary retention at 1-3 days after PAE; for relief, a temporary bladder catheter was placed at the time for 3-6 days and the patients were able to void spontaneously before discharge. There were no incidences of ejaculatory disorders post-procedure. No other minor complications were observed.

Discussion

The surgical management of patients with prostate volumes >80 mL causing LUTS secondary to BPH presents a challenge [15]. TURP has been the 'gold standard' surgical procedure during the last 30 years, but its role in treating patients with prostate volumes >80 mL is limited, mainly because of intra-operative and postoperative morbidities (e.g., intraoperative and postoperative bleeding, postoperative hyponatremia, and urethral stricture) [16,17]. Despite the more recent development of new techniques such as endoscopic laser enucleation, plasma

Table 2 Prostatic artery origin: 109 patients (218 pelvic sides)

PA orign	Incidence
Gluteal-pudendal trunk	86 (39.5%)
Superior vesical artery	69 (31.7%)
Internal pudendal artery	60 (27.5%)
Middle rectal artery	3 (1.4%)

enucleation, and laparoscopic adenomectomy, in terms of efficacy, open prostatectomy (OP) is still considered the "gold standard" for the surgical treatment of BPH in patients with prostates > 80 mL [1,2]. However, OP is associated with a high morbidity rate, considerable blood loss, prolongedrecovery time, and heavy patient burden [2]. Serretta et al. [18] reported 8.2% blood transfusion in a large Italian series of open prostatectomy for large prostates. Gratzke et al. [19] performed open surgery on 902 BPH patients with an average prostate volume of 96.3 ± 37.4 mL and found that the total incidence of postoperative complications reached 17.3%. Thus, the new treatment options are necessary to meet this challenge. Recently, PAE is emerging and is a promising minimally invasive therapy that improves lower urinary tract symptoms related to BPH and is associated with a decrease in PV [9-11].

Our study demonstrates that PAE could be used safely and effectively as a alternative treatment for BPH in patients with large volume BPH. Consistent with the literatures [9-11,20], our experience showed that PAE is a safe procedure, even in patients who were unsuited for surgery, without significant increases in morbidity or mortality. In the studies by Carnevale FC et al. [10], Bagla S et al. [20], and Pisco JM et al. [21], the mean prostatic volume before PAE was 69.7 mL (range 43.5-92 mL), 64 mL, and 83.5 mL (range 24-269 mL), respectively. In our study the mean prostate volume before PAE (118 mL, range 86-164 mL) was larger than that of the previous studies.

Table 3 Clinical values over time of response variables after PAE

Variable	1 Mo (n = 105)	3 Mo (n = 105)	6 Mo (n = 105)	12 Mo (n = 94)	24 Mo (n = 84)	
	Mean ± SD	Mean ± SD	Mean ± SD	Mean ± SD	Mean ± SD	P Values
Age(year)	71.5 ± 12.5	71.5 ± 12.5	71.5 ± 12.5	72.5 ± 11.5	70.5 ± 11.0	–
IPSS(point)	9.5 ± 5.5	8.5 ± 3.0	7.5 ± 4.0	8.0 ± 4.5	9.0 ± 5.5	<0.01
QoL score	2.5 ± 1.0	3.0 ± 0.5	3.0 ± 1.0	2.5 ± 1.5	3.0 ± 1.0	<0.01
PV (mL)	103.8 ± 30.0	72.5 ± 25.0	70.0 ± 15.0	68.5 ± 15.0	69.0 ± 18.0	<0.01
Qmax (mL/s)	14.0 ± 3.5	15.0 ± 4.5	15.5 ± 6.5	14.5 ± 5.0	14.5 ± 3.5	<0.01
PVR (mL)	45.0 ± 20.0	40.0 ± 25.0	35.0 ± 15.0	40.0 ± 20.0	40.0 ± 15.0	<0.01
IIEF-5 (point)	11.0 ± 5.0	10.0 ± 4.0	12.0 ± 3.0	13.0 ± 2.0	10.0 ± 2.5	0.6

IIEF-5 = International Index of Erectile Function short form, IPSS = International Prostate Symptom Score, PSA = prostatic specific antigen, PV = prostate volume, PVR = postvoid residual urine, Q_{max}=peak urinary flow rate, QoL = quality of life.

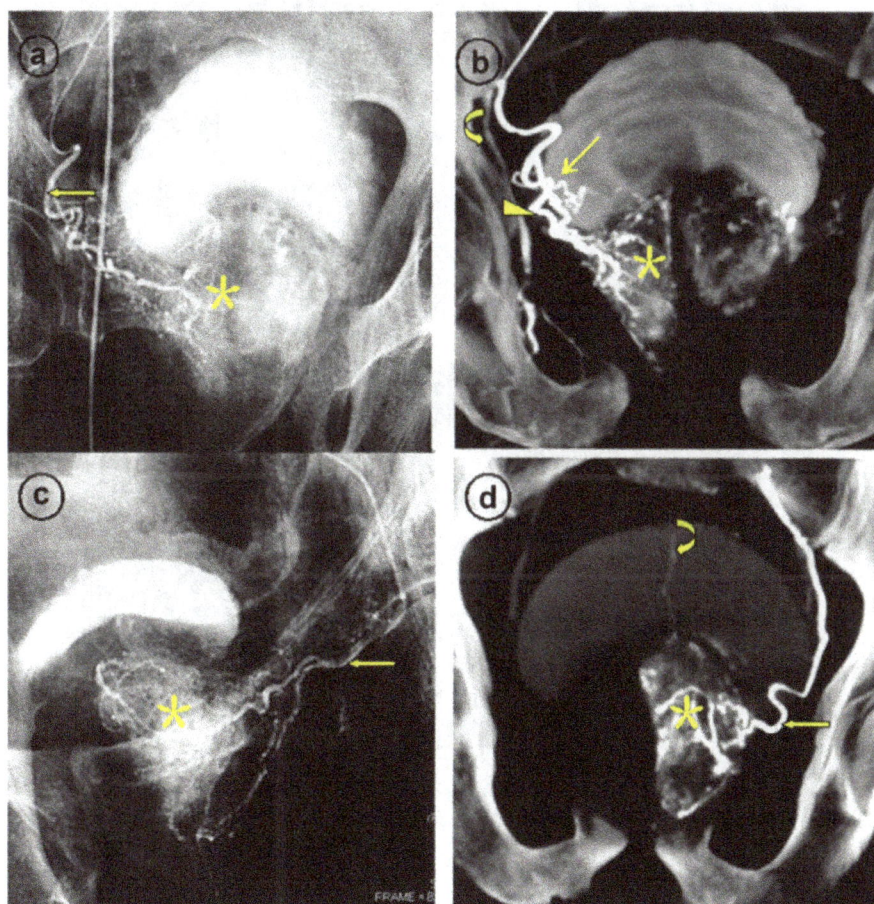

Figures 4 Images from a patient with lower urinary tract symptoms due to large benign prostatic hyperplasia (107 mL) underwent bilateral PAE. **a**. Angiography after selective catheterization of the riht prostatic artery (straight arrow) demonstrates contrast staining in the right prostate lobe (asterisk). **b**. Cone-beam CT image with coronal view after super-selective catheterization of the right prostatic artery demonstrates the the anterior-lateral prostatic branch (arrowhead), supplying to the central gland; the posterior-lateral prostatic branch (straight arrow), supplying to the peripheral and caudal gland. The asterisk indicates the contrast staining in the right prostate lobe and the curved arrow indicates the right internal pudendal artery. **c**. Angiography after super-selective catheterization of the left prostatic artery (straight arrow) demonstrates the corkscrew pattern of intra-prostate arteriola and contrast medium staining in the left prostate lobe (asterisk). **d**. Cone-beam CT image with coronal view after super-selective catheterization of the left prostatic artery (straight arrow) demonstrates contrast medium staining in the left prostate lobe (asterisk). The curved arrow indicates a branch of superior vesical artery, usually presented with high pressure injection of contrast medium through the anastomoses.

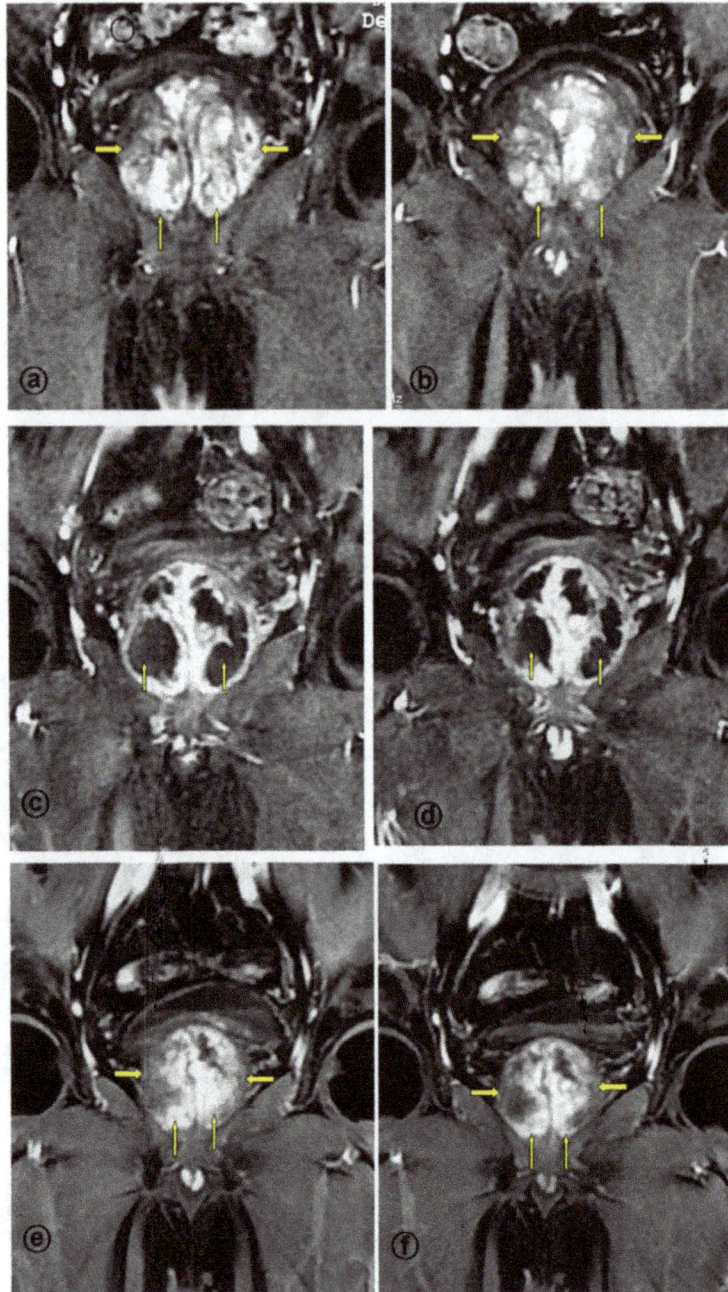

Figures 5 MR Images from a patient with lower urinary tract symptoms due to large benign prostatic hyperplasia underwent bilateral PAE, the same case as the Figure 4. **a-b**. Enhanced T1-weighted coronal MR images obtained before PAE shows a large benign prostatic hyperplasia (straight arrows). **c-d**. Enhanced T1-weighted coronal MR images obtained at 1-month after PAE shows significantly infarct areas on the both side of the prostate (straight arrows), with the volume reduction of 12%. **e-f**. Enhanced T1-weighted coronal MR images obtained at 12-month after PAE shows the prostate volume reduction of 62%; this patient experienced marked clinical improvement during 32 months follow-up, with IPSS improvement of 85%.

In the present study, the PV decreased from baseline to 24-month of follow-up (118.0 mL vs 69.0 mL, with a mean reduction of 41.5%, P <0.01), and Q_{max} increased (8.5 mL/s vs 14.5 mL/s, mean increase of 70.59%, P <0.01). This decrease in PV and increase in Q_{max} was accompanied by a significant reduction in BPH symptom burden as measured by IPSS (mean score, 26.0 at baseline, 9.0 in follow-up; P <0.01) and a commensurate improvement in patient QoL (mean index, 5.0 at baseline, 3.0 in follow-up; P <0.01). Many patients with LUTS due to large volume BPH are elderly, fragile patients with various comorbidities and therefore unsuited for surgery

Table 4 Total serum PSA values before and after PAE (n = 84)

	Values (ng/mL, Mean ± SD)	Range	P Values
Pre-PAE	4.0 ± 2.5	1.2-6.5	-
24 h	87.5 ± 45.0	30.0-145.0	<0.01
1 week	30.5 ± 20.0	9.5-57.0	<0.01
1-Month	4.2 ± 2.5	1.5-6.0	0.6
3-Month	3.7 ± 1.6	0.8-4.5	0.04
6-Month	3.1 ± 1.5	1.0-4.5	0.03
12-Month	3.9 ± 2.5	0.7-4.9	0.05
18-Month	4.1 ± 1.5	1.0-4.6	0.05
24-Month	3.7 ± 1.5	1.5-4.7	0.05

PAE = prostaic arterial embolization, PSA = prostatic specific antigen.

because of the operative risks involved [5,6]. The potential for PAE as an alternative treatment in patients with prostates > 80 mL is significant because TURP and laparoscopic prostatectomy are typically not considered for this population [1,2].

Comprehension of the functional arterial anatomy is crucial for an effective and a safe embolization, allowing better results and avoiding complications from untargeted embolization to surrounding organs (bladder, rectum, and penis) [22]. In a recent in vivo study by Bilhim T et al. [23], the authors reported that the origin of the prostatic artery is highly variable. PAs usually arise from the internal pudendal artery (35%), from a common origin with the superior vesical artery (20%), from the common anterior gluteal-pudendal trunk (15%), from the obturator artery (10%), or from a common prostato-rectal trunk (10%). Other origins are from the inferior gluteal artery, superior gluteal artery, or from an accessory pudendal artery (10%). Carnevale FC et al. [10] reported that the most common artery supplying the prostate was the inferior vesical artery, but branches from other arteries were also found to feed the gland. In the present study, we used the conventional DSA, combined with rotational angiography and CB-CT, for identifying the prostatic arteries and its origin; it may be

Table 5 Minor complications in the first week after PAE (n = 109)

Adverse event	Number of patients (%)
Urethral burning	19 (17.4%)
Hematuria	11 (10.9%)
Hematospermia	9 (8.1%)
Rectal bleeding	8 (7.3%)
AUR	31 (28.4%)
Inguinal hematoma	3 (2.8%)

PAE = prostate arterial embolization, AUR = acute urinary retention.

more accurate and more reliable than the conventional DSA alone for evaluation the pelvic vascular anatomy [21]. Our findings of the prostatic artery origins were somewhat different from previously published results [10,23]. In this study, we found that 95.0% of the internal iliac artery had only one prostatic artery, 5.1% (11/218) had two independent prostatic arteries, 39.5% originated from the gluteal-pudendal trunk,31.7% originated from the superior vesical artery (as a common pedicle with the superior vesical artery), and 27.5% of PA originated from the pudendal artery. Unlike reported by Bilhim T et al. [23] and others [10,24], we did not found that the prostatic arteries originated from the obturator artery, inferior gluteal artery, and superior gluteal artery.

A modified embolization protocol, which developed was based on others work [13] and our early clinical experience of PAE, was used in this study. We started embolization with smaller-sized PVA particles (50-μm) for the distal embolization, and ended with larger (100-μm) for the proximal embolization. Our data showed that the mean PV was decreased from 118.0 ± 35.0 mL to 69.0 ± 18.0 mL (a mean reduction of 41.5%) after PAE at 24-month follow up. The reduction rate was higher than those of previous reports by Bagla et al. [11] with a mean reduction of 18% and by Pisco et al. [9] with a mean reduction of 20%. Using the "standard technique" and 100-300 μm particles size, the infarcts have been seen in only 70.6% of the patients with a mean infarction rate of 30%-50% after PAE [9,25]. In the present study, we have observed infarcts area ≥50% in all patients with clinical success as measured by MRI. In addition, we have observed that serum total PSA values increased significantly at 24 h after embolization, with a mean 21.9 times relative to the mean baseline values; these also suggested that greater prostate infarction occurred after PAE with the smaller size particles.

It is reasonable to assume that smaller-sized particles may induce greater ischemia with a more distal penetration into the prostate microvasculature [13], and hence lead to a better clinical outcome. Because BPH develops primarily in the peri-urethral region of the prostate, therefore embolization of this part is important for improvement of LUTS. From previous studies [9,13], we knew that 100-μm PVA particles could be used safely for PAE without untargeted embolization. Anatomically, the prostatic part of the urethra is supplied by a branch of prostatic artery, both in dogs and in humans, with a diameter of 40–60 μm [26]. Based on these data, particles with 50-μm in size may penetrate into the peri-urethral region of the prostate, with a better result than that of particles ≥100-μm in size. However, untargeted embolization and injury of the urethral wall should be concerned using the small sized particles. In the present study, no major complications were observed from PAE in any patient treated, the minor complication rates were comparable to previously reported results [9-11], and all minor complications could be addressed with conservative care, showing that PAE with the combination of 50-μm and 100-μm particles is a safe procedure.

Bilateral PAE appears to produce better results than that of unilateral PAE. According to the reported by Bilhim T et al. [27], good clinical outcomes and improvements in urodynamic data could be achieved even in patients who underwent unilateral PAE. Another series reported by the same authors [28] showed that unilateral PAE might lead to moderate clinical relief with 8% PV reduction and 18% reduction in PSA. The authors suggested that the anastomoses between prostatic arteries from both pelvic sides, presented in as many as 20% of individuals, may partially explain these results [29]. In our study, of the 8 patients with unilateral PAE, Only two patients had clinical improvement during a 24-month follow-up. Carnevale FC et al. [30] reported one patient had unilateral PAE with continuous prostate reduction until 12 months follow-up (maximum of 27.8% reduction at the 6-month follow-up) and re-growth to the initial size at the 3-year follow-up. Therefore, the bilateral PAs and any other prostatic branches should be embolized to achieve optimal prostate ischemia, resulting in volume reduction for better long-term results.

No serious complications or adverse events in the performance of PAE were observed in the present series. The incidence of minor complications (ie., transient hematuria, hemospermia, and rectal bleeding) after PAE in the patients with large BPH was similar to those of previous reports [9-12]. In comparison with others reports [9,11,21], however, the acute urinary retention (AUR) after PAE was relatively high (28.4%) in our series; this may explained by the large volume BPH nature and edema in the periurethral prostatic tissue after embolization. For management of AUR, a temporary bladder catheter and antibiotics should be maintained for 1 week after PAE under the urologist's supervision.

There are some limitations to the present study. First, this study was a single-center experience with limited follow-up; however, continued follow-up is ongoing, and longer follow-up in our patients will bring additional information in the future. Second, the present study included only in patients with large-volume BPH and with unsuited for surgery; further analyses are necessary to establish the role of PAE in patients who are candidates for surgery, or the prostate volume less than 80 mL. Third, only PVA particle was used for our procedures; further investigation concerning different type of embolic agents are necessary. Finally, this is a non-randomised and non-comparative study. Although the results are promising more studies are needed, especially multicentre randomised controlled trials.

Conclusions

Our clinical results shows that PAE is a safe and effective treatment method for patients with severe LUTS due to large volume BPH. PAE may play an important role in patients in whom medical therapy has failed, who are not candidates for open surgery or TURP or refuse any surgical treatment. The prostatic artery origins in the present study population were different from previously published results. Larger case series, longer follow-up time, and comparative studies with standard TURP or holmium laser enucleation of the prostate (HoLEP) are needed, not as much to evaluate safety and efficacy of PAE, but to determine which patients should undergo which treatment.

Abbreviations

BPH: Benign prostatic hyperplasia; CB-CT: Cone-beam computed tomography; DSA: Digital subtraction angiography; HoLEP: Holmium laser enucleation of the prostate; IIEF-5: International index of erectile function short form; IPSS: International prostate symptom score; LUTS: Lower urinary tract symptoms; MRI: Magnetic resonance imaging; OP: Open prostatectomy; PAE: Prostatic arterial embolization; PAs: Prostatic arteries; PSA: Prostate specific antigen; PVA: Polyvinyl alcohol particles; PVR: Post-void residual volume; QoL: Quality of life; TURP: Transurethral resection of the prostate.

Competing interests

The authors declare that they have no competing interests.

Authors' contributions

All authors participated in creating the study design. MQW and ZJW drafted the manuscript. MQW, LPG, and GDZ obtained the funding of this study. MQW, YW, and HYK were responsible for clinical studies. KL, HYK, and JYY were responsible for data acquisition. DF and YK were responsible for the data analysis and statistical analysis. All authors read and approved the final manuscript.

Acknowledgments

This work was supported by grants from the National Scientific Foundation Committee of China (No. 81471769), the central health research project (2013BJ09) and Chinese PLA Scientific Foundation of the Twelve-Five Programme (BWS11J028). We thanks Dr. Xin Ma, from the Department of Urology, Chinese PLA General Hospital, for his consultations.

References

1. McVary KT, Roehrborn CG, Avins AL, Barry MJ, Bruskewitz RC, Donnell RF, et al. Update on AUA guideline on the management of benign prostatic hyperplasia. J Urol. 2011;85:1793–803.
2. Oelke M, Bachmann A, Descazeaud A, Emberton M, Gravas S, Michel MC, et al. European association of urology: EAU guidelines on the treatment and follow-up of non-neurogenic male lower urinary tract symptoms including benign prostatic obstruction. Eur Urol. 2013;64:118–40.
3. Auffenberg GB, Helfand BT, McVary KT. Established medical therapy for benign prostatic hyperplasia. Urol Clin North Am. 2009;36:443–59.
4. Kirby M, Chapple C, Jackson G, Eardley I, Edwards D, Hackett G, et al. Erectile dysfunction and lower urinary tract symptoms: a consensus on the importance of co-diagnosis. Int J Clin Pract. 2013;67:606–18.
5. Choi SY, Kim TH, Myung SC, Moon YT, Kim KD, Kim YS, et al. Impact of changing trends in medical therapy on surgery for benign prostatic hyperplasia over two decades. Korean J Urol. 2012;53:23–8.
6. Geavlete B, Stanescu F, Iacoboaie C, Geavlete P. Bipolar plasma enucleation of the prostate vs open prostatectomy in large benign prostatic hyperplasia cases - a medium term, prospective, randomized comparison. BJU Int. 2013;111:793–803.

7. Ahyai SA, Gilling P, Kaplan SA, Kuntz RM, Madersbacher S, Montorsi F, et al. Meta-analysis of functional outcomes and complications following transurethral procedures for lower urinary tract symptoms resulting from benign prostatic enlargement. Eur Urol. 2010;58:384–97.

8. Lourenco T, Pickard R, Vale L, Grant A, Fraser C, MacLennan G, et al. Benign prostatic enlargement team: minimally invasive treatments for benign prostatic enlargement: systematic review of randomised controlled trials. BMJ. 2008;337:a1662.

9. Pisco J, Campos Pinheiro L, Bilhim T, Duarte M, Rio Tinto H, Fernandes L, et al. Prostatic arterial embolization for benign prostatic hyperplasia: short- and intermediate-term results. Radiology. 2013;266:668–77.

10. Carnevale FC, da Motta-Leal-Filho JM, Antunes AA, Baroni RH, Marcelino AS, Cerri LM, et al. Quality of life and clinical symptom improvement support prostatic artery embolization for patients with acute urinary retention caused by benign prostatic hyperplasia. J Vasc Interv Radiol. 2013;24:535–42.

11. Bagla S, Martin CP, van Breda A, Sheridan MJ, Sterling KM, Papadouris D, et al. Early results from a United States trial of prostatic artery embolization in the treatment of benign prostatic hyperplasia. J Vasc Interv Radiol. 2014;25:47–52.

12. McWilliams JP, Kuo MD, Rose SC, Bagla S, Caplin DM, Cohen EI, et al. Society of interventional radiology position statement: prostate artery embolization for treatment of benign disease of the prostate. J Vasc Interv Radiol. 2014;25:1349–51.

13. Bilhim T, Pisco J, Campos Pinheiro L, Rio Tinto H, Fernandes L, Pereira JA, et al. Does polyvinyl alcohol particle size change the outcome of prostatic arterial embolization for benign prostatic hyperplasia? Results from a single-center randomized prospective study. J Vasc Interv Radiol. 2013;24:1595–602.

14. Angle JF, Siddiqi NH, Wallace MJ, Kundu S, Stokes L, Wojak JC, et al. Quality improvement guidelines for percutaneous transcatheter embolization: society of interventional radiology standards of practice committee. J Vasc Interv Radiol. 2010;21:1479–86.

15. Protogerou V, Argyropoulos V, Patrozos K, Tekerlekis P, Kostakopoulos A. An alternative minimally invasive technique for large prostates (>80 mL): transvesical prostatectomy through a 3-cm incision. Urology. 2010;75:184–6.

16. Seki N, Naito S. Instrumental treatments for benign prostatic obstruction. Curr Opin Urol. 2007;17:17–21.

17. Rassweiler J, Teber D, Kuntz R. Complications of transurethral resection of the prostate (TURP)–incidence, management, and prevention. Eur Urol. 2006;50:969–79.

18. Serretta V, Morgia G, Fondacaro L, Curto G, Lobianco A, Pirritano D, et al. Members of the sicilian-calabrian society of urology: open prostatectomy for benign prostatic enlargement in southern Europe in the late 1990s: a contemporary series of 1800 interventions. Urology. 2002;60:623–7.

19. Gratzke C, Schlenker B, Seitz M, Karl A, Hermanek P, Lack N, et al. Complications and early postoperative outcome after open prostatectomy in patients with benign prostatic enlargement: results of a prospective multicenter study. J Urol. 2007;177:1419–22.

20. Bagla S, Rholl KS, Sterling KM, van Breda A, Papadouris D, Cooper JM, et al. Utility of cone-beam CT imaging in prostatic artery embolization. J Vasc Interv Radiol. 2013;24:1603–7.

21. Pisco JM, Rio Tinto H, Campos Pinheiro L, Bilhim T. Embolisation of prostatic arteries as treatment of moderate to severe lower urinary symptoms (LUTS) secondary to benign hyperplasia: results of short- and mid-term follow-up. Eur Radiol. 2013;23:2561–72.

22. Moreira AM, Marques CF, Antunes AA, Nahas CS, Nahas SC, de Gregorio Ariza MA, et al. Transient ischemic rectitis as a potential complication after prostatic artery embolization: case report and review of the literature. Cardiovasc Intervent Radiol. 2013;36:1690–4.

23. Bilhim T, Tinto HR, Fernandes L, Martins Pisco J. Radiological anatomy of prostatic arteries. Tech Vasc Interv Radiol. 2012;15:276–85.

24. Garcia-Monaco R, Garategui L, Kizilevsky N, Peralta O, Rodriguez P, Palacios-Jaraquemada J. Human cadaveric specimen study of the prostatic arterial anatomy: implications for arterial embolization. J Vasc Interv Radiol. 2014;25:315–22.

25. Frenk NE, Baroni RH, Carnevale FC, Gonçalves OM, Antunes AA, Srougi M, et al. MRI findings after prostatic artery embolization for treatment of benign hyperplasia. AJR Am J Roentgenol. 2014;203:813–21.

26. Stefanov M. Extraglandular and intraglandular vascularization of canine prostate. Microsc Res Tech. 2004;63:188–97.

27. Bilhim T, Pisco J, Rio Tinto H, Fernandes L, Campos Pinheiro L, Duarte M, et al. Unilateral versus bilateral prostatic arterial embolization for lower urinary tract symptoms in patients with prostate enlargement. Cardiovasc Intervent Radiol. 2013;36:403–11.

28. Pisco JM, Pinheiro LC, Bilhim T, Duarte M, Mendes JR, Oliveira AG. Prostatic arterial embolization to treat benign prostatic hyperplasia. J Vasc Interv Radiol. 2011;22:11–9.

29. Bilhim T, Pisco JM, Rio Tinto H, Fernandes L, Pinheiro LC, Furtado A, et al. Prostatic arterial supply: anatomic and imaging findings relevant for selective arterial embolization. J Vasc Interv Radiol. 2012;23:1403–15.

30. Carnevale FC, da Motta-Leal-Filho JM, Antunes AA, Baroni RH, Freire GC, Cerri LM, et al. Midterm follow-up after prostate embolization in two patients with benign prostatic hyperplasia. Cardiovasc Intervent Radiol. 2011;34:1330–3.

17

Evaluation of noise hazard during the holmium laser enucleation of prostate

Huan Xu[†], Yan-bo Chen[†], Meng Gu, Qi Chen[*] and Zhong Wang[*]

Abstract

Background: To evaluate noise hazard during holmium laser enucleation of the prostate (HoLEP), we designed a study to detect such a risk in this procedure.

Methods: This study was conducted over a 12-month period on 223 patients with benign prostatic hyperplasia (BPH), 121 of whom underwent HoLEP while those remaining underwent transurethral resection of the prostate (TURP). A sound level meter was used to detect the exposure of surgeons to noise. The recordings used were in accordance with the standards set by the Occupational Safety and Health Administration (OSHA) and the United States Environmental Protection Agency. Moreover, each of the 43 surgeons participating in a BPH discussion conference answered the questionnaire on the influence of noise, and 33 surgeons in our department volunteered for blood pressure monitoring post-surgically.

Results: The sound level produced by a high-powered holmium laser emitter during HoLEP was 67.37 ± 0.13 dB, which was significantly higher than the sound heard during TURP (46.41 ± 0.29 dB, $P < 0.01$). The 65–70 dB noise during HoLEP was proved to be a safe level in accordance with the OSHA standards. However, this level was considerably greater than the stated 55 dB. Moreover, it exceeded the normal communication protective level of 60 dB. In the analysis of responses from the surgeons, the HoLEP group obtained an average score that reflected disturbance caused by the laser emitter and an increase in average systolic pressure relative to that in the TURP group.

Conclusions: The noise level during HoLEP is within hearing conservation levels. However, the noise disturbs intrateam communication and concentration during surgery. Some surgeons may experience discomfort post-surgically, but no significant difference among the groups is indicated. The findings suggest that measures should be taken to address the noise caused by the laser emitter during HoLEP.

Background

With the development of minimally invasive surgery, holmium laser enucleation of prostate (HoLEP) has been widely used worldwide and is considered as the "new golden standard" for benign prostate hyperplasia (BPH) [1]. A large number of studies have focused on the effects of surgery on patients, but few have evaluated the effects of surgery on surgeons. One of the potential risks of surgery for doctors is noise exposure. To reduce the negative effects of noise hazard, national and European community directives as well as United Nations guidelines recommend a 55 db threshold for work requiring concentration such as "decisions under time pressure," "decisions with severe consequences," or "examinations and operations by physicians, meetings, research, teaching." [2]. Ambient noise exhibits a tendency to affect performance during surgery, causing decreased concentration and mental loading during surgery; dexterity is also decreased, as shown in the simulation video [3, 4]. Noise volume is associated with surgical site infection, which may cause serious post-surgical complications [5]. In many medical areas, such as orthopedic and dental department, noise hazards have recently been reported and is given considerable attention [6, 7]. The present study is the first to evaluate the influence of noise produced during HoLEP on urological surgeons.

* Correspondence: qiqi_chenqi@yeah.net; zhongwang2000@sina.com
[†]Equal contributors
Department of Urology, Shanghai 9th People's Hospital, Shanghai Jiaotong University School of Medicine, 639 Zhi Zaoju Road, Shanghai 200011, China

Methods

This study was performed over a period of 12 months on 223 patients. Among the patients, 121 underwent

HoLEP using a high-powered holmium laser with a 100 W continuous flow and with power settings of 80–100 W at 2–1.5 J/s and 50–40 Hz. The remaining 102 patients underwent TURP. Average sound levels were recorded during surgery, and the sound range was measured during the procedure. The location chosen was 40 cm away from the surgeons' head. The sound level meter (Control Company, Friendswood, TX) produced by Thomas Scientific was used to measure the sound in decibels.

In addition, each of the 59 surgeons participating in a BPH operating conference responded to questionnaire regarding the effect of HoLEP noise on the performance of the surgeon, most of whom were skilled in both HoLEP and TURP. Excluding the incomplete questionnaires and those with logically erroneous responses, 43 of the 59 questionnaires were considered valid. The surgeons, aged 30–40 years, came from 4 different provinces in China. Among those participating in the HoLEP or TURP surgical procedures, 34 surgeons volunteered for blood pressure monitoring post-surgically. Ethical approval and written informed consent of the patients and the doctors were obtained.

All results obtained from the questionnaire were presented as means ± S.E.M. Statistically significant differences were assessed by 1-way ANOVA. All statistical analyses were performed using SPSS ver. 17.0. P value ≤0.05 was considered statistically significant.

Results

As presented in Table 1, the sound level produced by the high-powered holmium laser emitter during HoLEP is greater than that produced during TURP (67.37 ± 0.13 dB VS. 46.41 ± 0.29 dB, P < 0.01). The sound level produced during HoLEP against time is shown in Fig. 1. The harsh noise coming from the anesthesia alarm was 64.71 ± 0.73 dB, which is close to 67 dB. The sound during TURP was 46.41 ± 0.29 dB, which is close to the baseline at 45.38 ± 0.35 dB. The noise range of 65–70 dB during HoLEP verified the safety standard set by the Occupational Safety and Health Administration (OSHA), which allows 8 h of exposure to 90 dB per day. However, 65–70 dB was considerably louder than the stated 55 dB for work

requiring concentration. The range also exceeded the normal communication protective level of 60 dB.

Analysis of the responses from the surgeons indicated that in the HoLEP group, the laser emitter caused disturbance. As presented in Table 2, the score for the question "How strong was the disturbance of your communication/ concentration by noise?" was significantly higher in the HoLEP group than in the TURP group; however, no significant difference in hearing function damage was found between the 2 groups.

Analysis of results for systolic pressure (Table 3) indicated a slight increase in systolic pressure in the HoLEP group relative to that in the TURP group (140.9 ± 1.25 vs. 134.89 ± 1.01 mmHg, P < 0.01), whereas no significant difference was observed in the diastolic pressure results (89.5 ± 0.98 VS. 88.4 ± 1.67 mmHg, P = 0.562).

Discussion

Concern for the health of physicians has drawn increasing attention because of their high-pressure working environment. Noise during surgery negatively affects surgeons. However, studies on the noise levels produced by various surgical instruments have rarely been conducted. This study aims to evaluate the sound level during HoLEP. Thus, we determined whether the sound level in the operating room during surgery was hazardous to the surgeon. Our study confirmed that the noise produced by the high-powered holmium laser emitter, which falls within the range considered safe by OSHA, does not negatively affect the surgeons' audition in theory. Regardless, this matter should be given attention because the sound level beyond 60 dB is the upper threshold for normal communication, and 55 dB is the limit for "examinations and operations by physicians, meetings, research, and teaching."

The safe standard range set by OSHA is designed to measure sound health in various working areas. "Table G-16" by OSHA allows 8 h of exposure to 90 dB per day beyond which hearing protection is required [8]. Meanwhile, EPA and World Health Organization deliver the standard for normal communication and work requiring concentration [9]. The sound level within the range is comfortable for doctors in the operating room and similar professionals. As suggested, the ideal degree of loudness for normal communication is 45 dB, and the maximum is 60 dB.

As is known, noise exerts negative effects on surgeons and patients. Previous studies have reported on noise in the operating theater, which exerts deleterious effects [2, 6, 10, 11]. Kurmann et al. used an intraoperative noise volume associated with subsequent surgical site infection in 35 elective open abdominal procedures [5]. In addition, the high level of noise significantly increased the incidence of postoperative complications [2]. These complications were partly attributed to the disturbance caused by the noise on the

Table 1 Sound level measurements

Sound source	Average sound level (dB) ± S.E.M.	Sound range (dB)	P value
HoLEP	67.37 ± 0.13	65.00–70.00	
TURP	46.41 ± 0.29	42.10–51.82	<0.01
Anesthesia alarm	64.71 ± 0.73	63.07–69.31	0.73
Base Line	45.38 ± 0.35	44.21–49.76	<0.01

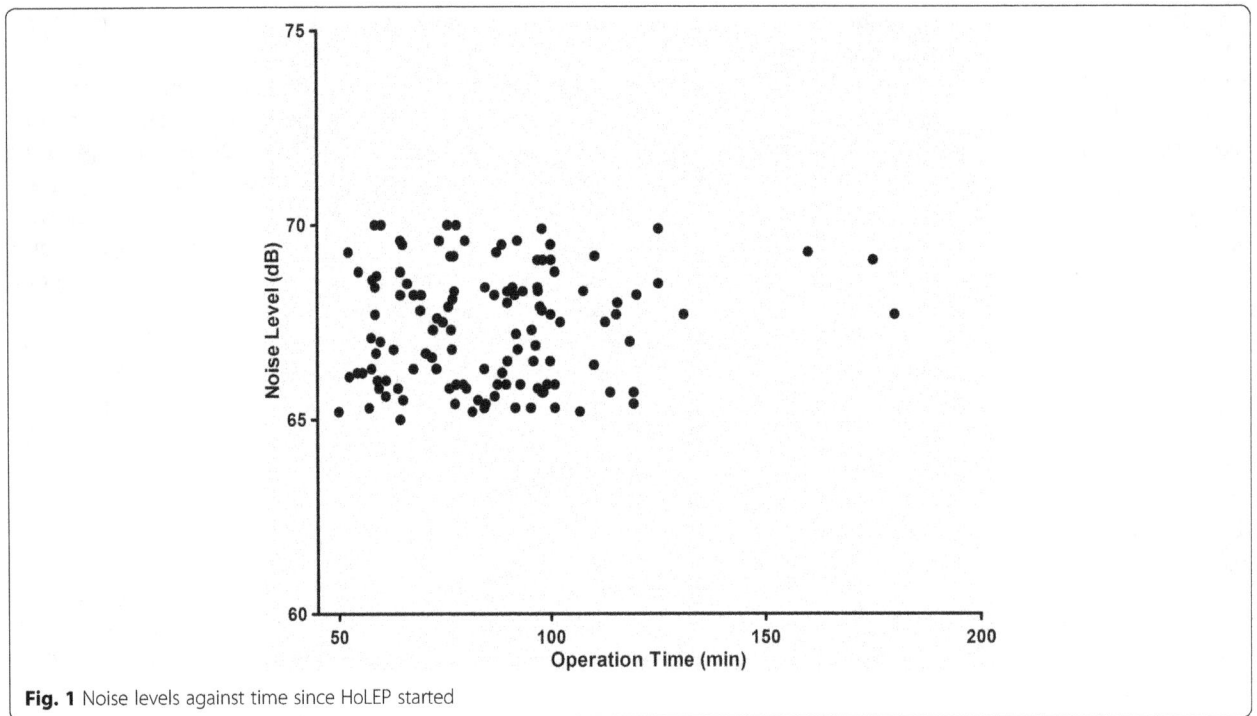

Fig. 1 Noise levels against time since HoLEP started

surgeon. A study found that surgeons surrounded by loud noise experienced decreased intrateam communication and interrupted conversations [2]. Another study reported that biometrically, the increased sound level enhanced both the pre- and post- operative cortisol levels and increased electrodermal potential in surgeons, which could be attributable to severe stress [12]. Thus, more effective technical and behavioral measures could be applied.

In urology, several studies suggested that the noise produced by extracorporeal shock wave lithotripsy (ESWL) can harm the hearing of the operating room personnel and the patient, although other studies contradicted this finding [13]. The difference between ESWL and the surgical procedure is that in the latter, concentration must be expended by surgeons into the surgery itself. The use of

HoLEP in BHP has been increasingly prevalent because of its superior outcome and low risk of bleeding. HoLEP can potentially replace TURP as the new golden standard for BPH [1], but the noise caused by the laser emitter presents a problem. No studies have been reported on the subject; however many surgeons have complained about the upsetting side effects of the noise coming from the holmium laser emitter. To the best of our knowledge, this study is the first to report on the effect of noise produced during HoLEP on surgeons.

The results of our study showed that the baseline in the operating room was in the 45.38 ± 0.35 dB range. The sound produced during TURP, which is set as the control, was in the 46.41 ± 0.29 dB range. The noise levels produced during both procedures were considerably lower than the maximum noise for normal communication (60 dB). Although the noise of anesthesia alarm exceeded the normal communication threshold, it was transient and short-term. In the HoLEP group, the noise reached 70 dB, and the average level was about 67.37 ± 0.13 dB. The reading near the surgeon's station verified the safety of the level of exposure set by OSHA standards, which

Table 2 Investigation results and analysis

Question	Average score	
	HoLEP	TURP
How strong was the auditory threshold up-regulated post-surgically?	0.8 ± 0.5	0.0 ± 0.0
How strong was your sleep disorder or dizziness?	0.6 ± 0.5	0.0 ± 0.0
How strong was the disturbance of your communication by noise?	2.2 ± 0.2[a]	0.0 ± 0.0
How strong was the disturbance of your concentration by noise?	0.8 ± 0.4[a]	0.0 ± 0.0
How strong have you felt uncomfortable after surgery because of the noise?	0.8 ± 0.5	0.0 ± 0.0

[a]$P < 0.05$

Table 3 Blood pressure of surgeons

	SP (mmHg) ± S.E.M	P value	DP (mmHg) ± S.E.M	P value
HoLEP	140.9 ± 1.25		89.5 ± 0.98	
TURP	134.89 ± 1.01	<0.01	88.4 ± 1.67	0.562

SP systolic pressure, DP diastolic pressure

allows 8 h of exposure to 90 dB per day. For hearing conservation, the 67.37 ± 0.13 dB level exhibited no tendency to reach the 75 dB level. Thus, no hearing hazard was observed during HoLEP. Normal communication was disturbed by the laser emitter, as determined in the study. The period lasting almost 60 min was filled with 65–70 dB noise; this degree of loudness was much higher than that by normal communication standards. During our 1-year study, 2 surgeons who performed 5 HoLEP procedures in a single day complained about tinnitus during sleep on the same day. The noise produced by the laser emitter was in the form of pulses and mainly came from the cooling system. Thus, the laser machine could be enhanced to avoid the noise.

This study has potential clinical implications. The noise level during HoLEP was within hearing conservation, but it disturbed intrateam communication and individual concentration during surgery. The noise produced by the laser emitter during HoLEP disturbed communication and concentration during surgery but did not affect hearing. In addition, post-surgical discomfort might be experienced. The major limitation of this study is its small sample size, which precludes multivariable analysis. Further studies should be conducted. Measures must also be taken to address the disturbance caused by HoLEP noise and to protect the surgeon.

Conclusions

The noise coming from the laser emitter during HoLEP disturbs intrateam communication and the concentration of surgeons working in the operating room; however, no hearing injury is detected. Some surgeons may also experience discomfort post-surgically. Measures must be taken to resolve the disturbance caused by the noise produced during HoLEP.

Abbreviations
BPH: Benign prostatic hyperplasia; EPA: Environmental protection agency; HoLEP: Holmium laser enucleation of the prostate; OSHA: Occupational Safety and Health Administration; TURP: Transurethral resection of the prostate

Acknowledgements
We gratefully acknowledge the urologists making great contributions to the prostatic enucleation, especially to Yinghao Sun and Peter Gilling. Authors' Information: Huan Xu, Yan-bo Chen, Meng Gu, Qi Chen, Zhong Wang. Department of Urology, Shanghai 9th People's Hospital, Shanghai Jiaotong University School of Medicine, Shanghai 200011, China.

Funding
Data collection and analysis: key disciplines group construction project of pudong health bureau of shanghai (PWZxq2014-11) and key project of science and technology of Shanghai (No. 134119a9800).

Authors' contributions
Study design: HX, ZW, QC, Data collection: YBC, data analysis: MG, HX, writing paper: HX. All authors read and approved the final manuscript.

Competing interests
The authors declare that they have no competing interests.

References
1. van Rij S, Gilling PJ. In 2013, holmium laser enucleation of the prostate (HoLEP) may be the new 'gold standard'. Curr Urol Rep. 2012;13(6):427–32.
2. Engelmann CR, Neis JP, Kirschbaum C, Grote G, Ure BM. A noise-reduction program in a pediatric operation theatre is associated with surgeon's benefits and a reduced rate of complications: a prospective controlled clinical trial. Ann Surg. 2014;259(5):1025–33.
3. Arora S, Sevdalis N, Nestel D, Woloshynowych M, Darzi A, Kneebone R. The impact of stress on surgical performance: a systematic review of the literature. Surgery. 2010;147(3):318–30. 330 e311-316.
4. Sevdalis N, Healey AN, Vincent CA. Distracting communications in the operating theatre. J Eval Clin Pract. 2007;13(3):390–4.
5. Kurmann A, Peter M, Tschan F, Muhlemann K, Candinas D, Beldi G. Adverse effect of noise in the operating theatre on surgical-site infection. Br J Surg. 2011;98(7):1021–5.
6. Holzer LA, Leithner A, Kazianschutz M, Gruber G. Noise measurement in total knee arthroplasty. Noise Health. 2014;16(71):205–7.
7. Tay BD, Prabhu IS, Cousin CH, Cousin GC. Occupational exposure to noise in maxillofacial operating theatres: an initial prospective study. Br J Oral Maxillofac Surg. 2015;
8. OSHA. OSHA Stanadard 29 CFR 1910.95. 2008. http://oshagov/pls/oshaweb/owadispshow_document?p_table=STANDARDS&pid=9735.
9. WHO. WHO guidelines for community noise. 1999. http://apps.who.int/iris/handle/10665/66217.
10. Ginsberg SH, Pantin E, Kraidin J, Solina A, Panjwani S, Yang G. Noise levels in modern operating rooms during surgery. J Cardiothorac Vasc Anesth. 2013;27(3):528–30.
11. Tsiou C, Efthymiatos G, Katostaras T. Noise in the operating rooms of Greek hospitals. J Acoust Soc Am. 2008;123(2):757–65.
12. Kirschbaum C, Hellhammer DH. Noise and Stress - Salivary Cortisol as a Non-Invasive Measure of Allostatic Load. Noise Health. 1999;1(4):57–66.
13. Terlecki RP, Triest JA. A contemporary evaluation of the auditory hazard of extracorporeal shock wave lithotripsy. Urology. 2007;70(5):898–9.

18

The evaluation of nocturia in patients with lower urinary tract symptoms suggestive of benign prostatic hyperplasia and the analysis of the curative effect after medical or placebo therapy for nocturia

Zhigang Xue[1,2], Yunhua Lin[1], Yongguang Jiang[1*], Nengbao Wei[2] and Jinwen Bi[2]

Abstract

Background: To study nocturia in patients with lower urinary tract symptoms (LUTS) suggestive of benign prostatic hyperplasia (BPH) after medical or placebo treatment.

Methods: Patients with LUTS suggestive of BPH from several community clinics were included. Patients completed the International Prostate Symptom Score (I-PSS) questionnaire and a 3-day voiding diary. Urinalysis, prostate-specific antigen (PSA) measurement, and prostate ultrasonography were performed. Nocturnal polyuria (NP) was defined as a nocturnal urine fraction exceeding one third of the daily urine output in elderly men. A total of 148 outpatients were randomized to drug treatment (tamsulosin) or placebo treatment. After 8 weeks of treatment, they were re-evaluated using a 3-day voiding diary, PSA measurement, prostate volume (PV), I-PSS, etc.

Results: The average I-PSS score was 20.3, storage symptom score was 11.7, voiding symptom score was 8.6, quality of life (QoL) score was 3.7, PV was 40.4 ± 19.4 ml, and nocturnal urine volume (NUV) was 845.7 ± 339.0 ml. The mean frequency of nocturia was 2.3 ± 1.1 per day, and 94% of the patients had a nocturia frequency of more than two times per day. Of these patients, 76.5% had NP. A significant correlation was found between NUV and the amount of water intake at night and 4 h before sleep ($r = 0.419, P = 0.002$; $r = 0.302, P = 0.031$). Eighty patients were randomized to drug treatment (tamsulosin) and 68 patients were randomized to placebo treatment. The I-PSS score was 16.8 ± 4.9 to 19.3 ± 5.0 ($p = 0.002$), the storage symptom score was 10.3 ± 3.4 to 10.7 ± 3.4 ($p = 0.007$), and the voiding symptom score was 7.5 ± 2.4 to 8.6 ± 2.3 ($p = 0.003$). The frequency of daytime urination was 7.5 ± 2.6 to 8.1 ± 2.6 ($p = 0.002$), maximum urine volume (ml) was 372.8 ± 103.3 to 302.8 ± 119.3 ($p = 0.007$), and morning urine volume (ml) was 280.5 ± 111.7 to 259.5 ± 100.7 ($p = 0.003$). However, the frequency of nocturia score was 2.8 ± 0.7 to 3.0 ± 0.6 ($p = 0.306$) and the nocturnal urine volume (ml) was 800.7 ± 323.0 to 845.7 ± 303.5 ($p = 0.056$), which did not change significantly. There were significant differences between the NP and non-NP groups in the duration of LUTS, first voided urine volume, daytime urination frequency, and the amount of water intake at night and 4 h before sleep.

(Continued on next page)

---

* Correspondence: jyg_doctor@sina.com
[1]Department of Urology, Beijing Anzhen Hospital, Capital Medical University, Beijing 100029, China
Full list of author information is available at the end of the article

(Continued from previous page)

Conclusions: Among the symptoms of LUTS, the improvement rates for nocturia were the lowest after medical treatment for BPH. The α-blockers did not improve nocturia, which was a common symptom accompanying LUTS suggestive of BPH. Our results showed that the prevalence of NP was 76.5% and that NP was significantly related to the amount of water intake during the evening and before sleep.

Keywords: Benign prostatic hyperplasia, Nocturia, Nocturnal polyuria, α-Adrenoceptor antagonists

Background

Nocturia, is perceived as one single symptoms of all lower urinary tract symptoms (LUTS) by most men, which is highly prevalent and the most bothersome component [1]. It has led to significant morbidity and, occasionally, mortality. Scholars have pointed out that, this bothersome symptom is related to cause arousal from sleep, and two or more voids per night are usually considered lead to a decreased health-related quality of life [2]. Nocturia could result from many others disease and conditions (including urological and non-urological diseases) [3]. However, the various causes are not differentiated excluded in men with LUTS/BPH, and none of the individual α_1-adrenoceptor antagonists without subtype selectivity have obvious benefit. The medical therapy have not shown a significant reduction in frequency of nocturia so far. There are also not equal amounts of studies showing positive or negative results on nocturia [4]. For all of these reasons, nocturia is often multifactorial in etiology, and many medical conditions are associated with nocturia. Therefore, we aim to explore nocturia in patients with lower urinary tract symptoms suggestive of benign prostatic hyperplasia, and we analyzed the curative effect after medical therapy for nocturia.

Methods

Patients

From January 2015 to May 2016, 148 patients were admitted to Beijing Huairou Community Health Service Center, with a median age of 69.0 years, a mean ± standard deviation (SD) age of 62.1 ± 13.6 years, LUTS/BPH duration of 5.0 ± 3.1 years, and absence of treatment using α-blockers and/or 5α-reductase inhibitors. The common inclusion criteria for all participants were age ≥ 50 years and diagnosis of BPH. All patients provided their written informed consent and the program was accepted by the hospital ethics committee. The exclusion criteria were prostate cancer, PSA > 10 ng/ml, urinary tract infection, nervous system disease, urolithiasis, medical therapy that could affect the function of urination, prostatic surgery, or pelvic surgery.

Methods

Based on the literature [5], we estimated that 74 patients will need to be recruited in order to detect a clinically significant difference of 25% between the 2 groups (with a power of 80%). Based on past clinical trial experience, we estimated that 20% of randomized participants will be lost in follow up, therefore 88 patients will need to be recruited, and 170 participants who will complete the item in our study.

The patients included in the study were randomly divided (1:1) into two groups (drug treatment and placebo treatment) by use of a computer generated random number table. But some patients of the two groups had lost in follow-up because of financial status, phone lost, language barriers, individual patient factors, etc.

At last all 148 patients with LUTS suggestive of BPH were divided into two random groups, which either received α-adrenoceptor antagonist (tamsulosin 2 mg qd po) or placebo for 8 weeks. IPSS, QoL index questionnaire, 3-day frequency volume charts (FVCs), PSA, urinalysis, PV, and uroflowmetry (Qmax) were assessed before and after medical therapy. Serum PSA and urinalysis were evaluated at Beijing Huairou Hospital. The specific instrument for the evaluation of nocturia was a 1000 ml graduated glass. This study was approved by the ethics committee of Beijing Huairou Hospital. Each patient was informed of the study and signed an informed consent form and had the right to withdraw from the study at any time.

Nocturia evaluation index

Nocturia, specifically, was the number of voids recorded during the nighttime [3]. The first morning void was excluded from the count because it is not followed by sleep. Nocturnal urine volume describes the amount of urine excreted during the nighttime and includes the volume of the first morning void because this urine has been produced during the nighttime [3]. Nocturnal polyuria is an abnormally large urine volume produced during the nighttime. The ICS classifies nocturnal polyuria as the nocturnal urine volume divided by the 24-h urine volume (i.e., nocturnal polyuria index, NPi) [3]. The ICS defines nocturnal polyuria as NPi > 33% in the elderly [3].

Statistical analysis

SPSS 22.0 statistical software was used for data analysis. All variables were expressed as the mean ± SD values. The numerical data were compared using the unpaired *t*-test. An analysis of the difference in the number of patients with nocturia before and after treatment was performed using McNemar's test. A multivariate analysis was performed. A *P-value* of 0.05 or less was considered significant.

Results

The clinical index and results of 3-day frequency-volume charts from patients with LUTS/BPH (Table 1)

The relationship between NUV, NPi, and evening drinking volume 4 h before bedtime drinking volume and other indices (Fig. 1 and Fig. 2)

The relationship between NUV and evening drinking volume ($r = 0.419$, $p = 0.002$) and 4 h before bedtime drinking volume ($r = 0.302$, $p = 0.031$) were related. NPi and maximum urination volume ($r = 0.440$, $p = 0.001$) and morning urine volume ($r = 0.445$, $p = 0.001$) were related, but there was no correlation between NPi and prostate volume, age, LUTS duration, or I-PSS score.

Table 1 Clinical indices and nocturia-related parameters in patients with BPH

Variable	Median (mean ± SD)
Number of patients	148
Age (years)	69.5 ± 5.6
LUTS/BPH duration (years)	6.3 ± 3.1
I-PSS	20.3 ± 5.0
Storage symptom score	11.7 ± 3.4
Voiding symptom score	8.6 ± 2.3
QoL score	3.7 ± 1.0
Nocturia score	3.0 ± 1.0
Serum PSA (ng/ml)	2.0 ± 1.7
Prostate volume (ml)	40.4 ± 19.4
NPi	0.43 ± 0.12
24-h drinking volume (ml)	1565.4 ± 624.8
4-h before bedtime drinking volume (ml)	123.9 ± 109.9
Frequency of nocturia	3.3 ± 1.1
Frequency of daytime urination	8.1 ± 2.6
Maximum urination volume (ml)	352.8 ± 119.3
Morning urine volume (ml)	260.5 ± 109.7
24-h total urine volume (ml)	1996.5 ± 637.5
Nocturnal urine volume (ml)	845.7 ± 339.0

LUTS lower urinary tract symptoms, *BPH* benign prostatic hyperplasia, *PSA* prostate-specific antigen, *I-PSS*, international prostate symptom score, *NPi* nocturnal polyuria index, *QoL* quality of life

The comparison of evaluation indices between drug treatment and placebo treatment groups for patients with BPH (Table 2)

Eighty patients were randomized to the drug treatment (tamsulosin) and 68 patients were randomized to the placebo treatment. The I-PSS score, storage symptom score, voiding symptom score, quality of life score, frequency of daytime urination, maximum urine volume, and morning urine volume were statistically significant between both groups. However, the frequency of nocturia score and nocturnal urine volume did not change significantly.

Data statistics between the NP group and the non-NP group (Table 3)

In the indices of age, 24-h drinking volume, bladder function, PV, and PSA level, there were no significant differences between the groups. While in LUTS duration, nocturnal urine volume, morning urine volume, and daytime voiding frequency, the differences between the two groups were statistically significant.

Discussion

Nocturia, one of the most bothersome symptoms of LUTS, has been the focus of a high volume of rapidly evolving research. The purpose of this study was to describe the relevant recent research in the field of nocturia in China, with particular emphasis on its evaluation and management. Nocturia is a complicated clinical entity that is often multifactorial in etiology. Experts of the International Continence Society (ICS) define nocturia as the general complaint when an individual (independent of age, gender, cause(s) and associated bother) must wake up at night one or more times to void [1, 2].

Epidemiological studies showed that the prevalence of nocturia in the < 30-year-old population was approximately 3%, in the 60- to 69-year-old population was 30%, and in the > 70-year-old population was 40% [6]. The survey regarding > 60-year-old men in the United States demonstrated that up to 65.2% of old men would get up at night to urinate, of whom 25% of elderly males woke up at night to urinate ≥2 times [7]. A Chinese questionnaire study showed that in patients living in the national scope, the storage symptoms of I-PSS were the most troubling symptoms of BPH in patients, in which nocturia was the most affecting [8]. Schatzl reported that more than 60% of old people thought nocturia would negatively affect their quality of life [6]. Recently, a study showed that the mortality rate of the elderly with nocturia was significantly higher (more than 3 times) than that of the elderly without nocturia (less than 3 times) [9].

Nocturia has been identified as the leading cause for sleep disturbance and sleep fragmentation; it causes daytime fatigue, impacts daily activities, and deteriorates psychomotor

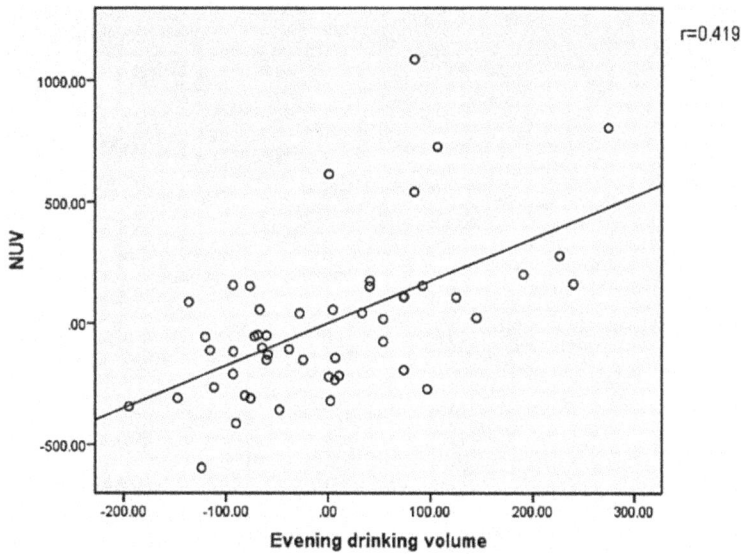

Fig. 1 The relationship between NUV and Evening drinking volume. 1) X axis caption: "Evening drinking volume (ml)". 2) Y axis caption: "NUV (ml)"

performance, cognitive function, and mood [10–12]. Nocturia can also cause depression and immunosuppression, and it increases the vulnerability for cardiovascular diseases and the development of diabetes mellitus [11, 13–15].

In these analyses, LUTS/BPH patients with nocturia had some urinary system diseases, such as lower urinary tract obstruction and overactive bladder, as well as cardiovascular diseases, diabetes, diabetes insipidus, and other awakening factors of urination (such as anxiety and sleep disorders). In this study, patients had hypertension, coronary heart disease, diabetes, and other diseases. Thus, nocturia may be caused by the combined effects of a

variety of conditions. Kupelian et al. demonstrated that while increased odds of the metabolic syndrome were observed with mild to moderate degrees of nocturia [16]. In this way, the etiology of nocturia, especially, nocturnal polyuria can be further analyzed by evaluating LUTS patients with metabolic syndrome.

BPH is a common disease in elderly men, not only with voiding symptoms such as dysuria but also with storage symptoms such as urinary frequency, urgency, and nocturia. Clinical studies showed that the application of α-blockers and 5α-reductase inhibitors could effectively relieve lower urinary tract symptoms caused

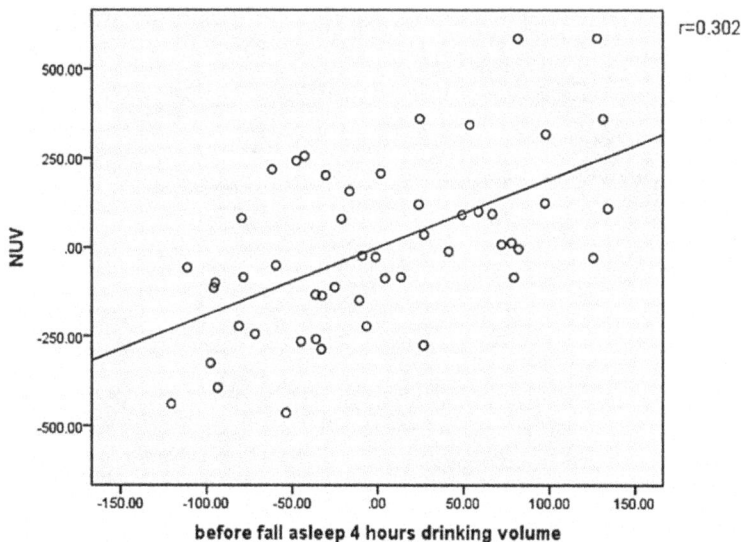

Fig. 2 The relationship between NUV and before fall asleep 4 h drinking volume. 1) X axis caption: "4-h before bedtime drinking volume (ml)". 2) Y axis caption: "NUV (ml)"

Table 2 Comparison of evaluation indices after treatment (drug or placebo) in patients with BPH and nocturia

Variable	Drug reatment	Placebo Treatment	P value
Number of patients	80	68	
Age (years)	69.5 ± 5.6	68.5 ± 5.3	0.450
I-PSS	16.8 ± 4.9	19.3 ± 5.0	0.002
Storage symptom score	10.3 ± 3.4	10.7 ± 3.4	0.007
Voiding symptom score	6.5 ± 2.4	8.6 ± 2.3	0.003
QoL score	3.1 ± 0.6	3.8 ± 1.0	0.005
Serum PSA (ng/ml)	2.2 ± 1.7	2.1 ± 1.6	0.355
Prostate volume (ml)	39.4 ± 19.4	41.4 ± 20.1	0.235
Qmax	14.0 ± 2.4	16.5 ± 2.6	0.043
24-h drinking volume (ml)	1465.4 ± 624.8	1505.4 ± 610.8	0.356
4-h before bedtime drinking volume (ml)	115.8 ± 100.9	106.6 ± 97.9	0.452
Frequency of nocturia	2.8 ± 0.7	3.0 ± 0.6	0.306
Frequency of daytime urination	7.5 ± 2.6	8.1 ± 2.6	0.002
Maximum urination volume (ml)	372.8 ± 103.3	302.8 ± 119.3	0.007
Morning urine volume (ml)	280.5 ± 111.7	259.5 ± 100.7	0.003
24-h total urine volume (ml)	1965.5 ± 623.5	1896.5 ± 637.5	0.231
Nocturnal urine volume (ml)	800.7 ± 323.0	845.7 ± 303.5	0.056

LUTS lower urinary symptom, PSA prostate-specific antigen

by BPH, but the efficacy in improving nocturia was not obvious [17, 18].

Tacklind thought that doxazosin and terazosin were significantly more effective than finasteride in improving nocturia, while no difference was found with tamsulosin [19]. This lack of specificity precluded prostatic surgery, such as transurethral resection of the prostate (TURP), from being the first-line therapy for nocturia. The symptoms of nocturia could not be improved in most patients. Nonetheless, various groups had reported decreases in nocturia after surgery in specific patient populations. In another study, Wada et al. evaluated the effect of TURP on nocturia in patients with LUTS/BPH. Nocturnal voids reduced from 3.0 to 1.9 per night after

Table 3 Comparison of evaluation indices in NP and non-NP patients

Variable	Median (mean ± SD)		P value
	NPi ≥0.33	NPi < 0.33	
Number of patients	113	35	
Percentage (%)	76.50	23.50	
Age (years)	69.6 ± 6.0	69.1 ± 4.0	0.746
LUTS duration (years)	5.8 ± 2.7	7.9 ± 4.0	0.043
24-h drinking volume (ml)	1931.9 ± 680.6	2206.5 ± 429.1	0.195
4-h before bedtime drinking volume (ml)	140.8 ± 135.8	132.9 ± 102.4	0.029
Nocturnal urine volume (ml)	922.4 ± 342.6	596.5 ± 168.2	0.003
Morning urine volume (ml)	278.3 ± 116.5	202.5 ± 55.0	0.004
Frequency of daytime urination	7.4 ± 2.2	10.6 ± 2.4	0.005
Bladder capacity index	0.8 ± 0.6	0.8 ± 0.6	0.963
Maximum urination volume (ml)	369.1 ± 126.0	299.4 ± 75.7	0.076
Prostate volume (ml)	41.9 ± 25.3	39.5 ± 24.8	0.198
Peak flow rate (ml/s)	13.2 ± 10.0	13.9 ± 9.9	0.12
Residual volume (ml)	21.8 ± 20.0	20.6 ± 18.7	0.087
Serum PSA (ng/ml)	4.7 ± 4.1	4.5 ± 4.0	0.102

NPi nocturnal polyuria index

surgical treatment, which showed significant difference [5]. Yoshimura et al. reported that 505 cases of patients with BPH after drug treatment of tamsulosin and TURP surgery decreased the frequency of nocturia in patients by 17.9 and 32.2%, respectively, but the efficacy in improving nocturia was not obvious [20]. Additional studies were warranted to validate and substantiate these findings. Though such treatments were unlikely to benefit most patients with nocturia, they could be tried in select cases.

In our study, 80 patients were randomized to drug treatment (tamsulosin) and 68 patients were randomized to placebo treatment. The scores and the data (include I-PSS score, storage symptom score, voiding symptom score, quality of life score, frequency of daytime urination, maximum urine volume, and morning urine volume) were all statistically significant. However, the frequency of nocturia score and the nocturnal urine volume did not change significantly. The traditional tool for evaluating nocturia was the I-PSS in nocturia subtype score, which was not described in detail [21]. Whatsmore, the important and detailed information of nocturia may not be fully captured by the I-PSS questionnaire alone. Michel et al. thought that the I-PSS (QoL and Nocturia score) can't show how nocturia decreases sleep quality [22]. Therefore, a thorough evaluation of any treatment of nocturia requires using a method for measuring the treatment impact on sleep quality and QoL [18]. The international consultation on incontinence questionnaire (ICIQ) N-QoL is developed by Abraham et al., and it is a validated questionnaire that can measure the deterioration of health-related quality of life (HRQoL) due to nocturia in general [23]. In our study, we also found it was just a basic assessment of the patient's own quality of life use I-PSS (QoL) score. On the one hand we worried about patients' coordination and understanding, on the other hand we ignored the importance of nocturia to quality of life. The (ICIQ) N-QoL et al. should be used to evaluate nocturia on quality of life in further study.

We used a 3-day urinary frequency voiding diary, including a 24-h urination, nocturnal urine volume, urine volume, total sleeping time, and amount of water intake for a detailed assessment of patients with nocturia to understand the correlation between nocturia and other factors. Therefore, the data that was obtained was in detail.

Koseoglu et al. reported 58 cases of patients with BPH, of whom 95% had NP. The frequency of nocturia was 2.73 ± 1.44 times/day, which confirmed that patients with BPH and NP had a relationship between LUTS duration and 3-h drinking of water before falling asleep [24]. In this study, patients with BPH were diagnosed as BPH/LUTS, which led to the decrease of a certain degree of bladder function, and all patients received treatment (drug treatment such as tamsulosin or placebo treatment). To some extent, medications could alleviate lower urinary tract symptoms in patients with BPH, including storage symptoms such as urinary frequency and urgency. However, according to the analysis on 3-day voiding diary results, NP was reported in 76.5% of patients with nocturia, which is lower than that reported for 95% of the patients with NP type nocturia. However, the proportion is still higher than other types of nocturia. Our results showed that there was no association between nocturnal urine volume and LUTS duration, PV, serum PSA, or I-PSS. However, there was a significant correlation between the amount of drinking water at night ($r = 0.419$, $p = 0.002$) and before falling asleep 4-h drinking water ($r = 0.302$, $P = 0.031$). Hence, we thought that the improvement of α-blockers treatment for nocturia was poor.

In this study, between the NP group and the non-NP group, there was a significant difference in LUTS duration, maximum urine volume, morning urine volume, nocturnal urine volume, daytime urination, and 4-h before falling asleep drinking water volume. The frequency of daytime micturition and LUTS duration were the indices between the NP group and the non-NP group. A long disease history and more frequent daytime urination were considered the non-NP type, and α-blocker drug treatment could improve this type of nocturia. Nocturia could also be alleviated by treating the other causes, such as increased water drinking before going to bed.

This study had some limitations, including a small sample size and the assessment with regard to short-term use of medication. Future studies of patients with LUTS/BPH and nocturia should, therefore, also include nocturia-specific instruments to correctly classify the underlying pathologies for nighttime voiding, and hence, provide a rationale for the treatment of all LUTS/BPH causes.

Conclusions

In conclusion, patients with lower urinary tract symptoms improved, to some extent, after receiving medication. However, the nocturia was not obviously improved and the incidence was still high. The patients could not achieve satisfactory results, and NP was highly prevalent among patients. The correlation between the frequency of nocturia and nighttime water intake and drinking water before going to bed were significant. We could control water intake to ease nocturnal urination.

Abbreviations

BPH: Benign prostatic hyperplasia; I-PSS: International Prostate Symptom Score; NP: Nocturnal polyuria; Npi: Nocturnal polyuria index

Acknowledgements

Not applicable.

Authors' contributions

ZGX, YHL, NBW and JWB obtained the data. ZGX and YGJ participated in designing of the study and performed the statistical analysis, and wrote the draft in the manuscript. All authors read and approved the final manuscript.

Competing interests

All authors' declare that they have no competing interests.

Author details

[1]Department of Urology, Beijing Anzhen Hospital, Capital Medical University, Beijing 100029, China. [2]Department of Urology, Beijing Huairou Hospital, Beijing 101400, China.

References

1. Austin PF, Bauer SB, Bower W, et al. The standardization of terminology of lower urinary tract function in children and adolescents: update report from the standardization committee of the international Children's continence society. Neurourol Urodyn. 2016;35(4):471–81.
2. Bosch JL, Weiss JP. The prevalence and causes of nocturia. J Urol. 2010; 184(2):440–6.
3. Van Kerrebroeck P, Abrams P, Chaikin D, et al. The standardisation of terminology in nocturia: report from the standardisation sub-Committee of the International Continence Society. Neurourol Urodyn. 2002;21(2): 179–83.
4. Asplund R. Nocturia: consequences for sleep and daytime activities and associated risks. Eur Urol Suppl. 2005;3(6):24–32.
5. Wada N, Numata A, Hou K, et al. Nocturia and sleep quality after transurethral resection of the prostate. Int J Urol. 2014;21(1):81_5.
6. Schatzl G, Temml C, Schmidbauer J, et al. Cross-sectional study of nocturia in both sexes: analysis of a voluntary health screening project. Urology. 2000;56(1):71–5.
7. Matthiesen TB, Ritting S, Norgaard JP, et al. Nocturnal polyuria and natriuresis in male patients with nocturia and lower urinary tract symptons. J Urol. 1996;156(4):1292–9.
8. Wang W, Chen S, Liu YX, et al. Understanding Chinese patient attitude toward BPH and BPH treatment: results from PHELP 2006 study. Urology. 2009;74(4):S48–8.
9. Asplund R, Aberg H. Health of the elderly with regard to sleep and nocturnal micturition. Scand J Prim Health Care. 1992;10(2):98–104.
10. Stanley N. The physiology of sleep and the impact of ageing. Eur Urol Suppl. 2005;3(6):17–23.
11. Abrams P. Nocturia: the effect on sleep and related health consequences. Eur Urol Suppl. 2005;3(6):1–7.
12. Torimoto K, Hirayama A, Matsushita C, et al. Evaluation of sleep quantity and quality in older adults with nocturia using portable electroencephalogram acquisition device. J Urol. 2013;189(4):e557–8.
13. Akerstedt T, Nilsson PM. Sleep as restitution: an introduction. J Intern Med. 2003;254(1):6–12.
14. Asplund R. Mortality in the elderly in relation to nocturnal micturition. BJU Int. 1999;84(3):297–301.
15. Bonnet MH, Arand DL. Clinical effects of sleep fragmentation versus sleep deprivation. Sleep Med Rev. 2003;7(4):297–310.
16. Kupelian V, McVary KT, Kaplan SA, et al. Association of lower urinary tract symptoms and the metabolic syndrome: results from the Boston area community health survey. J Urol. 2013;189(1 Suppl):S107–14.
17. Johnson TM, Burrows PK, Kusek JW, et al. Medical therapy of prostatic symptoms research group. The effect of doxazosin, finasteride and combination therapy on nocturia in men with benign prostatic hyperplasia. J Urol. 2007;178(5):2045–50.
18. Johnson TM, Williford WO, Kutner MH. Changes in nocturia from medical treatment of benign prostatic hyperplasia: secondary analysis of the Department of Veterans Affairs Cooperative Study Trial. J Urol. 2003;170(1):145–8.
19. Tacklind J, Fink HA, Macdonald R, et al. Finasteride for benign prostatic hyperplasia. Cochrane Database Syst Rev. 2010. https://doi.org/10.1002/14651858.CD006015.pub3.
20. Yoshimura K, Ohara H, Ichioka K, et al. Nocturia and benign prostatic hyperplasia. Urology. 2003;61(4):786–90.
21. Barry MJ, Fowler FJ, O'Leary MP, et al. The American urological association symptom index for benign prostatic hyperplasia. The Measurement Committee of the American Urological Association. J Urol. 1992;148(5):1549–57.
22. Michel MC, Chapple CR. Comparison of the cardiovascular effects of tamsulosin oral controlled absorption system (OCAS) and alfuzosin prolonged release (XL). Eur Urol. 2006;49(3):501–8.
23. Abraham L, Hareendran A, Mills IW, et al. Development and validation of a quality-of-life measure for men with nocturia. Urology. 2004;63(3):481–6.
24. Koseoglu H, Aslan G, Ozdemir I, et al. Noctural polyuria in patients with lower urinary tract symptoms and response to alpha-blocker therapy. Urology. 2006;67(6):1188–92.

Resource utilization and costs associated with the addition of an antimuscarinic in patients treated with an alpha-blocker for the treatment of urinary symptoms linked to benign prostatic hyperplasia

Antoni Sicras-Mainar[1*], Ruth Navarro-Artieda[2], Ana Mª. Mora[3] and Marta Hernández[3]

Abstract

Background: There has been a change in the focus of attention from prostate to bladder, as the etiology of lower urinary tract symptoms (LUTS) makes the bladder an additional therapeutic target. This study aims to evaluate the use of resources and costs associated with the addition of an antimuscarinic (AM) in patients receiving an alpha-adrenergic-blocker (AAB) for the treatment of LUTS linked to benign prostatic hyperplasia (BPH).

Methods: A multicentre, retrospective study was conducted using patient records from the databases of six primary care centers in Spain. Men with moderate-to-severe LUTS (IPSS > 7) who were initiated on AM treatment between January 2010 and December 2012 without previous treatment with an AM or 5-alpha reductase inhibitor (5-ARI) and had been on treatment with an AAB for a minimum of 6 months prior to the addition of the AM with a minimum of two records in the database were included. Comorbidity, treatment persistence, and use of resources and costs (direct and indirect) during monotherapy (AAB alone) and following the introduction of combination therapy (AAB + AM) over a treatment period of up to a year were compared. A paired sample Student t-test was performed where $p < 0.05$ were considered significant.

Results: One hundred and ninety-one patients (mean age (SD): 70 (10.4) years) were treated with combination therapy. Treatment persistence on combination therapy after 12 months was 65.4% (95% CI: 58.8-72.2%). Use of resources was numerically lower after initiation of combination therapy vs pre-treatment (AAB alone) period for medical visits (/year/patient) (13.4 (4.6) vs 15.4 (4.4) $p < 0.010$), percentage of patients using concomitant medication (13.3% vs 19.1%) and use of pads (9.7% vs 13.4%) among others analyzed. Comparing AAB vs AAB + AM, there were a numeric reduction in total cost/year (€2399 vs €2011; $p = 0.135$) and a reduction of costs due to medical visits (€645 vs. €546; $p = 0.003$) and concomitant medication (€181 vs. €101; $p = 0.009$).

Conclusions: The addition of an AM agent in patients treated for LUTS with AAB is associated with a lower use of healthcare resources in terms of number of medical visits, and concomitant medications required, thereby leading to reduction of overall costs to the healthcare system.

Keywords: Lower urinary tract symptoms, Benign prostatic hyperplasia, Antimuscarinics, Resource utilization, Costs

* Correspondence: asicras@bsa.cat
[1]Dirección de Planificación, Badalona Serveis Assistencials SA, Via Augusta, 9, 08911 Badalona, Barcelona, Spain
Full list of author information is available at the end of the article

Background

Benign prostatic hyperplasia (BPH) is a common condition and a major source of morbidity in older men [1–3]. Its prevalence increases with age, and it presents in more than 50% of men above 50 years old and in up to 80% of males above 90 years old [4–6]. The *International Continence Society* proposed the term Lower Urinary Tract Symptoms (LUTS) to describe symptoms associated with the storage and voiding phases of the urinary cycle [1]. Male LUTS have traditionally been attributed to the prostate, but breakthroughs in the knowledge of *bladder dysfunction* and its physiopathology have led to the understanding that the storage symptoms of male LUTS may be due to co-existing overactive bladder or bladder malfunction secondary to bladder outlet obstruction of prostatic origin [1, 3, 7].

The insufficient response in alleviating LUTS related to BPH in some cases, together with the increasing recognition of the complexity of the pathophysiology of the lower urinary tract as a functional unit, has helped to shift the focus of attention from the prostate to the bladder as a possible cause of LUTS, thus making it an additional therapeutic target [8–10]. This change of perspective, acknowledging the multifactorial etiology of male LUTS, and accepting that not all of the symptoms are necessarily related to the prostate, is mirrored in the current guidelines of Scientific Societies [1, 3, 5–7]. The main treatment objectives are to reduce symptoms, improve quality of life and prevent the development of complications [1, 2, 7–10]. In this regard, and as a step prior to treatment selection, the severity of symptoms should be assessed with the International Prostate Symptom Score (IPSS) [11, 12]. Drug treatment is indicated in patients with moderate-to-severe symptoms who do not present an absolute indication for surgery [13], and the combination of an antimuscarinic with an alpha-blocker is justified in patients with BPH and LUTS compatible with co-existing overactive bladder [7, 9, 10, 13, 14]. There are several reasons that have led to this treatment rationale, particularly: a) the profile of patients with mixed storage and voiding LUTS with an important storage symptom component; b) the recommendations of the EAU guidelines [1]; and c) the scientific evidence on the effectiveness of alpha-blocker and antimuscarinic combination in this patient population. However, there is limited data on the impact these treatments have on resource utilization and costs.

The limited evidence in clinical practice available on the combined use of alpha-blockers and antimuscarinics in patients with LUTS and its impact on resource utilization and costs makes this study particularly relevant. The main objective of the study was to compare the level of resource utilization and both direct and indirect costs before and after the addition of an antimuscarinic in patients receiving an alpha-blocker for the treatment of LUTS associated with BPH in routine clinical practice.

Methods

Study design and population

This was an observational, multicentre, retrospective study on the use of resources and costs associated with lower urinary tract symptoms(LUTS) suggestive of benign prostatic hyperplasia (BPH) according to different clinical profiles in routine clinical practice. This study was based on a review of computer-based medical records of patients identified from the databases of six primary care centers [PCC] managed by Badalona Serveis Assistencials SA. Information on secondary care health resource utilization by these patients was obtained from the two reference hospitals: The Municipal Hospital and Hospital Universitari Germans Trías i Pujol de Badalona (specialized care).

Inclusion and exclusion criteria

All male patients suffering from LUTS who started add-on therapy with an AM between January 2010 and December 2012 were included in the study if they fulfilled the following criteria: a) aged ≥45 years; b) assigned to the geographical reference area; c) no previous treatment with AM or 5-ARI; d) current treatment with an AAB (for a minimum of six months prior to the addition of the AM); e) moderate-to-severe LUTS (IPSS > 7); f) regular follow-up was likely (defined as having presented two or more times according to health records), and g) on a chronic treatment prescription program with a proven record of the daily dose, timeframe and the duration in each administered treatment. The following patients were excluded: a) those transferred and/or moved from other geographic areas; b) permanently institutionalized patients; c) patients with grade III-IV prostate volume by digital rectal examination (DRE) (>40 ml); and d) coexistence of other urological conditions (prostate, bladder or kidney cancer, chronic urinary tract infection, calculi, urethral stricture, chronic pelvic pain syndrome and pelvic organ surgical record). The index date was the date the patient started on an antimuscarinic and the follow-up was one year from the index date.

Treatment description and persistence

Patients being treated for BPH were identified according to the Anatomical Therapeutic Chemical Classification System (ATC) code G04C [15]. The choice of medication for a specific patient was based on the doctor's judgment during clinical practice. Persistence was defined as the time, measured in months, without the patient dropping out of the initial treatment or without switching to another medication at least 30 days after the initial prescription. A patient was classified as being persistent if they had no treatment discontinuation or switch to another medication during the 12-month follow-up period.

Identification of patients with LUTS associated with BPH

The diagnosis of BPH was based on the International Classification of Primary Care (ICPC-2), component 7, diseases and health problems [16] (Y85), and the hospital discharge and emergency coding according to the International Classification of Diseases, 9th Revision, Clinical Modification; ICD-9-MC [600]). The following disease-related variables were also obtained from the database records: a) years of disease progression (BPH); b) symptom profile (storage, voiding and post-micturition symptoms); c) score on the IPSS scale, d) prostate volume: volume I (<20 ml) and volume II (20-40 ml) by DRE; e) body mass index (BMI, kg/m^2) and other lab test parameters (systolic and diastolic blood pressure (mmHg), total cholesterol (mg/dL) and serum creatinine (mg/dL)) f) prostate-specific antigen (PSA) (ng/mL); and g) concomitant medication related with LUTS (antidepressants, anxiolytics and antibiotics).

Sociodemographic and comorbidity data

Patient demographics including age, occupational status, and concomitant diseases were assessed. The level of comorbidity was assessed based on the Charlson comorbidity index [17], which measures the level of severity of the patient's conditions; and the number of chronic conditions. Comorbidity was adjusted using the Adjusted Clinical Groups (ACG) system, which is a patient classification system that measures the expected-consumption of healthcare resources according to a particular disease pattern, age and sex [18]. The ACG application provides the resource utilization bands (RUB), and each patient, depending on their general morbidity, is grouped into one of the 5 mutually exclusive categories (1: healthy or very low morbidity users, 2: low morbidity, 3: moderate morbidity, 4: high morbidity, and 5: very high morbidity).

Use of resources and cost analysis

Direct healthcare costs were those associated with BPH-related healthcare activity by health professionals (primary care visits, secondary care visits and hospital emergencies, days of hospitalization, emergencies and diagnostic and/or therapeutic requests). Indirect costs related to lost occupational productivity (days off work) were also obtained. The cost was expressed as mean cost per patient and year. The different study concepts and their economic evaluation are detailed in Table 1 (corresponding to 2012). The different rates were obtained from the centers' analytical accounting, except medication and days off work. Medical prescriptions were quantified according to the recommended retail price on the container at the time of prescription. The cost of days off work or lost activity was quantified according to the mean interprofessional wage

Table 1 Breakdown of unit costs and lost occupational productivity (2012)

Health and non-health resources	Unit costs (€)
Medical visits	
Primary care medical visit	23.19
Hospital emergency medical visit	117.53
Hospitalization (day)	380.00
ICU/coronary hospitalization (day)	850.00
Specialized Care medical visit	104.41
Complementary tests	
Laboratory Tests	22.30
Radiology[a]	18.50
Diagnostic/therapeutic tests[b]	97.12
Pharmaceutical prescription[c]	RRP VAT
Occupational productivity – indirect costs	
Cost per day not worked[d]	101.21

Source of the health resources: own analytical accounting
Values expressed in Euros (€). RRP VAT: Recommended retail price plus VAT; ICU: Intensive Care Unit
[a]Includes: simple conventional radiology
[b]Includes: radiology with contrast, ultrasound, TC scan, NMR, uroflowmetry, cystoscopy, cytology
[c]Includes: pads for incontinence and concomitant medication (anxiolytics, antidepressants and antibiotics)
[d]Source: National Statistics Institute (INE)

(source: National Statistics Institute-INE) [19]. This study did not provide for the calculation of non-health direct costs, i.e. those regarded as "out-of-pocket expenses" or paid for by the actual patient/family, as they are not recorded in the database and direct access to the patient was not possible. Cost calculation was based on the use of pads for urinary incontinence and the concomitant medication associated with the clinical consequences of BPH. Costs were determined during the 12 months prior to (pre-treatment) and the 12 months following (treatment) the date that the AM add-on therapy was started (index date).

Confidentiality of information

Confidentiality of medical records of patients identified from the databases was observed in agreement with Spanish Data Protection Law. The study was classified by the Spanish Agency for Medicines and Medical Devices (EPA-OD) and was subsequently approved by the Clinical Research Ethical Committee of the Hospital Universitari Germans Trías y Pujol de Badalona.

Statistical analysis

The mean, standard deviation and 95% confidence intervals (CI) were produced for normally distributed variables; and median and interquartile intervals (percentiles) for other variables. The Student t-test (for paired groups) was used to compare pretreatment versus combination treatment period, and Pearson's linear correlation according to data distributed and calculated for all the variables.

The comparison of the use of resources and their corresponding costs, between the first period of treatment with AAB and the second period after starting add-on therapy (AAB + AM), was performed according to Thompson and Barber's (2000) recommendations [20]' using a general linear model (analysis of covariance -ANCOVA-). Continuous and categorical independent variables: age, RUB, the Charlson index and number of years of disease evolution were included in the model as covariables (procedure: estimated marginal means; Bonferroni correction).

Data was presented as adjusted mean differences between treatments with the corresponding 95% confidence intervals calculated, using re-sampling techniques (bootstrapping) corrected for bias, given the non-normal distributions of the variables with respect to resource utilization and costs. All data were entered and analyzed in the SPSSWIN statistics application, version 17 Safety.

This was a non-interventional study. According to the regular clinical practice of the participating physicians, suspected adverse reactions detected during the course of the study had to be reported by the investigators as promptly as possible to the competent authority in matters of pharmacovigilance of the Autonomous Community corresponding to the healthcare area. For this purpose, the individual reporting form for suspected adverse reactions ("yellow card") had to be used, following article 7 of Law 1344/2007, of 11 October.

During the conduct of the study, the sponsor was not made aware of any potential safety information.tics applicationtics application

Results

The population from the database was comprised of 26,690 subjects ≥45 years of age, 21,352 of whom requested care during the recruitment period. A total of 6528 patients were diagnosed with BPH. Between 2010 and 2012, 1650 patients began/modified treatment, 575 of whom initiated combination treatment (AAB + AM). Of these, 66.8% (n = 384) were given treatment with an AAB and 5-ARI, and 33.2% (n = 191) with an AAB and AM (Fig. 1).

Table 2 shows the baseline characteristics, the clinical profile (LUTS) and the biochemical and anthropometric parameters of the 191 patients (mean age 70.0 (10.4)) receiving an AAB and AM combination. Patients receiving a combination of AAB and AM, had a high predominance of storage symptoms (87.4%) and post-micturition symptoms (91.1%), and co-existence of voiding

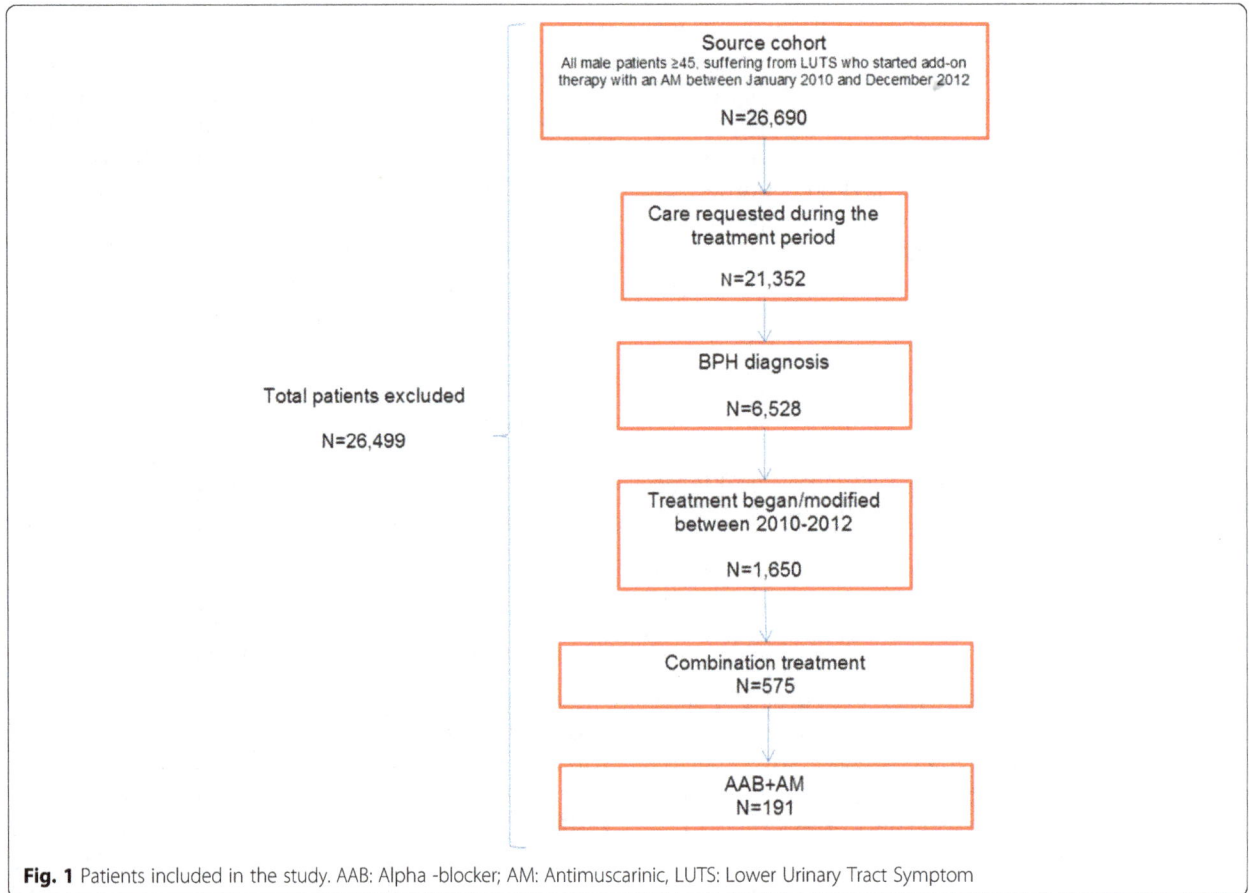

Fig. 1 Patients included in the study. AAB: Alpha -blocker; AM: Antimuscarinic, LUTS: Lower Urinary Tract Symptom

Table 2 Baseline characteristics of the population on combination (AAB + AM)

Subjects	N = 191
Demographic characteristics	
Mean age, years	70.0 (10.4)
Ranges: 45-64 years	29.8%
65-74 years	33.5%
≥ 75 years	36.6%
Pensioner	88.0%
General comorbidity	
Number of diagnoses	7.7 (4.2)
Charlson Comorbidity Index	0.6 (0.7)
RUB (morbidity)	3.0 (0.7)
1 (very low)	4.7%
2 (low)	10.1%
3 (moderate)	69.2%
4 (high)	15.4%
5 (very high)	0.6%
Specific comorbidity	
Arterial hypertension	59.8%
Dyslipidemia	51.3%
Cardiovascular event	32.8%
Diabetes mellitus	27.5%
Active smoker	22.2%
Vasculocerebral accident	22.2%
Organ failures	19.6%
COPD	18.5%
Obesity	18.0%
Ischemic heart disease	17.5%
Depressive syndrome	14.8%
Malignant neoplasms	13.2%
Alcoholism	5.3%
Asthma	4.8%
Neuropathies	4.8%
Dementias	2.6%
Clinical profile (symptoms)	
Storage	87.4%
Voiding	47.6%
Post-micturition	91.1%
Prostate volume (%)	
Volume I (<20 ml)	93.2%
Volume II (>20-40 ml)	6.8%
IPSS scale score	
Moderate symptoms (8-19 points)	71.2%
Severe symptoms (20-35 points)	28.8%
Biochemical/anthropometric parameters	

Table 2 Baseline characteristics of the population on combination (AAB + AM) *(Continued)*

Systolic blood pressure, mmHg	129.4 (15.0)
Diastolic blood pressure, mmHg	72.5 (10.6)
Body mass index kg/m^2	29.0 (4.0)
Total cholesterol, mg/dL	186.6 (42.1)
Serum creatinine, mg/dL	1.1 (0.4)
PSA (ng/mL)	0.9 (0.9)
Low PSA (<1.5 g/L)	79.3%
High PSA (≥1.5 g/L)	20.7%

Values expressed as a percentage or mean (standard deviation)
AAB alpha-blocker, *AM* antimuscarinic, *COPD* chronic obstructive pulmonary disease, *IPSS* international prostate symptom score, *PSA* prostate-specific antigen, *RUB* resource utilization bands

symptoms in (47.6%). There was also a high percentage of patients with prostate volume lower than 20 cm^3 (93.2%), a low percentage of patients with a prostate volume 20-40 cm^3 (6.8%) and a high percentage of patients with PSA <1.5 ng/ml (79.3%) in those receiving a combination of AAB and AM.

According to the IPSS, 71.2% of those receiving an AAB plus AM presented moderate symptoms (8-19 points) and 28.8% presented severe symptoms (20-35 points). The most frequent comorbidity reported in this patient population was arterial hypertension (59.8%).

Table 3 shows the treatment description and persistence rate of the 191 subjects analyzed in this study. The mean (SD) duration of the treatment with single therapy (AAB) prior to adding on AM was 15.7 (13.5) months. Treatment persistence on combination therapy (AAB + AM) after 12 months was 65.4%.

The comparison of pre-treatment (AAB alone) and combination treatment (AAB + AM) healthcare resource use and costs per patient per year is shown in Table 4. Use of resources was lower after initiation of AM + AAB vs pre-treatment (AAB alone) period for medical visits in general (13.4 (4.6) vs 15.4 (4.4) $p < 0.010$), primary care (10.6 (7.3) vs 12.1 (7.5) and hospital emergency visits (0.4 (0.8) vs 0.7 (0.7)) (p < 0.010 both). Concomitant medication (13.3% vs 19.1%) and use of pads (9.7% vs 13.4%) present a numerical (not statistically significant) reduction in use of resources with AAB + AM versus AAB alone. During the combination treatment period (AAB + AM), 84.3% of the total cost was healthcare related vs 80.2% on the pre-treatment period (AAB alone) and 15.7% was non-healthcare related vs 19.8% on the pre-treatment period (AAB alone). During the pre-treatment period (AAB alone), the total cost per patient per year was €2399 versus €2011 in the treatment period, despite including the cost of the AM. However, this numerical difference was not statistically significant ($p = 0.135$). A reduction in cost was also

Table 3 Description and persistence of the treatment administered from the series studied (CI 95%)

Subjects	N = 191
Time since diagnosis, years	
Mean (SD)	8.0 (3.7)
Median (P25 - P75)	9.0 (4.5-10.5)
Duration of the treatment (single therapy), months	
Mean (SD)	15.7 (13.5)
Median (P25 - P75)	14.1 (2.0-23.3)
Duration of the treatment (double therapy), months	
Mean (SD)	10.2 (7.1)
Median (P25 - P75)	9.0 (4.0-11.5)
Treatment persistence[a]	
Persistence on double therapy, 12 months	65.4%
CI 95%	58.8-72.2%

Values expressed as mean (SD: standard deviation) or percentage,
P: percentiles
[a]*Persistence* was defined as the time, measured in months, without the patient dropping out of the initial treatment or without switching to another medication at least 30 days after the initial prescription. A patient was classified as being persistent if they had no treatment discontinuation or switch to another medication during the 12-month follow-up period. CI: Confident Interval

Table 4 Use of resources and healthcare costs per patient/year of the series studied

Periods	Pretreatment (AAB)	Treatment[a] (AAB + AM)
Use of resources		
Medical visits (all)	15.4 (4.4)	13.4 (4.6)[†]
- Primary Care	12.1 (7.5)	10.6 (7.3)[†]
- Specialists	2.6 (4.3)	2.4 (3.0)
- Hospital emergencies	0.7 (0.7)	0.4 (0.8)[‡]
Laboratory	1.4 (1.6)	1.6 (1.7)
Radiology	1.0 (1.9)	0.7 (1.2)
Complementary tests	0.3 (0.9)	0.2 (0.5)
Concomitant medication[b]	19.1%	13.3%
Pads	13.4%	9.7%
Hospital stays	2.0 (7.7)	2.0 (6.1)
Occupational disability, days	4.7 (17.9)	3.1 (17.1)
Costs (in €)		
Medical visits (all)	645 (460)	546 (420)[†]
Laboratory	32 (55)	35 (39)
Radiology	19 (25)	13 (22)
Complementary tests	20 (42)	17 (46)
Hospital stays	750 (2.449)	746 (2.337)
Specific medication		
Alpha-adrenergic blockers	195 (174)	190 (159)
Antimuscarinics	–	398 (117)
Concomitant medication[b]	181 (99)	101 (75) [‡]
Pads	82 (144)	47 (138)
Healthcare cost	1924 (2478)	1695 (2542)
Occupational disability cost	475 (1677)	316 (1744)
Total cost	2399 (3113)	2011 (3026)

Values expressed as mean (SD: standard deviation) or percentage, p: statistical significance
AAB alpha-blocker, AM antimuscarinic, € euros
[a]Period of combined treatment (12 months after the index date)
[b]Concomitant medication (anxiolytics, antidepressants and antibiotics)
Non-statistically significant difference when it is not indicated between the comparison by pairs (pretreatment vs. treatment), [‡]p < 0.001, [†]p < 0.01

shown from the pre-treatment (AAB alone) to the treatment period (AAB + AM) for medical visits (from €645 to €546 ($p < 0.01$)) and concomitant medication (from €181 to €101 ($p < 0.001$)). Differences in mean costs are shown in Fig. 2.

Discussion

This study using data from the Spanish National Health System shows that patients with LUTS associated with BPH who were on treatment with an AAB and initiate a new pharmacological treatment with an AM have lower use of healthcare resources as compared to previous pretreatment with AAB alone and incur lower costs in terms of concomitant medication and medical visits. This is a valuable contribution as there is a lack of information about the use of healthcare resource and costs related to the use of this combination. Few observational studies which address the use of these drugs in real life conditions have compared resource utilization before and after the addition of an AM in men on AAB therapy for the treatment of LUTS [21]. Most of the published studies are based on economic assessment models [22], the cost of treatment given [23] and/or different modalities of surgery [24].

A meta-analysis recently published by Filson and colleagues [13] compared the efficacy of combined treatment with an AAB and an AM versus monotherapy with an AAB in men with storage symptoms associated with BPH. Combination treatment was shown to be associated with significantly greater reductions in the storage symptom subscale score of the IPSS and in micturition frequency. Furthermore, this therapeutic approach was associated with only a minimal risk of either increased post-void residual volume, reduction in maximum urinary flow rate or acute urinary retention. Therefore, the authors concluded that combination therapy with AM is a reasonable treatment option for men with LUTS associated with BPH, particularly when their symptoms have a major storage component. A systematic review by Athanasopoulos et al. suggest that in men with persistent storage symptoms consistent with OAB, clinically meaningful improvements can be achieved through the addition of an antimuscarinic therapy to an a-blocker and that

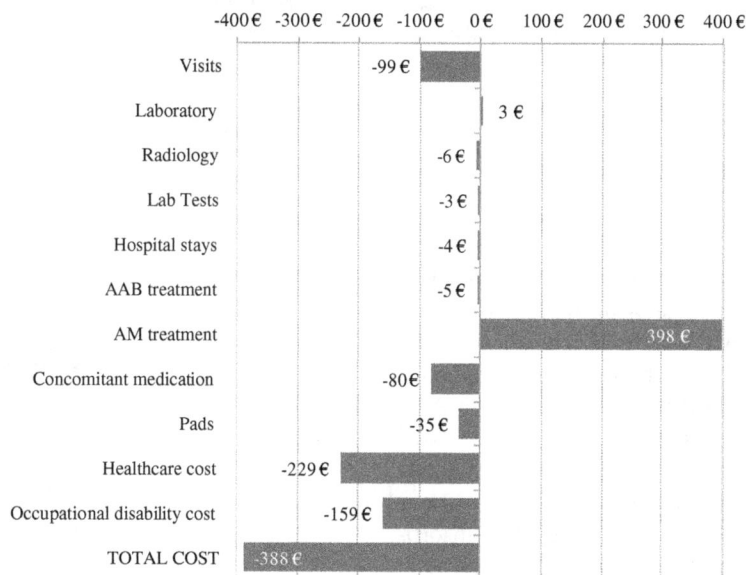

Fig. 2 Differences in mean cost after adding an AM agent. Values in Euros (€); AAB:Alpha-blockers; AM: Antimuscarinics

monotherapy with an antimuscarinic alone in this patient group is controversial, given the results of the few existing trials [25].

The results of this study supports that adding an AM agent (in combination with an AAB) leads to a reduction in the use of healthcare resources and related costs. One possible explanation could be that combination therapy provides better outcomes on storage and voiding LUTS, resulting in a reduction in the use of concomitant medication (anxiolytics, antidepressants and antibiotics) and health services (medical visits). However further investigation is required to ascertain this conclusively given the low number of patients on concomitant treatment in this study and the lack of baseline data (prior to initiating AAB treatment) of these patients. Furthermore, although there was not statistical significance in all the studied variables, a numerical reduction was observed in the majority of them. Despite these limitations, we think these findings are valuable and can help guide future investigations.

The differences in cost persisted despite the greater cost for combined treatment. In our opinion, this reduction in unit costs is important from the standpoint of efficiency in the clinical management of this group of patients, especially considering the high percentage of patients with mixed clinical symptoms with a predominance of the storage component [2]. In a meta-analysis by Xin and coworkers [26], based on 15 clinical trials (N = 4556), combination therapy (AAB and AM) improved LUTS with a low incidence of adverse effects. These findings are also in line with a recent meta-analysis (Gong et al.) [27] (N = 3063) that evaluated the efficacy and safety of tamsulosin and solifenacin combination therapy compared with tamsulosin

monotherapy for male LUTS (including fixed-dose combination evidence), which concluded that this combination may be a reasonable option for male LUTS patients, especially for those who have significant storage symptoms.

It is remarkable that from the initial sample size of 26,690 subjects only 191 were on combination treatment with AAB + AM. There could be several reasons for this finding. One, only patients diagnosed with BPH according to ICPC-2 and ICD-9CM were evaluated. Additionally, during the time of the observation period for this study (2010-2012), the combination treatment with AAB + AM was already recommended in the EAU guidelines. However, the fixed dose combination, was not licensed and marketed in Spain until 2015. In contrast, the 5-ARI + AAB combination was marketed as a fixed dose combination in Spain during this time. Therefore, AAB + AM combination was recommended and could be used as a free dose combination at the time of this study. However, the extent by which the EAU recommendations were followed at this time is uncertain. None-the-less the level of use of this combination was an interesting point to assess in our study as literature about combination therapy in this profile of patients was emerging.

The limitations of the current study are those typical of retrospective studies, such as under-reporting of disease, the possible variability in clinicians' practice and assessment of patients due to the observational design. The cost system used and/or the possible existence of a classification bias are also limitations that must be taken into account. In this regard, the possible inaccuracy of the diagnostic coding in terms of the diagnosis of BPH and other comorbidities, the reliability of the evaluation of the IPSS criteria, or the lack of a variable that might impact the final results (response to treatment, prescribed doses, etc.), must be considered.

Due to the retrospective design of the study, we cannot determine if this cost reduction is a consequence of the AM addition to the treatment with AAB or if other confounding factors could exist.

In conclusion, despite the possible limitations, this study showed that patients with LUTS associated with BPH with predominant storage symptoms who are on combination treatment with an AAB and an AM display a lower use of healthcare resources (medical visits and concomitant medication),than treatment with AAB alone,.leading to lower costs for the Spanish National Health System Further studies are warranted to determine whether the fixed-dose combination of AM + AAB (solifenacin + tamsulosin oral-controlled absorption system (TOCAS)) for the treatment of men with moderate to severe storage and voiding symptoms (available in the market after this study) reinforces or optimizes these results.

The future perspectives offered by this study could be on the potential replication of this model to better assess how treatments impact cost and resource use in other health institutions, to assist in reporting recommendations on the use of antimuscarinics to healthcare professionals.

Conclusions
In our study, males treated with AAB monotherapy for LUTS related to BPH had a mean (SD) cost per year of 2399 (3113) € per patient. After the addition of an AM to the treatment, the mean (SD) annual cost was reduced to 2011 (3026) € per patient. The lower cost was associated with the lower use of medical visits and concomitant medication.

Abbreviations
5ARI: 5-Alpha reductase inhibitors; AAB: Alpha-Adrenergic Blockers; ACG: Adjusted clinical groups; AM: Antimuscarinic; ANCOVA: ANalysis of COVAriance; ATC: Anatomical therapeutic chemical; BMI: Body Mass Index; BPH: Benign prostatic hyperplasia; BSA: Badalona Serveis Assistencials; CI: Confidence Interval; EAU: European association of urology; ICD-9-CM: International classification of diseases, 9th revision, clinical modification; ICPC-2: International classification of primary care; ICU: Intensive care unit; INE: Instituto Nacional de Estadística; IPSS: International prostatic symptom score; LUTS: Lower urinary tract symptoms; OR: Odds-ratio; PCC: Primary care centres; PSA: Prostatic specific antigen; RUB: Resource utilization bands; SD: Standard deviation; SPSS: Statistical product and service solutions; TOCAS: Tamsulosin oral controlled absorption system

Acknowledgements
We thank the BSA healthcare professionals who aided this study.

Funding
This study was funded by Astellas Pharma, Spain.

Availability of data and materials
The data contained within the manuscript and the datasets supporting the conclusion of this article are available from the corresponding author upon reasonable request.

Authors' contributions
ASM, RNA and AMM participated in the design and idea of the original study. ASM, RNA, AMM and MH contributed to the data interpretation, and draft writing, review and approval of the submitted manuscript.

Authors' information
Not applicable.

Ethics approval and consent to participate
The study was governed by the basic ethical principles contained in the Declaration of Helsinki. The study, its design and procedures were classified by the Spanish Medicines Agency (AEMPS) as a Post-Authorisation Study – Other Designs (EPA-OD) trial type and was subsequently approved by the Clinical Research Ethics Committee of Hospital Germans Trias i Pujol. Based on its design, it was exempt under Spanish law from requiring written informed consent (Law 29/2006 of 26 July and Royal Decree 1344/2007 of 11 October).

Competing interests
This study was sponsored by Astellas Pharma S.A. AMM y MH are employees of Astellas Pharma S.A. ASM and RNA have no conflicts of interests to declare.

Author details
[1]Dirección de Planificación, Badalona Serveis Assistencials SA, Via Augusta, 9, 08911 Badalona, Barcelona, Spain. [2]Documentación Médica, Hospital Germans Trias i Pujol, Badalona, Barcelona, Spain. [3]Medical Department, Astellas Pharma S.A, Madrid, Spain.

References
1. Gravas S, Bach T, Bachmann A, Drake M, Gacci M, Gratzke C,et al. Male lower urinary tract symptoms (LUTS), incl.Benign prostatic obstruction (BPO). 2016 [available online: https://uroweb.org/guideline/treatment-of-non-neurogenic-male-luts/].
2. Cambronero J, Arlandis S, Errando C, Mora AM. Profile of lower urinary tract symptoms in the male and their impact on quality of life. Actas Urol Esp. 2013;37:401–7.
3. Cózar-Olmo JM, Hernández-Fenández C, Miñana-López B, Amón-Sesmero JH, Montlleó-González M, Rodríguez-Antolín A, et al. Consenso sobre el impacto clínico de la nueva evidencia científica disponible sobre hiperplasia benigna prostática. Actas Urol Esp. 2012;36:265–75.
4. Bushman W. Etiology, epidemiology, and natural history of benign prostatic hyperplasia. Urol Clin North Am. 2009;36:403–15.
5. Brenes Bermúdez FJ, Cozar Olmo JM, Esteban Fuertes M, Fernández-Pro Ledesma A, Molero García JM. Urine incontinence referral criteria for primary care. Aten Primaria. 2013;45:263–73.
6. Grupo Español de Urodinámica y de SINUG. Consenso sobre terminología y conceptos de la función del tracto urinario inferior. Actas Urol Esp. 2005;29:16–30.
7. Liao CH, Kuo YC, Kuo HC. Predictors of successful first-line antimuscarinic monotherapy in men with enlarged prostate and predominant storage symptoms. Urology. 2013;81:1030–3.
8. Ventura S, Oliver VI, White CW, Xie JH, Haynes JM, Exintaris B. Novel drug targets for the pharmacotherapy of benign prostatic hyperplasia (BPH). Br J Pharmacol. 2011;163:891–907.
9. Ruiz Cerdá JL. Use of antimuscarinics in patients with LUTS-BPH and OAB symptoms: clinical expertise and resistance to lose the fear to urinary retention risk. Actas Urol Esp. 2008;32:957–60.
10. Hakimi Z, Johnson M, Nazir J, Blak B, Odeyemi IA. Drug treatment patterns for the management of men with lower urinary tract symptoms associated with benign prostatic hyperplasia who have both storage and voiding

Resource utilization and costs associated with the addition of an antimuscarinic in patients treated...

165

symptoms: a study using the health improvement network UK primary care data. Curr Med Res Opin. 2015 Jan;31(1):43–50.

11. Castiñeiras Fernández J, Cozar Olmo JM, Fernández-Pro A, Martín JA, Brenes Bermúdez FJ, Naval Pulido E, et al. Sociedad Española de Médicos de Atención Primaria; Sociedad Española de Medicina General; Sociedad Española de Medicina de Familia y Comunitaria; Asociación Española de Urología. Referral criteria for benign prostatic hyperplasia in primary care. Sociedad Española de Médicos de Atención Primaria, Sociedad Española de Medicina General, Sociedad Española de Medicina de Familia y Comunitaria, Asociación Española de Urología. Actas Urol Esp. 2010;34:24–34.

12. Kaplan SA, Roehrborn CG, Chancellor M, Carlsson M, Bavendam T, Guan Z. Extended-release tolterodine with or without tamsulosin in men with lower urinary tract symptoms and overactive bladder: effects on urinary symptoms assessed by the international prostate symptom score. BJU Int. 2008;102:1133–9.

13. Filson CP, Wei JT, Hollingsworth JM. Trends in medical management of men with lower urinary tract symptoms suggestive of benign prostatic hyperplasia. Urology. 2013;82:1386–92.

14. Verheggen BG, Lee R, Lieuw On MM, Treur MJ, Botteman MF, Kaplan SA, Trocio JN. Estimating the quality-of-life impact and cost-effectiveness of alpha-blocker and anti-muscarinic combination treatment in men with lower urinary tract symptoms related to benign prostatic hyperplasia and overactive bladder. J Med Econ. 2012;15:586–600.

15. WHO; 1991. The anatomical therapeutic chemical classification system.

16. Lamberts H, Wood M, Hofmans-Okkes ÍM, editors. The international classification of primary Care in the European Community. With a multi-language layer. Oxford: Oxford University Press; 1993.

17. Charlson ME, Pompei P, Ales KL, Mackenzie CR. A new method of classifying prognostic comorbidity in longitudinal studies: development and validation. J Chronic Dis. 1987;40:373–83.

18. Weiner JP, Starfield BH, Steinwachs DM, Mumford LM. Development and application of a population-oriented measure of ambulatory care case-mix. Med Care. 1991;29:452–72.

19. Instituto Nacional de Estadística 2010. Encuesta de costes laborales del año 2010. http://www.ine.es/prensa/np671.pdf. Accessed Sept 2013.

20. Thompson SG, Barber JA. How should cost data in pragmatic randomised trials be analysed? BMJ. 2000;320:1197–200.

21. Kirby RS, Kirby M, Fitzpatrick JM. Benign prostatic hyperplasia: counting the cost of its management. BJU Int. 2010;105:901–2.

22. Walker A, Doyle S, Posnett J, Hunjan M. Cost-effectiveness of single-dose tamsulosin and dutasteride combination therapy compared with tamsulosin monotherapy in patients with benign prostatic hyperplasia in the UK. BJU Int. 2013;112:638–46.

23. Carballido J, Ruiz-Cerdá JL, Unda M, Baena V, Campoy P, Manasanch J, Slof J. Economic evaluation of medical treatment of benign prostatic hyperplasia (BPH) in the specialised care setting in Spain. Application to the cost-effectiveness of two drugs frequently used in its treatment. Actas Urol Esp. 2008;32:916–25.

24. Frieben RW, Lin HC, Hinh PP, Berardinelli F, Canfield SE, Wang R. The impact of minimally invasive surgeries for the treatment of symptomatic benign prostatic hyperplasia on male sexual function: a systematic review. Asian J Androl. 2010;12:500–8.

25. Athanasopoulos A, Chapple C, Fowler C, Gratzke C, Kaplan S, Stief C, et al. The role of antimuscarinics in the management of men with symptoms of overactive bladder associated with concomitant bladder outlet obstruction: an update. Eur Urol. 2011;60:94–105.

26. Xin Z, Huang Y, Lu J, Zhang Q, Chen C. Addition of antimuscarinics to alpha-blockers for treatment of lower urinary tract symptoms in men: a meta-analysis. Urology. 2013;82:270–7.

27. Gong M, Dong W, Huang G, Gong Z, Deng D, Qiu S. Tamsulosin combined with solifenacin versus tamsulosin monotherapy for male lower urinary tract symptoms: a meta-analysis. Curr Med Res Opin. 2015;31(9):1781–92.

20

Cone-beam CT findings during prostate artery embolization for benign prostatic hyperplasia-induced lower urinary tract symptoms

Chia-Bang Chen[1], Chen-Te Chou[1,2,5] and Yao-Li Chen[3,4,5,6]*

Abstract

Background: Cone-beam computed tomography (CBCT) is a new and useful technique for angiographic procedures. Prostatic artery embolization (PAE) has emerged as a promising treatment modality for lower urinary tract symptoms (LUTS) caused by benign prostatic hyperplasia (BPH). CBCT can be helpful for PAE to determine the correct arteries for embolization, and to show any occlusion of these arteries.

Case presentation: Herein, we report on a patient who underwent CBCT-guided PAE as treatment for BPH-induced LUTS, present the imaging findings, and provide technical suggestions.

Conclusions: PAE is an effective, minimally invasive modality for the treatment of LUTS due to BPH, and contrast CBCT can help visualize and demonstrate occlusion of the prostatic arteries.

Keywords: Cone-beam computed tomography, Prostatic artery embolization, Benign prostatic hyperplasia, Lower urinary tract symptoms

Background

Benign prostatic hyperplasia (BPH) is a very common benign disease in elderly men, with a prevalence rate ranging from 50 to 90% [1]. Acute urinary retention and lower urinary tract symptoms (LUTS) are common complications of BPH, and many different treatment modalities are available. Surgical therapies are indicated for patients with severe LUTS or for non-responders to medical treatment. Transurethral resection of the prostate (TURP) is the most common surgical modality for patients with LUTS due to BPH; however, many patients develop complications after the operation. Prostatic artery embolization (PAE) is a minimally invasive technique that has been shown to be effective at relieving LUTS in patients with BPH. Cone-beam computed tomography (CBCT) is a new imaging technique for angiographic procedures. The modality provides high resolution three-dimensional and cross-sectional images. Administration of intravascular contrast medium results in good enhancement of the vessels and target lesion after which the CBCT images can be reconstructed into images that resemble angiographic images. Herein, we present the first case in Taiwan of BPH-related LUTS that was treated using CBCT-guided PAE. CBCT was used to visualize and show total occlusion of the prostatic arteries. The technical aspects of the procedure are also provided.

Case presentation

An 85-year-old man presented with a two-year history of progressive urinary frequency, urgency, nocturia, and acute urinary retention. Sonography revealed an enlarged prostate gland measuring about 127 mL in volume. Based on the symptoms and sonographic findings, the diagnosis of BPH with LUTS was made, and a Foley catheter was inserted immediately to provide short-term relief of acute urinary retention. Surgical treatment

* Correspondence: ylchen.cch@gmail.com
[3]Transplant Medicine and Surgery Research Centre, Changhua Christian Hospital, No. 135, Nan-Hsiao Street, Changhua 500, Taiwan
[4]School of Medicine, Chung Shan Medical University, Taichung City 40201, Taiwan
Full list of author information is available at the end of the article

rather than medical therapy was provided considering the time it would have taken for medical therapy to take effect and the patient's wish to avoid having an indwelling Foley catheter for a prolonged period. PAE rather than TURP was attempted because of the patient's advanced age. Before the procedure, the patient's score on the symptom index of the international prostate symptom score (IPSS) was 21 and his score on the quality of life index was 4. Prostate gland volume (162 mL) was estimated on axial T2-weighted magnetic resonance (MR) images.

Before the embolization procedure, 10 mL of diluted iodinated contrast medium (a mixture of 50% iodinated contrast medium plus 50% normal saline solution) was injected into the balloon of the Foley catheter to help localize the prostate gland under fluoroscopy. The left common and internal iliac arteries were accessed using a 4 Fr. J-curve catheter (Terumo, Tokyo, Japan) via the right femoral approach. Angiography of the left common and internal iliac arteries was performed, with 10 mL pure contrast medium injected by power injector at a rate of 2 mL/s, and with an image intensifier at a left anterior oblique (LAO) projection angle of 55 degrees to visualize the vascular anatomy (Fig. 1). A 1.98 Fr. coaxial microcatheter (Asahi INTECC CO, Nagoya, Japan) was used to access the left prostatic artery (LPA), which in our patient arose from the left pudendal artery. Contrast CBCT was performed from the left internal iliac artery, with 20 mL of a 67%:33% saline-to-contrast medium mixture injected by power injector at a flow rate of 1 mL/s and with an image delay of 6 s, and also from

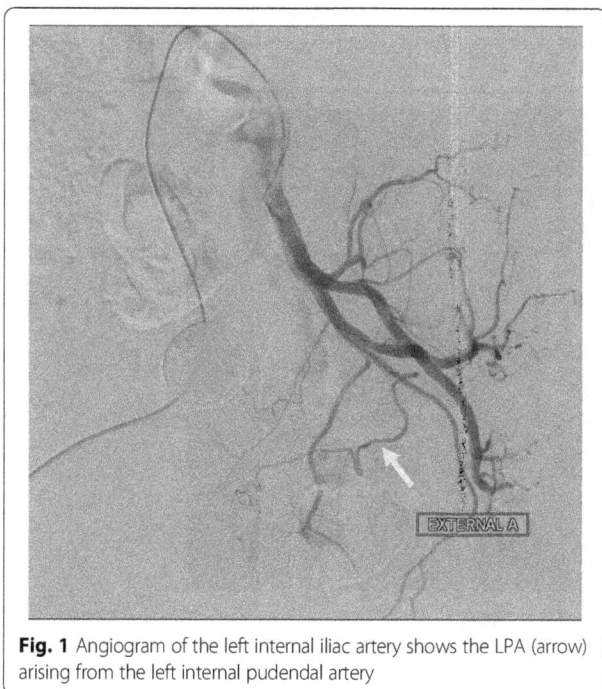

Fig. 1 Angiogram of the left internal iliac artery shows the LPA (arrow) arising from the left internal pudendal artery

the superselected LPA with 10 mL of diluted contrast medium injected by power injector at a flow rate of 0.5 mL/s and with an image delay of 6 s, to provide a three-dimensional view of the detailed vascular anatomy and to visualize the parenchymal enhancement of the left aspect of the prostate gland without filling defect (Fig. 2). Embozene Color-Advanced Microspheres measuring 250 μm in diameter (Celonova Biosciences Inc., San Antonio, USA) were slowly delivered after dilution with 5 mL contrast medium, until near stasis was achieved. Non-contrast CBCT demonstrated retention of the contrast medium without filling defect, and contrast CBCT revealed no further enhancement of the left aspect of the prostate gland parenchyma (Fig. 3).

A 5 Fr. RIM catheter (Cook Medical, Bloomington, Indiana) and a 1.98 Fr. coaxial microcatheter were used to access the right prostatic artery (RPA), which arose from the anterior division of the right internal iliac artery. Conventional angiography with a right anterior oblique (RAO) projection of 55 degrees was performed to demonstrate the vascular anatomy. Contrast CBCT was performed both from the right internal iliac artery and super selected RPA to demonstrate the vascular anatomy and to visualize parenchymal enhancement of the right aspect of the prostate gland without filling defect. In addition, decreased retention of contrast medium in the left aspect of the prostate gland parenchyma was depicted, as compared with the CBCT during embolization of the LPA. The contrast CBCT also clearly demonstrated that some small distal branches of the RPA supplied the right aspect of the rectum (Fig. 4). Embolization of these branches using microcoils could not be performed because they were too small to access. Embolization of the RPA was also performed with Embozene microspheres (250 μm) diluted with 5 mL contrast medium, and contrast CBCT was performed to ensure occlusion of the RPA, by visualizing retention of the contrast medium without filling defects and without further enhancement of the right aspect of the prostate gland parenchyma. Only 1 mL of the Embozene microspheres was delivered during this procedure.

There were no postprocedural complications. The patient was discharged the day after the procedure and the Foley catheter was removed 4 days after discharge. The patient reported a several-day history of passing mucus-containing stool after the procedure, but the side effect was self-limiting. His symptom index score on the IPSS decreased from 21 before the procedure to 5 about 3 weeks after the procedure and his quality of life index score decreased from 4 to 0. At the two-month follow-up, the prostate volume as measured on MR images was 76 mL.

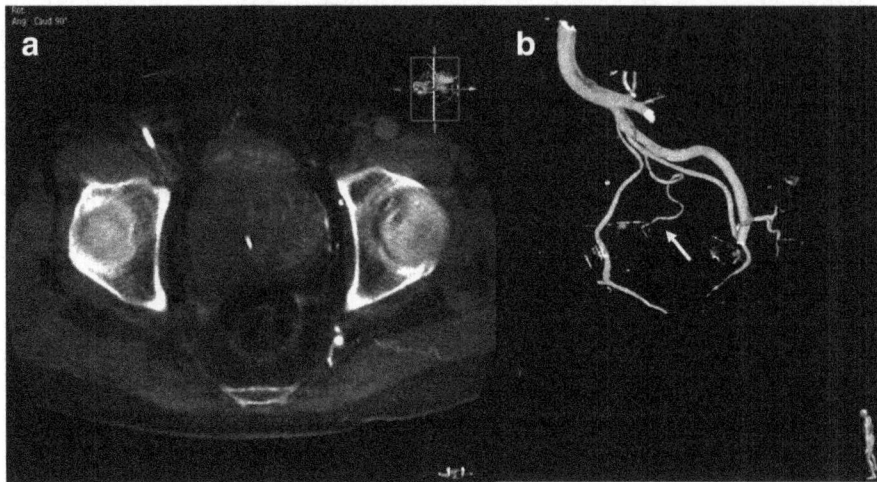

Fig. 2 Contrast CBCT of the left internal iliac artery. **a** Good parenchymal enhancement of the left aspect of the prostate gland was visualized. **b** Three-dimensional reconstructed image demonstrates the vascular anatomy of the LPA (arrow)

Discussion

In the previous literature, computed tomography angiography (CTA) was recommended before the embolization procedure to evaluate the pelvic vascular anatomy [2]. However, contrast CBCT has been shown to clearly demonstrate the vascular anatomy during the embolization procedure [3], and thus it is no longer necessary to perform CTA before the procedure. Furthermore, CBCT can demonstrate filling defects of the prostate gland due to accessory or collateral arterial supplies, and demonstrate occlusion of the prostatic arteries, by showing retention of contrast medium in the prostatic parenchyma without filling defects, and revealing no further parenchymal enhancement.

The contrast Foley balloon catheter can be used as a landmark of urinary bladder and prostate under fluoroscopic guidance [4], since the prostate is radiolucent. When accessing the prostatic arteries under fluoroscopy, the prostatic arteries can be located easily because they run just under the contrast Foley balloon, along a course to the midline of the pelvis. After successfully catheterizing the prostatic arteries, contrast CBCT can be used for confirmation, by demonstrating enhancement of the prostatic parenchyma, and also to detect arteries supplying adjacent organs to avoid non-target embolization.

In our patient, microspheres of 250 μm were used for embolization. After near stasis had been achieved, non-contrast CBCT showed retained contrast medium in the prostatic gland parenchyma without filling defect.

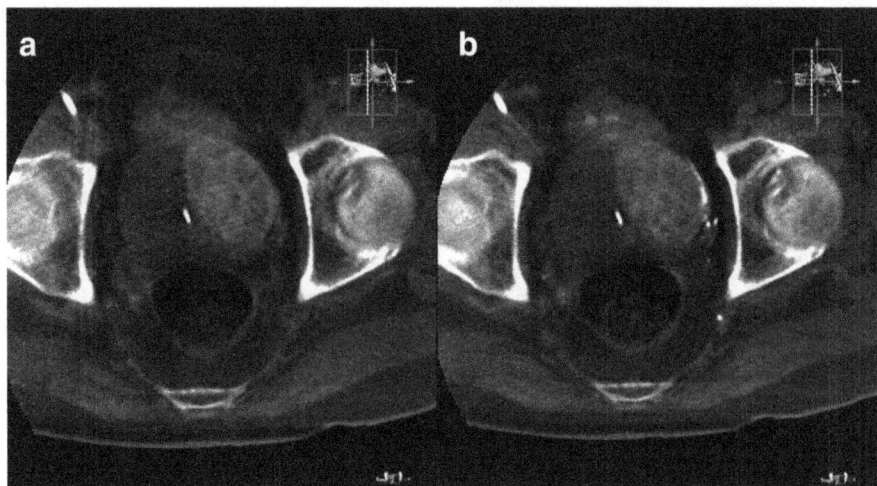

Fig. 3 a Non-contrast CBCT after embolization of the LPA shows retention of contrast medium in the left aspect of the prostatic parenchyma without filling defect. Some contrast medium was excreted from the kidneys and accumulated in the urinary bladder. **b** Contrast CBCT after embolization of the LPA shows no further enhancement of the left aspect of the prostatic parenchyma, suggesting adequate embolization

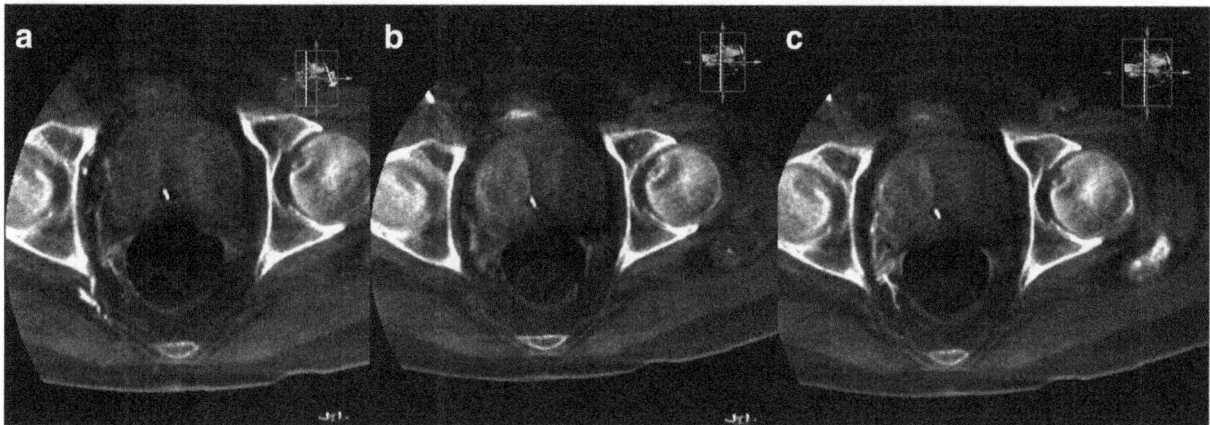

Fig. 4 a Contrast CBCT of the RPA shows small distal branches supplying the right aspect of the rectum. Decreased contrast medium retention in the left aspect of the prostate gland can be seen, as compared with Fig. 3(a). **b** Non-contrast CBCT after embolization of the RPA shows retention of contrast medium in the right aspect of the prostatic parenchyma and the distal branches, without filling defect. **c** Contrast CBCT after embolization of the RPA shows no further enhancement of the right aspect of the prostate gland

However, decreased retention of the contrast medium in the left prostate gland parenchyma after embolization of the LPA was noted on contrast CBCT images, probably because much of the contrast medium had been flushed out by the blood flow from the RPA. This finding suggests that there are tiny collateral vessels connecting the LPA and RPA. Pisco et al. [5] reported that embolization of the bilateral prostatic arteries should be attempted because unilateral embolization results in a higher rate of treatment failure. In our patient, contrast CBCT revealed no further enhancement, and non-contrast CBCT showed no filling defects of retained contrast medium in the prostatic parenchyma, both indicating occlusion of the prostatic arteries. There were some small vessels branching from the RPA to the rectum and embolization of these branches using microspheres larger than 200 μm in diameter has been shown to be safe [6].

Conclusions
In conclusion, PAE is an effective, minimally invasive modality for the treatment of LUTS due to BPH, and contrast CBCT can help visualize the prostatic arteries and detect accessory or collateral supplying vessels. Embolization of the prostatic arteries can be visualized using non-contrast and contrast CBCT by showing retention of contrast medium without filling defect and no further enhancement of the prostatic gland parenchyma. However, embolization in the bilateral prostatic arteries should be attempted to achieve a better clinical outcome.

Abbreviation
BPH: benign prostatic hyperplasia; CBCT: cone-beam computed tomography; LUTS: lower urinary tract symptoms; PAE: prostate artery embolization

Acknowledgements
None.

Funding
None.

Availability of data and materials
The data and materials are available from the authors.

Authors' contributions
CBC and CTC designed the study. CBC performed the treatment. CBC and YLC wrote the manuscript. All authors have read and approved the final manuscript.

Competing interests
The authors declare that they have no competing interests.

Author details
[1]Department of Radiology, Changhua Christian Hospital, No. 135, Nan-Hsiao Street, Changhua 500, Taiwan. [2]Department of Biomedical Imaging and Radiological Science, National Yang-Ming Medical University, No.155, Sec. 2, Linong Street, Taipei 112, Taiwan. [3]Transplant Medicine and Surgery Research Centre, Changhua Christian Hospital, No. 135, Nan-Hsiao Street, Changhua 500, Taiwan. [4]School of Medicine, Chung Shan Medical University, Taichung City 40201, Taiwan. [5]School of Medicine, Kaohsiung Medical University, Kaohsiung, Taiwan. [6]Department of General Surgery, Changhua Christian Hospital, No. 135, Nan-Hsiao Street, Changhua 5006, Taiwan.

References
1. Ziada A, Rosenblum M, Crawford ED. Benign prostate hyperplasia: an overview. Urology. 1999;53(3 Suppl 3A):1–6.
2. Bilhim T, Pereira JA, Fernandes L, et al. Angiographic anatomy of the male pelvic arteries. AJR. 2014;203:373–82.

3. MQ Wang, F Duan, K Uyan, et al. Benign prostate hyperplasia: cone-beam
    CT in conjunction with DSA for identifying prostateic arterial anatomy.
    Radiol (on-line on 28 Jul 2016).
4. Carnevale FC, Antunes AA. Prostatic artery embolization for enlarged
    prostates due to benign prostatic hyperplasia. How I do it. Cardiovasc
    Intervent Radiol. 2013;36(6):1452–63.
5. Pisco JM, Pinheiro LC, Bilhim T, et al. Prostatic arterial embolization for
    benign prostatic hyperplasia: short- and intermediate-term results.
    Radiology. 2013;266:668–77.
6. Pisco JM, Peteira J, Tinto HR, et al. How to perform prostatic artery
    embolization. Tech Vasc Interventional Rad. 2016;15:286–9.

21

Efficacy and safety of PDE5-Is and α-1 blockers for treating lower ureteric stones or LUTS

Xifeng Sun[1,2†], Wei Guan[1†], Haoran Liu[1,2], Kun Tang[1,2], Libin Yan[1,2], Yangjun Zhang[1,2], Jin Zeng[1,2], Zhiqiang Chen[1,2], Hua Xu[1,2*] and Zhangqun Ye[1,2]

Abstract

Background: Lower ureteric stones and lower urinary tract symptoms are common in urology.Drug treatment is one of standard therapy,but the efficacy was controversial.Thus we aimed to investigate the efficacy and safety of monotherapy or combination therapy of adrenoceptor1 blockers and phosphodiesterase5 inhibitors for treatment.

Methods: Randomized controlled trials up to November 2016 were retrieved from PubMed, the Cochrane Library, Web of Science and Embase. A total of 17 studies were included. We analyzed data through random or fixed effect models. The heterogeneity between studies was assessed by the I^2 test statistic.

Results: As for lower ureter stones, our analysis demonstrated tadalafil had a significantly lower incidence of abnormal ejaculation than adrenoceptor1 blockers (2.31 95%CI 0.22to0.84, $P = 0.01$),while combination therapy had a higher expulsion rate (2.49 95%CI 1.44to4.29, $P = 0.001$) and shorter expulsion time (− 1.98 95%CI -3.08to0.88, $P = 0.0004$) than tamsulosin. As for lower urinary tract symptoms, our analysis indicated adrenoceptor1 blockers was more effective than phosphodiesterase5 inhibitors on decreasing International Prostate Symptom Score (1.96 95%CI 0.03to3.89, $P = 0.05$) and Post-Void Residual (9.41 95%CI 1.40to14.41, $P = 0.02$) and phosphodiesterase5 inhibitors showed a greater effect than adrenoceptor1 blockers on improving Erectile Dysfunction (2.23 95%CI 1.24to3.22, $P<0.0001$).Combination therapy had a significantly better effect on International Prostate Symptom Score (1.47 95%CI 1.25to1.69, $P<0.0001$), Maximum flow rate (0.87 95%CI 0.71to1.04, $P<0.0001$), Post-Void Residual (10.74 95%CI 3.53to17.96,$P = 0.004$) and Quality of life (0.59 95%CI 0.22to0.97, $P = 0.002$) but was associated with higher incidences of adverse events (3.40 95%CI 1.82to6.36, $P = 0.0001$) than adrenoceptor1 blockers. Combination therapy had a significantly better effect on International Prostate Symptom Score (4.19 95%CI 3.34to5.04, $P<0.0001$), Maximum flow rate (1.86 95%CI 1.32to2.39, $P<0.0001$), Post-Void Residual (22.58 95%CI 9.13to36.04, $P = 0.001$) and Quality of life (0.68 95%CI 0.37to1.00, $P<0.0001$) without higher incidences of adverse events than PDE5-Is.

Conclusions: In conclusion, this meta-analysis suggested combination therapy had a best efficacy of therapy for lower ureteric stones or lower urinary tract symptoms correlated with benign prostatic hyperplasia than monotherapy. Adrenoceptor1 blockers was more effective than phosphodiesterase5 inhibitors on International Prostate Symptom Score and Post-Void Residual. Both monotherapy and combination therapy were safe.

Keywords: Adrenergic alpha-1 receptor antagonists, Phosphodiesterase 5 inhibitors, Ureteral calculi, Lower urinary tract symptoms, Prostatic hyperplasia

* Correspondence: xuhuawhu@163.com
†Equal contributors
[1]Department of Urology, Tongji Hospital, Tongji Medical College, Huazhong University of Science and Technology, Wuhan 430030, China
[2]Institute of Urology of Hubei Province, Wuhan 430030, China

Background

Benign prostatic hyperplasia (BPH) is characterized by nonmalignant hyperplasia of prostatic tissue and is caused by proliferation of smooth muscle (SM) and epithelial cell in the transition zone of prostate.BPH is common in aging men and could result in bothersome lower urinary tract symptoms correlated with BPH (LUTS/BPH) which decrease Quality of life (QoL) by interrupting sleep and daily activities [1, 2]. In the US, approximately 75% of males from 60 to 69 years old and 83% of men aged 70 years or older are estimated to have got LUTS/BPH, and the annual direct medical cost due to management is more than $1.1 billion [3].

Each year, about 0.1% of the adult population of the US are admitted to hospital for treating urinary stones, leading to direct medical costs of more than $2 billion per year [4]. Stone incidence varies by race, ethnicity, geographic region and is higher in mountainous areas and deserts located in the southern US and Central European areas [5]. Nowadays, kidney stones are most prevailing from 20 to 40 years old and the incidence of men are 2 to 3 times higher as compared with women, which may due to less calcium and more citrate excreted by women. About 22% of all urinary calculus locate in the ureter, of which about 68% are found in the distal ureter [6].

In the past 20 years, various therapy methods for LUTS/BPH and lower ureteric stones were developed, which included observation, drug treatment and surgical procedures [7–10]. At present, drug treatment has become standard therapy and is widely recommended by clinical guidelines for LUTS/BPH and lower ureteric stones after series randomized controlled trials (RCTs) revealing the obvious effect of adrenoceptor blockers(ABs) [8]. α-1adrenergic receptors play significant roles in the contraction of SMs of the urinary tract and mainly centralize in the distal ureter, and relaxation of these SMs by blocking the receptors will improve LUTS/BPH and cause ureter dilatation contributing to stone expulsion [11].

Recently, the phosphodiesterase5 inhibitors (PDE5-Is) such as tadalafil, have shown up which could relax the SMs of ureter and prostate by working on nitric oxide cyclic-guanine monophosphate (NO/cGMP) signaling pathway [12–14]. Because of this character, tadalafil was approved by FDA in treating LUTS/BPH, erectile dysfunction (ED) and pulmonary arterial hypertension [15] and PDE5-Is were acknowledged in the guidelines published by the Japanese Urological Association (JUA) and the European Association of Urology (EAU). There is Level 1 evidence supporting the efficacy of PDE5-Is for treating LUTS/BPH [16]. By combining drugs acting through different mechanisms, better relaxation of SMs could be achieved [17]. Like ABs, PDE5-Is have an onset

of action that occurs within weeks. However, the two classes of drugs are associated with adverse events (AEs) such as headache, dizziness and hypotension leading to the relatively limited clinical application.

Nowadays, a few meta-analyses had compared the effect of PDE5-Is with ABs in the therapy of LUTS/BPH but meta-analyses about lower ureteric stones were rare. In 2012, Gacci et al. [18] performed a meta-analysis of PDE5-Is plus ABs verse ABs for treating LUTS/BPH. They declared that PDE5-Is might be a treatment option with great promise for patients with LUTS/BPH. Then several clinical trials analyzed the effect of PDE5-Is for LUTS/BPH vs ABs. In 2015, XH Wang et al. [19] conducted an meta-analysis to summarize the comparative effect and safety of monotherapy and combination therapy of PDE5-Is and ABs for LUTS/BPH, in which they suggested that PDE5-Is used alone was effective except for Post-Void Residual (PVR) than ABs and was more effective than ABs on increase of International Index Of Erectile Function (IIEF) score while combination therapy had the best effect. Moreover, either monotherapy or combination therapy was safe. However, the literature searches weren't extensive enough in the two studies.

Recently, researchers focused on investigating the comparative effect and safety of monotherapy and combined use of PDE5-Is and ABs for treating LUTS/BPH and lower ureteric stones. However, the conclusions were still very controversial. Thus, our study aimed to comprehensively compare efficiency and safety of monotherapy with combination therapy of PDE5-Is and ABs for treating LUTS/BPH and lower ureteric stones based on existing RCTs.

Methods

All methods for this systematic review and meta-analysis are outlined in a prospectively registered protocol available online [20] (PROSPERO identifier CRD42017059295), and reporting follows Preferred Reporting Items for Systematic Reviews and Meta-Analysis (PRISMA) guidelines.

Search strategy

According to the PRISMA statement [21], we performed an extensive search of a database of PubMed, the Cochrane Library, Web of Science and Embase up to November 2016. The search terms included the following keywords: ("lower urinary tract symptom" OR "LUTS" OR "benign prostatic hyperplasia" OR "BPH" OR "ureter stone" OR "ureteric stone") AND ("a-adrenoceptor antagonist" OR "a-adrenoceptor inhibitor" OR "α-blocker" OR "alfuzosin" OR "doxazosin" OR "tamsulosin" OR "silodosin" OR "terazosin") AND ("phosphodiesterase type 5 inhibitor" OR "sildenafil" OR "tadalafil" OR "mirodenafil" OR "avanafil" OR "udenafil" OR "vardenafil" OR "lodenafil"). Furthermore, the references of selected articles and the abstracts presented at related conferences were also checked by hand to identify additional potential studies. The languages were limited to English.

Inclusion and exclusion criteria

The inclusion criteria for the studies were as follows: (1) human studies; (2) reporting original research;(3) enrolling patients of LUTS/BPH or lower ureteric stone; (4) reporting evaluation indexes of LUTS/BPH such as IPSS, Qmax, PVR, QoL, IIEF before and after treatment; (5) reporting evaluation indexes of stones such as expulsion rate, expulsion time. Additionally, reviews, superficial abstracts, studies with a sample size< 10 were excluded.

Selection of studies

Two authors (XFS and WG) respectively screened the title, abstract and results, keywords and conclusion of every single study to identify included articles. Any discrepancies were resolved by discussing together. Full texts were screened to further evaluate whether the article had met the inclusion criteria.

Data extraction

Two authors (XFS and WG) respectively extracted the required data from the included articles through using a designed tabulation based on the Inclusion criteria and a third author verified the data. Data of different aspects were classified into the corresponding column. Based on the Cochrane Handbook, missing or vague information was imputed and was required from the authors of original articles or other relevant articles when necessary.

Quality assessment

Two investigators independently assessed the quality levels of the included studies according to the Jadad score, which is based on the following aspects: randomized allocation sequence, allocation concealment, blinding and quitting. Studies with scores of 4 points or higher were considered to be of high quality.

Statistical analysis

All analyses were conducted applying Cochrane Collaboration review manager software (RevMan5.3). The pooled effects were calculated as weighted mean difference (WMD) for continuous variable and odds ratio (OR) for dichotomy variable, as well as 95% confidence intervals (Cls). We chose two-sided in all test and $P < 0.05$ were considered statistical significance. The heterogeneity was determined by the Cochrane's Q-statistic test [22], and the inconsistency was quantified with the I^2 statistic. When $I^2 > 50\%$ or $P_Q \le 0.1$, which suggested substantial heterogeneity, the random-effects model (DerSimonian-Laird method) was applied [23]; otherwise, the fixed-effects model (Mantel-Haenszel method) was applied [24]. Sensitivity analyses were conducted by sequentially excluding each study to validate the reliability of the results and analyse the heterogeneity. Evaluation of safety was conducted via comparing the AEs, and the indexes could be calculated when at least 2 studies contained relevant data.

Results

Search results

Figure 1 displayed the study selection process. Of 127 retrieved articles in initial search, 17 RCTs finally met full inclusion criteria via full-text evaluation from 33 potentially eligible articles for this systematic review and meta-analysis.

Study characteristics and quality assessment

Tables 1 and 2 list the characteristics of the included studies in the meta-analysis. Regarding the lower ureteric stones, 5 studies [6, 13, 25–27] including a total of 861 patients were available. Regarding the LUTS/BPH, 12 studies [28–39] including a total of 1052 patients were available. As for bias, we gave positive appraise for all the selected studies. Additionally, 13 [6, 13, 25–30, 33, 35, 37, 38, 40] included studies were of high quality and 4 [31, 32, 34, 36] were of low quality according to the Jadad scores [41].

Quantitative synthesis

PDE5-is versus ABs for lower ureteric stones

As displayed in Fig. 2 and Additional file 1: Table S1, baseline characteristics, treatment outcomes and AEs were not statistically different except for the abnormal ejaculation between the two groups. There was a trend that ABs had a lower incidence of headache, dizziness and backache. Combining the results of included studies, PDE5-Is was comparable on the efficacy of lower ureter stones passage and had a significantly lower rate of abnormal ejaculation (2.31[1.19 to 4.50]; $P = 0.01$) than ABs. Sensitivity analysis was conducted by excluding each of the 4 studies.When excluding the study of Kumar (2015′) et al. [13] the pooled odds ratio (OR) of expulsion rate and expulsion time was 0.37 (95%CI: 0.21–0.65, $P = 0.0005$) and 1.90 (95%CI: 0.98–2.82, $P < 0.0001$), respectively, demonstrating tadalafil might have better expulsion effect and shorter expulsion time than tamsulosin.

Tadalafil plus tamsulosin versus tamsulosin for lower ureteric stones

As displayed in Fig. 3 and Additional file 1: Table S1, the pooled WMD for expulsion time, no. of hospital visits, no. of colic episodes and analgesic use was − 1.98 (95%CI: -3.08–0.88, $P = 0.0004$), − 0.71 (95%CI: -0.92–0.50, $P < 0.0001$), − 1.15 (95%CI: -1.34–0.96, $P < 0.0001$) and − 1.03 (95%CI: -1.23–0.83, P < 0.0001), respectively and the pooled OR for expulsion rate and Improvement in ED was 2,49

Table 1 Characteristics of the included studies of lower ureteric stones in meta-analysis

Author	Year	Country	Characteristics of participants		Design	Intervention	No.	Study interval	Comparable index	Jadad score
			location	size						
Kumar	2015	India	distal ureteric stones	5-10 mm	RCT	tamsulosin 0.4 mg qd tadalafil 10 mg qd silodosin 8 mg qd	90 90 90	4 weeks	age,gender,stone size,expulsion rate,expultion time,analgesic use,AEs	6
KC	2016	Nepal	distal ureteric stones	5-10 mm	RCT	tamsulosin 0.4 mg qd tadalafil 10 mg qd	41 44	2 weeks	age,gender, stone size, expulsion rate, expulsion time,analgesic use,AEs	4
Puvvada	2016	India	distal ureteric stones	5-10 mm	RCT	tadalafil 10 mg qd tamsulosin 0.4 mg qd	100, 100	4 weeks	age, gender, stone size, expulsion rate, expulsion time, analgesic use, AEs	6
Kumar	2014	India	distal ureteric stones	5-10 mm	RCT	tamsulosin 0.4 mg qd + tadalafil 10 mg qd tamsulosin 0.4 mg qd	31 31	6 weeks	age,gender,stone size, expulsion rate, expulsion time,analgesic use, AEs	4
Jayant	2014	India	distal ureteric stones	5-10 mm	RCT	tamsulosin 0.4 mg qd + tadalafil 10 mg qd tamsulosin 0.4 mg qd	122 122	4 weeks	age, gender,stone size, expulsion rate, expulsion time, analgesic use, AEs	5

/ not available, *AEs* adverse events, *RCT* randomized controlled trial

(95%CI: 1.44–4.29, $P = 0.001$) and 22.92 (95%CI: 3.02–173.82, $P = 0.002$), respectively. The resultsindicated the combination therapy of tadalafil and tamsulosin was more effective on treating ED and lower ureteric stones without higher rate of AEs than tamsulosin. Sensitivity analysis was not performed because only 2 studies were included.

PDE5-is versus ABs for LUTS/BPH

As displayed in Fig. 4 and Additional file 1: Table S1, ABs was significantly more effective than PDE5-Is on decreasing PVR (– 9.41 [– 17.41 to – 1.40]; $P = 0.02$) and

IPSS (– 1.96 [– 3.89 to – 0.03]; $P = 0.05$), while PDE5-Is showed greater effect than ABs on increasing IIEF score (2.23 [1.24 to 3.22]; $P < 0.0001$). Sensitivity analysis was conducted, and when ruling out the study of Kim et al. [29] the pooled WMD of change of Qmax was – 0.78 (95%CI:-1.41–0.15,P = 0.02) which meant ABs might have a better effect in increasing Qmax. The pooled WMD of the change of PVR was – 8.58 (95%CI: -19.34-2.19, $P = 0.12$) after excluding the low-quality study of Kaplan et al. [32] which indicated there might have no statistical significance on decreasing PVR. When ruling

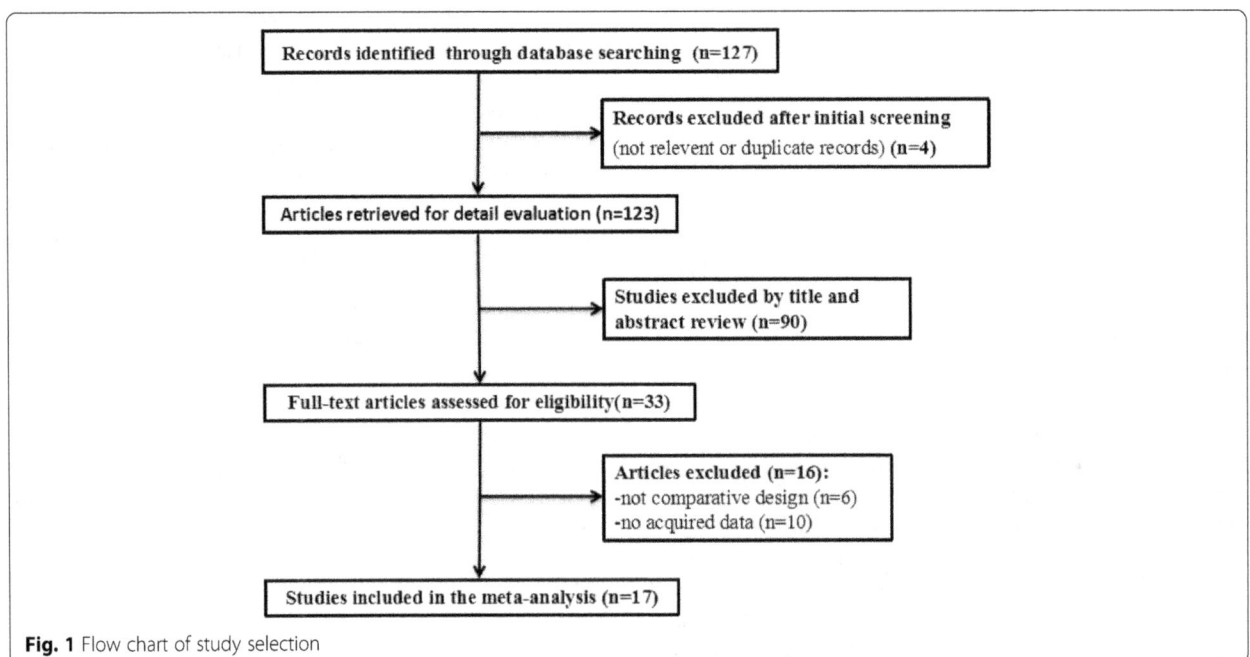

Fig. 1 Flow chart of study selection

out the three low-quality studies of Kaplan et al. [32],Singh et al. [31] and Liguori et al. [36] the pooled WMD of change of IPSS was − 1.24 (95%CI:-3.11–0.79,$P = 0.19$) which meant ABs might not have a better effect in decreasing IPSS.

PDE5-is plus ABs versus ABs for LUTS/BPH

As displayed in Fig. 5 and Additional file 1: Table S1, the pooled WMD for change of IPSS, QoL, IIEF score, Qmax and PVR was 1.47 (95%CI: 1.25–1.69, $P < 0.0001$), 0.59 (95%CI: 0.22–0.97, $P = 0.002$), 2.83 (95%CI: 2.08–3.58, $P < 0.0001$), 0.87 (95%CI: 0.71–1.04, $P < 0.0001$) and 10.74 (95%CI: 3.53–17.96, $P = 0.004$), respectively, indicating PDE5-Is plus ABs had better effect on improving LUTS/BPH than ABs alone. PDE5-Is plus ABs had higher incidences of AEs (3.69 [2.38 to 5.74]; $P < 0.0001$), headache (4.87 [2.28 to 5.74]; $P < 0.0001$) and dyspepsia (6.67 [1.46 to 30.55]; $P = 0.01$) than ABs alone. Sensitivity analysis was conducted and there was no significant change.

PDE5-Is plus ABs versusPDE5-Is for LUTS/BPH

As displayed in Fig. 6 and Additional file 1: Table S1, the pooled WMD for change of IPSS, QoL, Qmax and PVR was 4.19 (95%CI: 3.34–5.04, $P < 0.0001$), 0.68 (95%CI: 0.37–1.00, $P < 0.0001$), 1.86 (95%CI: 1.32–2.39, $P < 0.0001$) and 22.58 (95%CI: 9.13–36.04, $P = 0.001$), respectively, indicating PDE5-Is plus ABs had a significantly better effect on improving LUTS/BPH and ED without increased incidences of AEs than PDE5-Is alone. Sensitivity analysis was conducted and there was no significant change.

Discussion

This is the first systematic review and meta-analysiscomparing the efficacy and safety of monotherapy and combination therapy of PDE5-Is and ABs for treating lower ureteric stones. Meanwhile, it is an update in LUTS/BPH. A few meta-analyses had analyzed the effect of PDE5-Is for treating LUTS/BPH when compared with ABs or placebo [42–44]. In 2015, XH Wang et al. worked out several different conclusions comparing with our analysis in LUTS/BPH which could mainly attribute

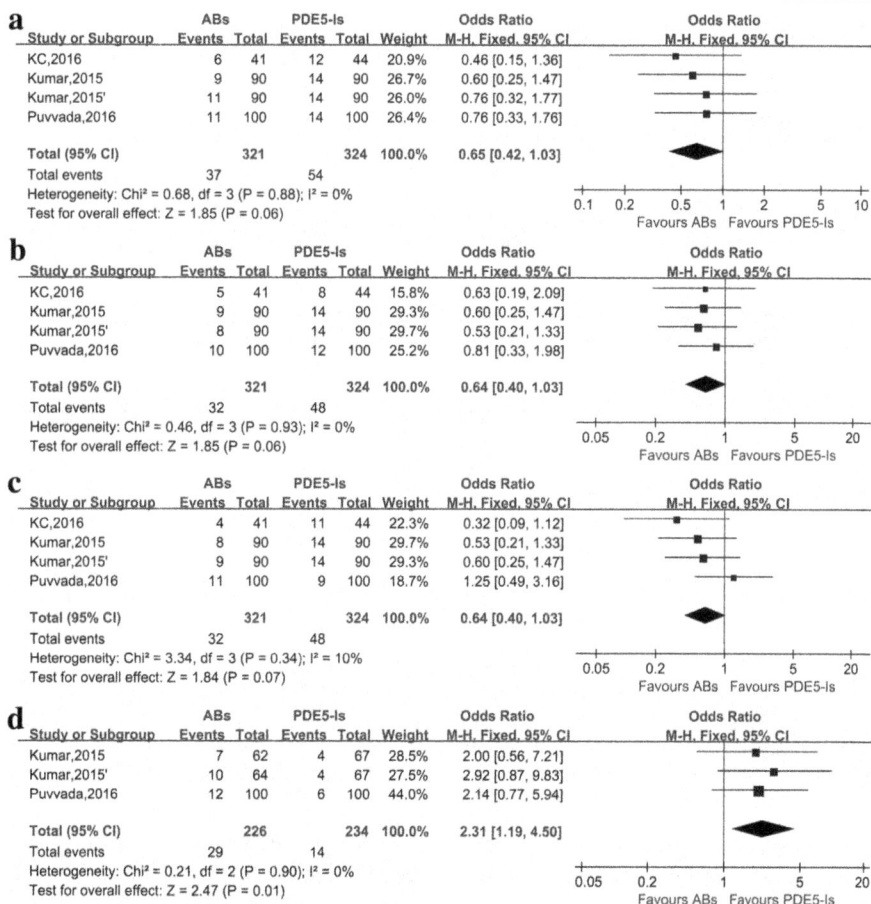

Fig. 2 The comparisons between PDE5-Is and ABs for treating lower ureteric stones **a** Headache **b** Dizziness **c** Backache **d** Abnormal ejaculation Kumar, 2015: tamsulosin vs tadalafil. Kumar, 2015': silodosin vs tadalafil

Table 2 Characteristics of the included studies of LUTS/BPH in meta-analysis

Author	Year	Country	Characteristics of participants					Design	Intervention	No.	Study interval	Comparable index	Jadad score
			Age	Cause of LUTS	IPSS	ED	Sick time						
Abolyosr	2013	Egypt	≥45	BPH	≥7	Yes	≥3 months	RCT	Doxazosin 2 mg qd Sildenafil 50 mg qd Combination	50 50 50	4 months	IPSS, PVR, Qmax, IIEF, QoL	4
Kaplan	2007	USA	50–76	BPH	17.4(mean)	Yes	/	RCT	Alfuzosin 10 mg qd Sildenafil 25 mg qd Combination	20 21 21	12 weeks	IPSS, Qmax, Nocturia, PVR, IIEF, AEs	3
KIM	2011	Korea	≥45	BPH	≥13	/	≥6 months	RCT	Tadalafil 5 mg qd Tamsulosin 0.2 mg qd	51 49	12 weeks	IPSS, QoL, Nocturia, Qmax, PVR, AEs	5
Singh	2014	India	≥45	BPH	> 8	/	≥6 months	RCT	Tamsulosin 0.4 mg qd Tadalafil 10 mg qd Combination	45 44 44	3 months	IPSS, Qmax, PVR, QoL, IIEF, AEs	3
Tuncel	2010	Turkey	47–77	BPH	> 12	Yes	≥6 months	RCT	Sildenafil 25 mg qd 4d/week Tamsulosin 0.4 mg qd Combination	20 20 20	8 weeks	IPSS, Qmax, PVR, QoL, IIEF	4
Bechara	2008	Argentina	> 50	BPH	> 12	/	≥6 months	RCCT	Tamsulosin 0.4 mg qd + tadalafil 20 mg qd Tamsulosin 0.4 mg qd + placebo	27 27	45 days	IPSS, Qmax, PVR, QoL, AEs	5
Liguori	2009	Italy	50–75	BPH	> 8	Yes	≥6 months	MRCT	Alfuzosin 10 mg qd Tadalafil 20 mg qd Combination	18 19 21	12 weeks	IPSS, Qmax, PVR, QoL, IIEF, AEs	3
Ng	2009	China	50–80	BPH	/	Yes	/	RCCT	Doxazosin0.4–0.8 mg qd + vardenafil 10 mg qd Doxazosin0.4–0.8 mg qd + placebo	37 37	2 days	AEs	6
Regadas	2013	Brazil	> 45	BPH	> 14	/	≥6 months	RCT	Tamsulosin 0.4 mg qd + tadalafil 5 mg qd Tamsulosin 0.4 mg qd	20 20	30 days	IPSS, Qmax, QoL, AEs	5
Gacci	2012	Italy	40–80	BPH	≥12	Yes/No	/	RCT	Vardenafil 10 mg qd + tamsulosin 0.4 mg qd Tamsulosin 0.4 mg qd + Placebo	30 30	2 weeks	IPSS, Qmax, PVR, QoL, IIEF, AEs	5
Kumar	2014	India	> 50	BPH	≥8	/	/	RCT	Alfuzosin 10 mg qd Tadalafil 10 mg qd Combination	25 25 25	12 weeks	IPSS, IIEF, Qmax, PVR, QoL	5
Jin	2011	China	50–75	BPH	≥10	Yes	/	MRCT	Doxazosin 4 mg qd + sildenafil 25–100 mg on demand Sildenafil 25–100 mg on demand	168 82	6 months	IPSS, QoL, IIEF, AEs	3

LUTS lower urinary tract symptom, *BPH* benign prostatic hyperplasia, *ED* erectile dysfunction, *Qmax* maximum flow rate, *IPSS* international prostase Symptom score, *PVR* postvoid residual urine, *QoL* quality of life, *IIEF* international index of erectile function, / not available, *AEs* adverse events, *RCT* randomized controlled trial, *MRCT* multicenter randomized controlled trial, *RCCT* randomized controlled crossover trial

to the incomplete literature search. However, we made an integrated and high-quality literature search and most of the included studies were high-quality RCTs.

As for LUTS/BPH, our pooled results suggested that ABs had a significantly better effect than PDE5-Is on the reduction of IPSS and PVR without significant difference of Qmax and QoL. Meanwhile, PDE5-Is had a statistically significant better effect than ABs on improving IIEF score. This suggested PDE5-Is could exert different therapeutic effect by relieving the obstruction of prostate

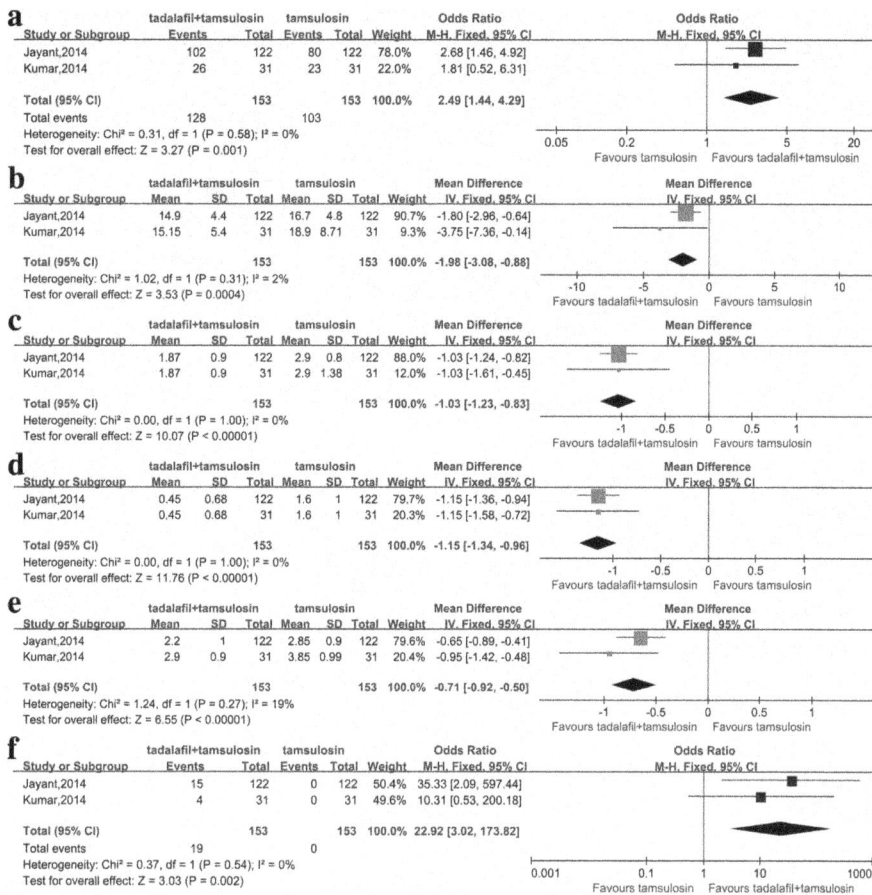

Fig. 3 The comparisons between combination therapy and tamsulosin monotherapy for treating lower ureteric stones **a** Expulsion rate **b** Expulsion time **c** Analgesic use **d** No. of colic episodes **e** No. of hospital visits **f** Improvement in ED

and relaxing the bladder SMs [45]. The relaxation of PDE5-Is in the detrusor muscle could withstand the relaxation of prostate and bladder neck, which lessen the effect of urodynamics, especially PVR and IPSS [46].We also found that combination therapy had the best effect on reducing IPSS, PVR, and on increasing Qmax and QoL compared with either of monotherapy, while the combination therapy was significantly more effective on improving IIEF score compared with ABs. The results might demonstrate the therapy of tadalafil daily don't have a negative impact on bladder contractility and outlet condition [47]. No significant difference on increasing IIEF score between combination therapy and monotherapy of PDE5-Is was found, which demonstrated that ABs had little power to improve ED. Significant heterogeneity was detected among treatment outcomes of all the three comparisons for treating LUTS/BPH, which might due to various methods and doses, quality, and duration of intervention.

It is important that our meta-analysis revealed that the combination therapy for treating LUTS/BPH showed better effect than either monotherapy on reducing IPSS

and PVR and increasing QoL and Qmax. The best effect may result from the synergistic function of NO-mediated relaxation effect by PDE5-Is, and reduction of the sympathetic tone mediated by α-adrenergic receptors blocking by ABs of the identical SMs in the bladder neck and prostate [32]. Also, our results corroborated the efficacy of combination therapy for patients suffered from LUTS and ED. In the comparison of PDE5-Is with ABs for LUTS/BPH, we found that ABs had significantly better effect on increasing Qmax than PDE5-Is after removing the study of Kim et al. and the pooled WMD for change of PVR turned to be non-significant after removing the study of Kaplan et al., which could be explained by large sample size and low quality, respectively. When ruling out all the three low-quality studies of Kaplan et al. [32], Singh et al. [31] and Liguori et al. [36], the pooled WMD of change of IPSS turned to be non-significant, which meant ABs might not have a better effect in decreasing IPSS.

Variations of the outcomes could also be explained by different baseline characteristics such as age, BMI, and initial risk factors for LUTS/BPH.

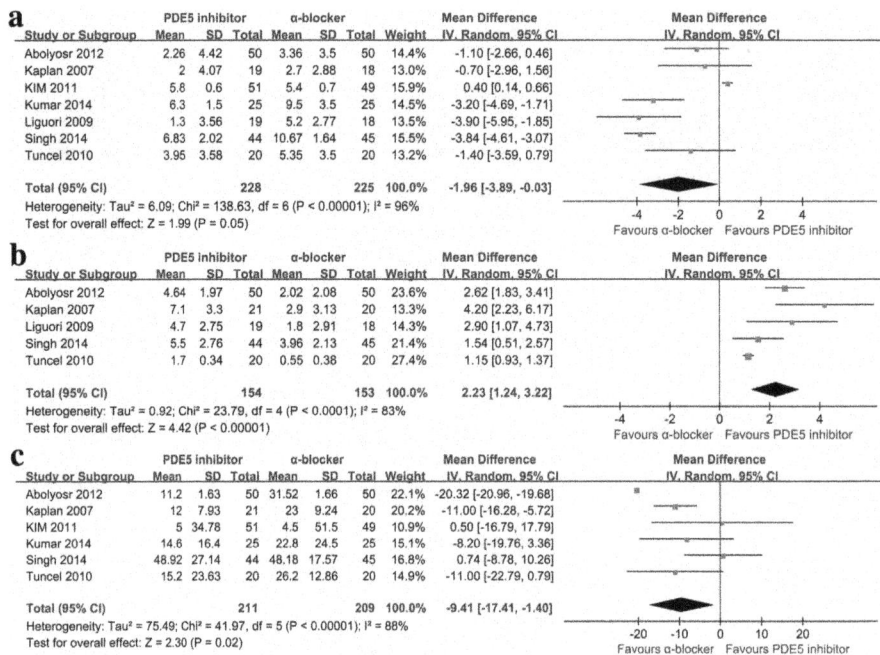

Fig. 4 The comparisons between PDE5-Is and ABs for treating LUTS/BPH **a** Change of IPSS **b** Change of IIEF score **c** Change of PVR

It is clear that substantial work has been conducted to verify the relationship between ED and LUTS/BPH. Both of them are highly prevailing in older men and are closely linked [48], independently of cardiovascular problems, as confirmed by numerous epidemiology researches [10, 49–51]. At present, the connection between ED and LUTS/BPH is supported by four primary mechanisms in the penis and prostate as followed: ①the rhokinase activation/endothelin pathway; ②the metabolic syndrome hypothesis and autonomic hyperactivity; ③the physiopathologic consequences of pelvic atherosclerosis; ④changes in the NO/cGMP pathway [52]. PDE5 isoenzymes play a role in the metabolisms and exist in the human bladder, prostate and urethra. Moreover, there is increasing evidence that PDE5-Is may be effective for LUTS/BPH [53–55].

As for AEs, our pooled results suggested that PDE5-Is plus ABs had a higher incidence of total AEs, headache and dyspepsia than ABs without significant difference in other two comparisons of LUTS/BPH, which suggested the addition of PDE5-Is to ABs could increase risks of the AEs in treating LUTS to some extent. It is wise to be prudent in comparing the AEs of similar medicines even though tiny differences in the mechanisms. In the study of XH Wang et al., the occurrence rate of AEs for the combination treatment was only numerically greater than either of monotherapy, and this might due to the inadequate size of the sample. Based on the present RCTs, most related AEs of cases were slight or moderate and only a few patients discontinued due to AEs.

Therefore, the overall safety profile of the two classes of drugs was good.

As for lower ureteric stones, the pooled results of this study indicated that tadalafil had better expulsion effect and shorter expulsion time than tamsulosin, and tadalafil had a lower incidence of abnormal ejaculation compared with ABs, which could be explained that tadalafil played a better role in relaxing SMs of posterior urethra than that of anterior urethra and bladder neck. This result reminds us that prescribing ABs for patients with lower ureteric stones and ejaculatory dysfunction should be prudent, and tadalafil may be a good substitute. And tadalafil plus ABs had significantly better improvement on IIEF score, higher expulsion rate, shorter expulsion time, less analgesic use and fewer hospital visits than ABs monotherapy without increased AEs. Our results demonstrated that tadalafil had an impressive improvement on expelling lower ureteric stones when combined with ABs and the combination therapy was safe for patients. Significant heterogeneity was observed among treatment outcomes of comparing ABs with PDE5-Is, which might due to various methods and duration of intervention.

At present, two convincing mechanisms of tadalafil in expelling lower ureteric stones are as followed: (1) slight-to-moderate relaxation of SMs; (2) extension of local blood vessels which increases blood perfusion [56–58]. Increased NO/cGMP concentration could relax the SMs in the prostate, urethra and bladder,and increased blood perfusion may relieve intraprostatic inflammation, ureter

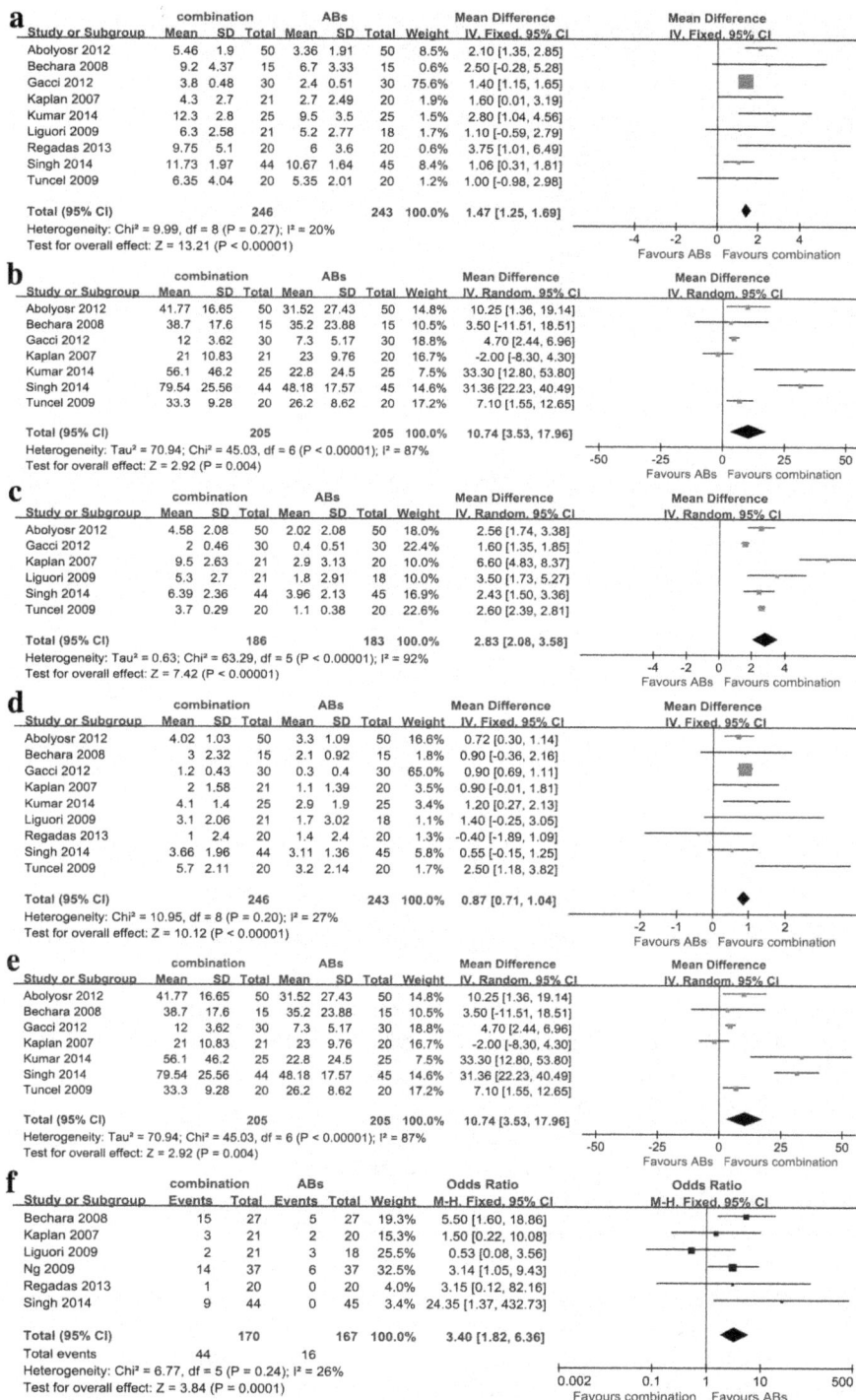

Fig. 5 The comparisons between combination therapy and ABs for treating LUTS/BPH **a** Change of IPSS **b** Change of QoL **c** Change of IIEF score **d** Change of Qmax **e** Change of PVR. **f** AEs

spasms and mucosal edema, which may contribute to the expulsion of lower ureteric stones.

Unfortunately, the important issue of PDE5-Is, the daily cost, has not been investigated, and none of the included RCTs had a performed cost analysis. The cost of drug therapy is directly related to the long-term

efficacy and safety profile, and the QoL of men treated with PDE5-Is alone or in combination with other drugs in continuous administration.

Nevertheless, there were several main limitations when analyzing and interpreting results in our present systematic review and meta-analysis. The major limitation was

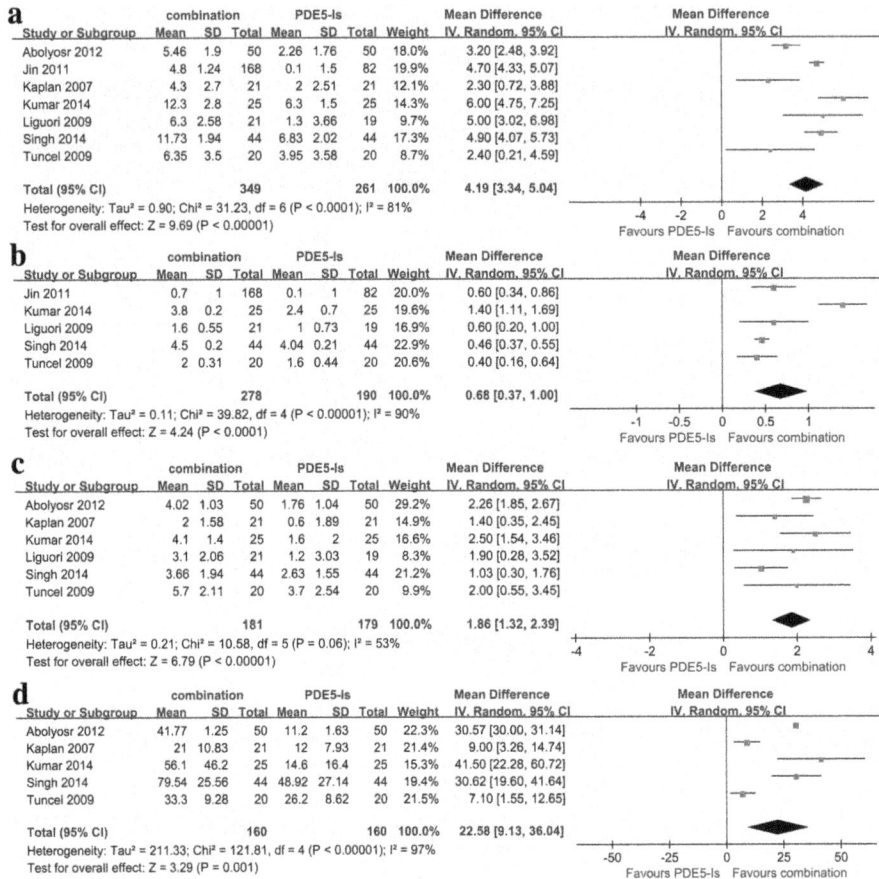

Fig. 6 The comparisons between combination therapy and PDE5-Is for treating LUTS/BPH **a** Change of IPSS **b** Change of QoL **c** Change of Qmax **d** Change of PVR

the quantity and various qualities and it was difficult to perform subgroup analysis to evaluate the heterogeneity among the included studies. In Table 1, we evaluated the quality by Jadad score and 4 RCTs had got 3 points which meant low-quality, which may limit the quality grade of evidence although other studies were evaluated as high-quality. Secondly, short duration and small populations also had a huge impact on the overall results. Thirdly, uncontrollable lifestyle modifications might influence the results. In our study, there were significant changes when removing some certain studies, which indicated there existed instability in our consequences, which might due to small sample size, inconsistent quality and the heterogeneity of the included original RCTs.

In the further, well-designed, prospective, multicenter randomized control studies with data of cost analysis, longer duration and larger sample size, and fundamental researches surveying mechanisms of PDE5-Is treating LUTS/BPH and lower ureteric stones, are required to help us better demonstrate the advantages as well as drawbacks of combination drug therapies. Clinical trials on the basis of the highest quality standard and method should be encouraged to ensure that the results have statistical significance and clinical relevance at the same time.

Conclusion

In conclusion, our study indicated that combination therapy of PDE5-Is and ABs had the best effect on improving LUTS/BPH or expulsing lower ureteric stones. As for monotherapy therapy, ABs had a better effect on improving LUTS/BPH and PDE5-Is were more effective on treating ED. Monotherapy use of PDE5-Is was effective on improving LUTS/BPH except for less reduction of PVR and IPSS as compared with ABs. Monotherapy of tadalafil had a better effect on expulsing lower ureteric stones than tamsulosin and had a lower incidence of abnormal ejaculation than ABs. What's more, monotherapy or combination therapy was safe and tolerant. Our results affirmed the therapeutic effect and safety of PDE5-Is and ABs, and provided evidences for drug treatment and update of guideline of LUTS/BPH or lower ureteric stones.

Additional file

Additional file 1: Table S1. Outcomes including baseline characteristics, treatment outcomes and adverse effects of this study. *ABs* α-1 blockers, *PDE5-Is* phosphodiesterase 5 inhibitors, *BPH* benign prostatic hyperplasia, *LUTS* lower urinary tract symptoms, *ED* erectile dysfunction, *OR* odds ratio, *WMD* weighted mean difference, *CI* confidence interval, *IPSS* International Prostate Symptom Score, *PVR* postvoid residual urine, *Qmax* maximum flow rate, *IIEF* International Index of Erectile Function, *QoL* quality of life, *AEs* adverse effects.

Abbreviations
ABs: Adrenoceptor1 blockers; AEs: Adverse events; BPH: Benign prostatic hyperplasia; cGMP: Cyclic-guanine monophosphate; CI: Confidence interval; EAU: European association of urology; ED: Erectile dysfunction; IIEF: International index of erectile function; IPSS: International prostate symptom score; JUA: Japanese urological association; LUTS: Lower urinary tract symptoms; NO: Nitric oxide; OR: Odds ratio; PDE5-Is: phosphodiesterase5 inhibitors; PVR: Post-void residual; Qmax: Maximum flow rate; QOL: Quality of life; RCT: Randomized controlled trials; SM: Smooth muscle; WMD: Weighted mean difference

Funding
This work was supported by the National Natural Science Foundation of China (81470935, 81370805, 81670645), the Chenguang Program of Wuhan Science and Technology Bureau (2015070404010199, 2015071704021644), and the National High Technology Research and Development Program 863 (2014AA020607).
No interferences occurred in carrying out the research project and in writing the manuscript that is the sole responsibility of the authors.

Authors' contributions
XFS, WG and KT: Study conception and design, data collection and management; HRL, LBY, JZ and YJZ: data collection and analysis, preparation of figures and tables; XFS, WG, KT, HX, ZQC and ZQY: Writing and revision of the manuscript. All authors read and approved the final manuscript.

Competing interests
The authors declare that they have no competing interests.

References
1. Nickel JC, Saad F. The American urological association 2003 guideline on management of benign prostatic hyperplasia: a Canadian opinion. Can J Urol. 2004;11:2186–93.
2. Welch G, Weinger K, Barry MJ. Quality-of-life impact of lower urinary tract symptom severity: results from the health professionals follow-up study. Urology. 2002;59:245–50.
3. Wei JT, Calhoun E, Jacobsen SJ. Urologic diseases in america project: benign prostatic hyperplasia. J Urol. 2008;179:S75–80.
4. Colella J, Kochis E, Galli B, et al. Urolithiasis/nephrolithiasis: what's it all about? Urol Nurs. 2005;25:427–48. 75, 49
5. Hollingsworth JM, Rogers MA, Kaufman SR, et al. Medical therapy to facilitate urinary stone passage: a meta-analysis. Lancet (London, England). 2006;368:1171–9.
6. Jayant K, Agrawal R, Agrawal S. Tamsulosin versus tamsulosin plus tadalafil as medical expulsive therapy for lower ureteric stones: a randomized controlled trial. Int J Urol. 2014;21:1012–5.
7. Stohrer M, Blok B, Castro-Diaz D, et al. EAU guidelines on neurogenic lower urinary tract dysfunction. Eur Urol. 2009;56:81–8.
8. Lepor H. Medical treatment of benign prostatic hyperplasia. Rev Urol. 2011; 13:20–33.
9. Speakman MJ, Kirby RS, Joyce A, et al. Guideline for the primary care management of male lower urinary tract symptoms. BJU Int. 2004;93:985–90.
10. Rosen RC, Giuliano F, Carson CC. Sexual dysfunction and lower urinary tract symptoms (LUTS) associated with benign prostatic hyperplasia (BPH). Eur Urol. 2005;47:824–37.
11. Porpiglia F, Vaccino D, Billia M, et al. Corticosteroids and tamsulosin in the medical expulsive therapy for symptomatic distal ureter stones: single drug or association? Eur Urol. 2006;50:339–44.
12. Wyllie MG. Monotherapy for comorbid erectile dysfunction and lower urinary tract symptoms: phosphodiesterase inhibitor or alpha-adrenoceptor antagonist? BJU Int. 2012;109:965–6.
13. Kumar S, Jayant K, Agrawal MM, et al. Role of tamsulosin, tadalafil, and silodosin as the medical expulsive therapy in lower ureteric stone: a randomized trial (a pilot study). Urology. 2015;85:59–63.
14. Gratzke C, Uckert S, Kedia G, et al. In vitro effects of PDE5 inhibitors sildenafil, vardenafil and tadalafil on isolated human ureteral smooth muscle: a basic research approach. Urol Res. 2007;35:49–54.
15. Capitanio U, Salonia A, Briganti A, et al. Silodosin in the management of lower urinary tract symptoms as a result of benign prostatic hyperplasia: who are the best candidates. Int J Clin Pract. 2013;67:544_51.
16. Oelke M, Bachmann A, Descazeaud A, et al. EAU guidelines on the treatment and follow-up of non-neurogenic male lower urinary tract symptoms including benign prostatic obstruction. Eur Urol. 2013;64:118–40.
17. Oelke M, Giuliano F, Mirone V, et al. Monotherapy with tadalafil or tamsulosin similarly improved lower urinary tract symptoms suggestive of benign prostatic hyperplasia in an international, randomised, parallel, placebo-controlled clinical trial. Eur Urol. 2012;61:917–25.
18. Gacci M, Corona G, Salvi M, et al. A systematic review and meta-analysis on the use of phosphodiesterase 5 inhibitors alone or in combination with alpha-blockers for lower urinary tract symptoms due to benign prostatic hyperplasia. Eur Urol. 2012;61:994–1003.
19. Wang XH, Wang X, Shi MJ, et al. Systematic review and meta-analysis on phosphodiesterase 5 inhibitors and alpha-adrenoceptor antagonists used alone or combined for treatment of LUTS due to BPH. Asian J Androl. 2015; 17:1022–32.
20. International Prospective Register of Systematic Reviews [http://www.crd.york.ac.uk/prospero]. Accessed 16 Mar 2017.
21. Moher D, Liberati A, Tetzlaff J, et al. Preferred reporting items for systematic reviews and meta-analyses: the PRISMA statement. Ann Int Med. 2009;151: 264–9. w64
22. Sterne JA, Juni P, Schulz KF, et al. Statistical methods for assessing the influence of study characteristics on treatment effects in 'meta-epidemiological' research. Stat Med. 2002;21:1513–24.
23. DerSimonian R. Meta-analysis in the design and monitoring of clinical trials. Stat Med. 1996;15:1237–48. discussion 49-52
24. Blunch NJ. Statistical analysis of data from clinical and retrospective studies. Ugeskr Laeger. 1976;138:401–7.
25. Kc HB, Shrestha A, Acharya GB, et al. Tamsulosin versus tadalafil as a medical expulsive therapy for distal ureteral stones: a prospective randomized study. Investig Clin Urol. 2016;57:351–6.
26. Puvvada S, Mylarappa P, Aggarwal K, et al. Comparative efficacy of tadalafil versus tamsulosin as the medical expulsive therapy in lower ureteric stone: a prospective randomized trial. Cent European J Urol. 2016;69:178–82.
27. Kumar S, Jayant K, Agrawal S, et al. Comparative efficacy of tamsulosin versus tamsulosin with tadalafil in combination with prednisolone for the medical expulsive therapy of lower ureteric stones: a randomized trial. Korean J Urol. 2014;55:196–200.
28. Regadas RP, Reges R, Cerqueira JB, et al. Urodynamic effects of the combination of tamsulosin and daily tadalafil in men with lower urinary tract symptoms secondary to benign prostatic hyperplasia: a randomized, placebo-controlled clinical trial. Int Urol Nephrol. 2013;45:39–43.
29. Kim SC, Park JK, Kim SW, et al. Tadalafil administered once daily for treatment of lower urinary tract symptoms in Korean men with benign

prostatic hyperplasia: results from a placebo-controlled pilot study using Tamsulosin as an active control. Low Urin Tract Symptoms. 2011;3:86–93.

30. Bechara A, Romano S, Casabe A, et al. Comparative efficacy assessment of tamsulosin vs. tamsulosin plus tadalafil in the treatment of LUTS/BPH. Pilot study. J Sex Med. 2008;5:2170–8.

31. Singh DV, Mete UK, Mandal AK, et al. A comparative randomized prospective study to evaluate efficacy and safety of combination of tamsulosin and tadalafil vs. tamsulosin or tadalafil alone in patients with lower urinary tract symptoms due to benign prostatic hyperplasia. J Sex Med. 2014;11:187–96.

32. Kaplan SA, Gonzalez RR, Te AE. Combination of alfuzosin and sildenafil is superior to monotherapy in treating lower urinary tract symptoms and erectile dysfunction. Eur Urol. 2007;51:1717–23.

33. Abolyosr A, Elsagheer GA, Abdel-Kader MS, et al. Evaluation of the effect of sildenafil and/or doxazosin on benign prostatic hyperplasia-related lower urinary tract symptoms and erectile dysfunction. Urol Ann. 2013;5:237–40.

34. Jin Z, Zhang ZC, Liu JH, et al. An open, comparative, multicentre clinical study of combined oral therapy with sildenafil and doxazosin GITS for treating Chinese patients with erectile dysfunction and lower urinary tract symptoms secondary to benign prostatic hyperplasia. Asian J Androl. 2011;13:630–5.

35. Tuncel A, Nalcacioglu V, Ener K, et al. Sildenafil citrate and tamsulosin combination is not superior to monotherapy in treating lower urinary tract symptoms and erectile dysfunction. World J Urol. 2010;28:17–22.

36. Liguori G, Trombetta C, De Giorgi G, et al. Efficacy and safety of combined oral therapy with tadalafil and alfuzosin: an integrated approach to the management of patients with lower urinary tract symptoms and erectile dysfunction. Preliminary report. J Sex Med. 2009;6:544–52.

37. Ng CF, Wong A, Cheng CW, et al. Effect of vardenafil on blood pressure profile of patients with erectile dysfunction concomitantly treated with doxazosin gastrointestinal therapeutic system for benign prostatic hyperplasia. J Urol. 2008;180:1042–6.

38. Gacci M, Vittori G, Tosi N, et al. A randomized, placebo-controlled study to assess safety and efficacy of vardenafil 10 mg and tamsulosin 0.4 mg vs. tamsulosin 0.4 mg alone in the treatment of lower urinary tract symptoms secondary to benign prostatic hyperplasia. J Sex Med. 2012;9:1624–33.

39. Kumar S, Kondareddy C, Ganesamoni R, et al. Randomized controlled trial to assess the efficacy of the combination therapy of Alfuzosin and Tadalafil in patients with lower urinary tract symptoms due to benign prostatic hyperplasia. Low Urin Tract Symptoms. 2014;6:35–40.

40. Mehrazmay A, Karambakhsh A, Salesi M. Reporting quality assessment of randomized controlled trials published in nephrology urology monthly journal. Nephrourol Mon. 2015;7:e28752.

41. Yuan JQ, Yang ZY, Mao C. Re: Mauro Gacci, Giovanni Corona, Matteo Salvi, et al. a systematic review and meta-analysis on the use of phosphodiesterase 5 inhibitors alone or in combination with alpha-blockers for lower urinary tract symptoms due to benign prostatic hyperplasia. Eur Urol. 2012;61:994–1003. European urology. 2012; 62:e35; author reply e6–8

42. Laydner HK, Oliveira P, Oliveira CR, et al. Phosphodiesterase 5 inhibitors for lower urinary tract symptoms secondary to benign prostatic hyperplasia: a systematic review. BJU Int. 2011;107:1104–9.

43. Liu L, Zheng S, Han P, et al. Phosphodiesterase-5 inhibitors for lower urinary tract symptoms secondary to benign prostatic hyperplasia: a systematic review and meta-analysis. Urology. 2011;77:123–9.

44. Fibbi B, Morelli A, Vignozzi L, et al. Characterization of phosphodiesterase type 5 expression and functional activity in the human male lower urinary tract. J Sex Med. 2010;7:59–69.

45. Tinel H, Stelte-Ludwig B, Hutter J, et al. Pre-clinical evidence for the use of phosphodiesterase-5 inhibitors for treating benign prostatic hyperplasia and lower urinary tract symptoms. BJU Int. 2006;98:1259–63.

46. Dmochowski R, Roehrborn C, Klise S, et al. Urodynamic effects of once daily tadalafil in men with lower urinary tract symptoms secondary to clinical benign prostatic hyperplasia: a randomized, placebo controlled 12-week clinical trial. J Urol. 2010;183:1092–7.

47. Braun M, Wassmer G, Klotz T, et al. Epidemiology of erectile dysfunction: results of the 'Cologne male Survey'. Int J Impot Res. 2000;12:305–11.

48. Gacci M, Bartoletti R, Figlioli S, et al. Urinary symptoms, quality of life and sexual function in patients with benign prostatic hypertrophy before and after prostatectomy: a prospective study. BJU Int. 2003;91:196–200.

49. Rosen R, Altwein J, Boyle P, et al. Lower urinary tract symptoms and male sexual dysfunction: the multinational survey of the aging male (MSAM-7). Eur Urol. 2003;44:637–49.

50. Vallancien G, Emberton M, Harving N, et al. Sexual dysfunction in 1,274 European men suffering from lower urinary tract symptoms. J Urol. 2003; 169:2257–61.

51. Uckert S, Oelke M, Stief CG, et al. Immunohistochemical distribution of cAMP- and cGMP-phosphodiesterase (PDE) isoenzymes in the human prostate. Eur Urol. 2006;49:740–5.

52. Kedia GT, Oelke M, Sonnenberg JE, et al. Phosphodiesterase isoenzymes in the human urethra: a molecular biology and functional study. Eur J Pharmacol. 2014;741:330–5.

53. Sairam K, Kulinskaya E, McNicholas TA, et al. Sildenafil influences lower urinary tract symptoms. BJU Int. 2002;90:836–9.

54. Vignozzi L, Gacci M, Cellai I, et al. PDE5 inhibitors blunt inflammation in human BPH: a potential mechanism of action for PDE5 inhibitors in LUTS. Prostate. 2013;73:1391–402.

55. Fusco F, di Villa Bianca R, Mitidieri E, et al. Sildenafil effect on the human bladder involves the L-cysteine/hydrogen sulfide pathway: a novel mechanism of action of phosphodiesterase type 5 inhibitors. Eur Urol. 2012; 62:1174–80.

56. Cohen PG. Intra-abdominal pressure, LUTS, and tadalafil. Re: Andersson K-E, et al. tadalafil for the treatment of lower urinary tract symptoms secondary to benign prostatic hyperplasia: pathophysiology and mechanism(s) of action. Neurourol urodyn 2011;30:292-301. Neurourol Urodyn. 2012;31:706.

57. Giuliano F, Uckert S, Maggi M, et al. The mechanism of action of phosphodiesterase type 5 inhibitors in the treatment of lower urinary tract symptoms related to benign prostatic hyperplasia. Eur Urol. 2013;63:506–16.

58. Morelli A, Sarchielli E, Comeglio P, et al. Phosphodiesterase type 5 expression in human and rat lower urinary tract tissues and the effect of tadalafil on prostate gland oxygenation in spontaneously hypertensive rats. J Sex Med. 2011;8:2746–60.

Permissions

The contributors of this book come from diverse backgrounds, making this book a truly international effort. This book will bring forth new frontiers with its revolutionizing research information and detailed analysis of the nascent developments around the world.

We would like to thank all the contributing authors for lending their expertise to make the book truly unique. They have played a crucial role in the development of this book. Without their invaluable contributions this book wouldn't have been possible. They have made vital efforts to compile up to date information on the varied aspects of this subject to make this book a valuable addition to the collection of many professionals and students.

This book was conceptualized with the vision of imparting up-to-date information and advanced data in this field. To ensure the same, a matchless editorial board was set up. Every individual on the board went through rigorous rounds of assessment to prove their worth. After which they invested a large part of their time researching and compiling the most relevant data for our readers.

The editorial board has been involved in producing this book since its inception. They have spent rigorous hours researching and exploring the diverse topics which have resulted in the successful publishing of this book. They have passed on their knowledge of decades through this book. To expedite this challenging task, the publisher supported the team at every step. A small team of assistant editors was also appointed to further simplify the editing procedure and attain best results for the readers.

Apart from the editorial board, the designing team has also invested a significant amount of their time in understanding the subject and creating the most relevant covers. They scrutinized every image to scout for the most suitable representation of the subject and create an appropriate cover for the book.

The publishing team has been an ardent support to the editorial, designing and production team. Their endless efforts to recruit the best for this project, has resulted in the accomplishment of this book. They are a veteran in the field of academics and their pool of knowledge is as vast as their experience in printing. Their expertise and guidance has proved useful at every step. Their uncompromising quality standards have made this book an exceptional effort. Their encouragement from time to time has been an inspiration for everyone.

The publisher and the editorial board hope that this book will prove to be a valuable piece of knowledge for researchers, students, practitioners and scholars across the globe.

List of Contributors

Maria Geitona
School of Social Sciences, University of Peloponnese, Corinth, Greece

Eleni Lyberopoulou, Eleftherios Bitros, Loukas Xaplanteris and Pinelopi Karabela
GlaxoSmithKline, Athens, Greece

Ioannis A Katsoulis, Hara Kousoulakou and Sotiria Papanicolaou
PRMA consulting, Athens, Greece

Mathew Y. Kyei, George O. Klufio, J ames E. Mensah, Samuel Gepi-Attee, Kwabena Ampadu, Bernard Toboh and Edward D. Yeboah
Department of Surgery and Urology, School of Medicine and Dentistry, College of Health Sciences, University of Ghana, Accra, Ghana

Livio Mordasini, Dominik Abt, Gautier Müllhaupt, Daniel S Engeler, Hans-Peter Schmid and Christoph Schwab
Department of Urology, Cantonal Hospital St. Gallen, Rorschacherstrasse 95, 9007 St. Gallen, Switzerland

Andreas Lüthi
Department of Anaesthesiology, Cantonal Hospital St. Gallen, Rorschacherstrasse 95, 9007 St. Gallen, Switzerland

Luca Cindolo and Luigi Schips
Department of Urology, "S.Pio da Pietrelcina" Hospital, via San Camillo de Lellis, 1-66054 Vasto, Italy

Luisella Pirozzi, Caterina Fanizza and Marilena Romero
Department of Clinical Pharmacology and Epidemiology, Fondazione "Mario Negri Sud", Santa Maria Imbaro, Italy

Petros Sountoulides
Department of Urology, General Hospital of Veria, Veria, Greece

Pietro Castellan
Department of Urology, "SS. Annunziata" Hospital, Chieti, Italy

Alessandro Antonelli and Claudio Simeone
Department of Urology, "Spedali Civili" Hospital, Brescia, Italy

Andrea Tubaro and Cosimo de Nunzio
Department of Urology, "Sant'Andrea" Hospital, University "La Sapienza", Rome, Italy

Kuan-Chou Chen
Department of Urology, Shuang Ho Hospital, Taipei Medical University, 291 Zhongzheng Rd.,, Zhonghe, Taipei 23561, Taiwan
Department of Urology, School of Medicine, College of Medicine, Taipei Medical University, 250 Wu-Shing St., Taipei 11031, Taiwan

Shian-Ying Sung
The Ph. D. Program for Translational Medicine, College of Medical Science and Technology, Taipei Medical University, Taipei, Taiwan

Yi-Ting Lin
Department of Urology, St. Joseph's Hospital, 74, Sinsheng Road, Huwei County, Yunlin Hsien 632, Taiwan
Research Institute of Biotechnology, Hungkuang University, 34 Chung-Chie Rd., Shalu County, Taichung Hsien 43302, Taiwan

Robert Y. Peng
Research Institute of Biotechnology, Hungkuang University, 34 Chung-Chie Rd., Shalu County, Taichung Hsien 43302, Taiwan

Chiu-Lan Hsieh
Graduate Institute of Biotechnology, Changhua University of Education, 1 Jin-De Rd., Changhua 50007, Taiwan

Kun-Hung Shen
Division of Urology, Department of Surgery, Chi-Mei Medical Center, 901 Chung Hwa Road, Yung Kang City, Tainan 701, Taiwan

Chiung-Chi Peng
Graduate Institute of Clinical Medicine, College of Medicine, Taipei Medical University, 250 Wu-Shing St., Xin-Yi District, Taipei 110, Taiwan

Simone Albisinni, Ibrahim Biaou, Quentin Marcelis, Fouad Aoun and Thierry Roumeguère
Urology Department, Erasme Hospital, Université Libre de Bruxelles, Route de Lennik 808, B-1070 Brussels, Belgium

Cosimo De Nunzio
Department of Urology, Ospedale Sant'Andrea, University "La Sapienza", Roma, Italy

Josephina G. Kuiper, Irene D. Bezemer, Fernie J. A. Penning-van Beest and Ron M. C. Herings
PHARMO Institute for Drug Outcomes Research, van Deventerlaan 30-40, 3528 AE Utrecht, Netherlands

Maurice T. Driessen
GlaxoSmithKline, 980 Great West Road, TW8 9 GS, Brentford, London, UK

Averyan Vasylyev
GlaxoSmithKline, 980 Great West RdBrentford, London, UK

Claus G. Roehrborn
Department of Urology, University of Texas Southwestern Medical Center, 5323 Harry Hines Bldv, TX 75390 Dallas, TX, USA

Shuyuan Yeh
Departments of Pathology and Laboratory Medicine, University of Rochester School of Medicine and Dentistry, Rochester, NY, USA
Department of Urology, University of Rochester School of Medicine and Dentistry, Rochester, NY, USA

Shalini Singh, Chunliu Pan, Kai Sha, John J. Krolewski and Kent L. Nastiuk
Departments of Pathology and Laboratory Medicine, University of Rochester School of Medicine and Dentistry, Rochester, NY, USA
Current address: Department of Cancer Genetics, Roswell Park Cancer Institute, Buffalo 14263NY, USA

Ronald Wood
Departments of Neurobiology and Anatomy and Obstetrics and Gynecology, University of Rochester School of Medicine and Dentistry, Rochester, NY, USA
Department of Urology, University of Rochester School of Medicine and Dentistry, Rochester, NY, USA

Chiuan-Ren Yeh
Department of Urology, University of Rochester School of Medicine and Dentistry, Rochester, NY, USA

Mauro Gacci, Arcangelo Sebastianelli, Matteo Salvi, Tommaso Jaeger, Tommaso Chini, Marco Carini and Sergio Serni
Department of Urology, University of Florence, Careggi Hospital, Florence, Italy

Cosimo De Nunzio and Andrea Tubaro
Department of Urology, Sant'Andrea Hospital, University "La Sapienza", Rome, Italy

Linda Vignozzi and Mario Maggi
Department of Clinical Physiopathology, University of Florence, Florence, Italy

Giovanni Corona
Endocrinology Unit, Maggiore-Bellaria Hospital, Bologna, Italy

Giorgio Ivan Russo and Giuseppe Morgia
Department of Urology, Policlinico Hospital, University of Catania, Catania, Italy

Jameel Nazir
Astellas Pharma Europe Ltd, Chertsey, UK

Lars Heemstra, Anke van Engen and Cristina Ivanescu
Quintiles Consulting, Hoofddorp, Netherlands

Zalmai Hakimi
Astellas Pharma Global Development, Leiden, Netherlands

Dominik Abt, Livio Mordasini, Hans-Peter Schmid and Daniel S Engeler
Department of Urology, Cantonal Hospital St. Gallen, Rorschacherstrasse 95, St. Gallen 9007, Switzerland

Lukas Hechelhammer
Department of Radiology and Nuclear Medicine, Cantonal Hospital St. Gallen, Rorschacherstrasse 95, St. Gallen 9007, Switzerland

Thomas M Kessler
Neuro-Urology, Spinal Cord Injury Centre & Research, University of Zürich, Balgrist University Hospital, Forchstrasse 340, Zürich 8008, Switzerland

Marcus J. Drake
Bristol Urological Institute and the School of Clinical Sciences, University of Bristol, Bristol, UK

Sally Bowditch, Emilio Arbe and Jameel Nazir
Astellas Pharma Europe Ltd, Chertsey, UK

Zalmai Hakimi
Astellas Pharma Europe B.V, Leiden, the Netherlands

Florent Guelfucci
Creativ-Ceutical Ltd, London, UK

Ikbel Amri
Creativ-Ceutical Ltd, Tunis, Tunisia

Yi-Ping Zhu, Bo Dai, Hai-Liang Zhang, Guo-hai Shi and Ding-Wei Ye
Department of Urology, Fudan University Shanghai Cancer Center, No. 270 Dong an Road, Shanghai 200032, People's Republic of China
Department of Oncology, Shanghai Medical College, Fudan University, No. 270 Dong an Road, Shanghai 200032, People's Republic of China

Sung Ryul Shim
Department of Epidemiology and Medical Informatics, Korea University, Seoul, South Korea

Jae Heon Kim
Department of Urology, Soonchunhyang University College of Medicine, Seoul Hospital, Seoul, South Korea

Hoon Choi and Jae Hyun Bae
Department of Urology, Korea University College of Medicine, Ansan Hospital, Ansan, South Korea

Soon-Sun Kwon
Biomedical Research Center, Seoul National University Bundang Hospital, Seongnam, South Korea

Hae Joon Kim, Byung Chul Chun and Won Jin Lee
Department of Preventive Medicine, College of Medicine, Korea University, Seoul, South Korea

Jin Huang and Hui-Zhen Zhang
Department of Pathology, Sixth People's Hospital affiliated to Shanghai Jiaotong University, Yishan Rd 600#, Xuhui District, Shanghai 200233, People's Republic of China

Kathleen H. Reilly
New York City, NY, USA

Hai-Bo Wang
Peking University Clinical Research Institute, Xueyuan Rd 38#, Haidian District, Beijing 100191, People's Republic of China

Mao Qiang Wang, Li Ping Guo, Guo Dong Zhang, Kai Yuan, Kai Li, Feng Duan, Jie Yu Yan, Yan Wang, Hai Yan Kang and Zhi Jun Wang
Department of Interventional Radiology, Chinese PLA General Hospital Beijing, 100853 Beijing, People's Republic of China

Huan Xu, Yan-bo Chen, Meng Gu, Qi Chen and Zhong Wang
Department of Urology, Shanghai 9th People's Hospital, Shanghai Jiaotong University School of Medicine, 639 Zhi Zaoju Road, Shanghai 200011, China

Yunhua Lin and Yongguang Jiang
Department of Urology, Beijing Anzhen Hospital, Capital Medical University, Beijing 100029, China

Zhigang Xue
Department of Urology, Beijing Anzhen Hospital, Capital Medical University, Beijing 100029, China
Department of Urology, Beijing Huairou Hospital, Beijing 101400, China

Nengbao Wei and Jinwen Bi
Department of Urology, Beijing Huairou Hospital, Beijing 101400, China

Antoni Sicras-Mainar
Dirección de Planificación, Badalona Serveis Assistencials SA, Via Augusta, 9, 08911 Badalona, Barcelona, Spain

Ruth Navarro-Artieda
Documentación Médica, Hospital Germans Trias i Pujol, Badalona, Barcelona, Spain

Ana Mª. Mora and Marta Hernández
Medical Department, Astellas Pharma S.A, Madrid, Spain

Chia-Bang Chen
Department of Radiology, Changhua Christian Hospital, No. 135, Nan-Hsiao Street, Changhua 500, Taiwan

Chen-Te Chou
Department of Radiology, Changhua Christian Hospital, No. 135, Nan-Hsiao Street, Changhua 500, Taiwan
Department of Biomedical Imaging and Radiological Science, National Yang-Ming Medical University, No.155, Sec. 2, Linong Street, Taipei 112, Taiwan
School of Medicine, Kaohsiung Medical University, Kaohsiung, Taiwan

Yao-Li Chen
Transplant Medicine and Surgery Research Centre, Changhua Christian Hospital, No. 135, Nan-Hsiao Street, Changhua 500, Taiwan
School of Medicine, Chung Shan Medical University, Taichung City 40201, Taiwan
School of Medicine, Kaohsiung Medical University, Kaohsiung, Taiwan

Department of General Surgery, Changhua Christian Hospital, No. 135, Nan-Hsiao Street, Changhua 5006, Taiwan

Wei Guan
Department of Urology, Tongji Hospital, Tongji Medical College, Huazhong University of Science and Technology, Wuhan 430030, China

Xifeng Sun, Haoran Liu, Kun Tang, Libin Yan, Yangjun Zhang, Jin Zeng, Zhiqiang Chen, Hua Xu and Zhangqun Ye
Department of Urology, Tongji Hospital, Tongji Medical College, Huazhong University of Science and Technology, Wuhan 430030, China
Institute of Urology of Hubei Province, Wuhan 430030, China

Index

Nocturnal Polyuria Index, 151-152, 154-155

O

Open Prostatectomy, 9-16, 18, 78, 81, 140, 144-145

Overactive Bladder, 30, 48, 54-57, 88, 90-92, 100, 108-110, 128, 153, 158, 165

P

Pathophysiology, 53, 55, 158, 182

Peri-operative Blood Transfusion, 10, 14

Perioperative Blood Loss, 111, 116

Pharmacokinetics, 48-49

Pharmacological Therapy, 25-27, 29, 31, 109

Polypharmacy, 53, 101, 104, 107

Prostate, 1-4, 6, 8-21, 23-24, 27, 31-32, 34-36, 38-40, 42-49, 51-60, 62-82, 84, 86-87, 89, 91, 93-98, 100, 108, 116-118, 123, 126-146, 154-159, 161, 164-172, 181-182

Prostate Cancer Gene 3, 129-131, 133-134

Prostatic Arterial Embolization, 98, 135, 137, 145, 170

Prostatic Artery, 94-95, 98, 135-136, 139-141, 143-145, 166-167, 170

Prostatic Artery Embolization, 94-95, 98, 145, 166, 170

Prostatic Specific Antigen, 34, 135, 137, 141, 143, 164

Puboprostatic Ligaments, 12

R

Randomized Controlled Trials, 94, 111, 171-172, 181-182

S

Segmentation, 68-71, 73-74

Solifenacin, 52, 57, 83-92, 99-100, 102, 104-109, 163-165

Spinal Anesthesia, 14, 22

Superior Vesical Artery, 139, 141, 143

Systolic Blood Pressure, 10, 13-15, 17, 77-80, 161

T

Tamsulosin Monotherapy, 1-2, 6-7, 31, 57, 91, 163, 165, 177

Testosterone, 2, 32-34, 38, 40-47, 59, 63, 82, 111, 117

Thulium Laser Vaporization, 19-20

Tolterodine, 52, 54, 56-57, 83-92, 99, 106, 108-109, 165

Transurethral Resection Syndrome, 19, 23-24

U

Ureteral Calculi, 171

Urethral Stenosis, 20, 95

Urgency, 20, 51-54, 56-57, 84-85, 90-92, 94, 100, 106, 108-109, 123-124, 153, 155, 166

Uroflowmetry, 20, 22, 97, 151, 159

V

Ventral Prostate, 44, 47, 68-71, 73, 75-76, 121

Voiding Symptoms, 52, 54, 78, 83-85, 88, 90-92, 100, 122, 128, 153, 164

X

Xenograft, 68, 71-76

www.ingramcontent.com/pod-product-compliance
Lightning Source LLC
Chambersburg PA
CBHW082012190326
41458CB00010B/3160